CONTEMPORARY AND INNOVATIVE PRACTICE IN PALLIATIVE CARE

Edited by **Esther Chang** and **Amanda Johnson**

Contemporary and Innovative Practice in Palliative Care
Edited by Esther Chang and Amanda Johnson

Published by InTech
Janeza Trdine 9, 51000 Rijeka, Croatia

Publishing Process Manager Martina Durovic

Technical Editor Teodora Smiljanic

Cover Designer InTech Design Team

Additional hard copies can be obtained from orders@intechopen.com

Contemporary and Innovative Practice in Palliative Care,
Edited by Esther Chang and Amanda Johnson
p. cm.
ISBN 978-953-307-986-8

For EU product safety concerns:
IN TECH d.o.o., Prolaz Marije Krucifikse Kozulić 3, 51000 Rijeka, Croatia,
info@intechopen.com or visit our website at intechopen.com.

Meet the editors

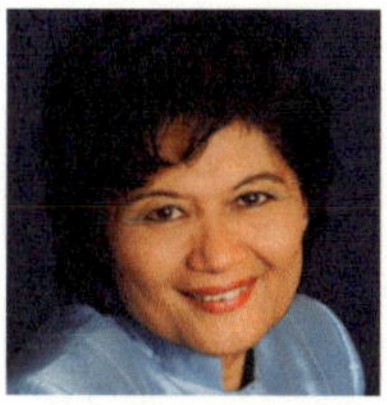

Professor Esther Chang is Director of Research, Head of Program for the Undergraduate Honours and Higher Research Degree programs in the School of Nursing and Midwifery, University of Western Sydney. She has worked in academia since 1986 with three tertiary institutions. She has been a Head of School, Dean of the Faculty of Health, and Acting Pro-Vice Chancellor Academic at the University of Western Sydney Hawkesbury. She is currently the President of the Lifestyle Medicine Institute, Australia. Professor Chang is committed to aged and palliative care. She received many large grants investigating, nursing and meeting health needs in older people; developed models of care for acutely ill elderly patients and clients with end-stage dementia. Professor Chang's international links have generated collaborative research into aged care across several countries. She has received partnership grants with industry and leads the School's Aged Care and Palliation (ACAP) research team.

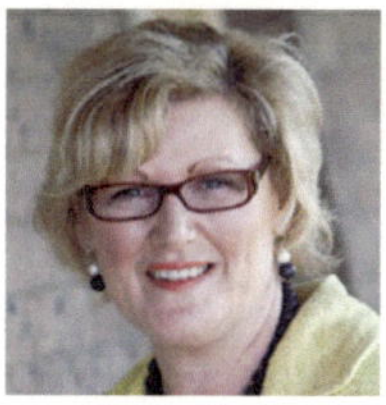

Dr. Amanda Johnson is Director of Undergraduate Studies, Head of Program for the Bachelor of Nursing in the School of Nursing and Midwifery, University of Western Sydney. She has worked in the tertiary sector since 1992. She is currently the Senior Lecturer in Aged Care for the school, and recently participated in a government reference group responsible for the translation of palliative care standards to the aged care sector. Dr. Johnson's PhD thesis is also in undergraduate palliative care education, and she is the recipient of a Vice Chancellor's Excellence award in the teaching of chronic illness and palliation in 2010. In the last 12 years, Dr. Johnson's research has been focused on aged care and palliation. She is committed to making a difference in the lives of older people, those who are dying and their families.

Contents

Preface

This book was developed to showcase the evolution of palliative care internationally in both developed and developing nations. It plays the vital role in alleviating suffering and promoting prosperity so that all people living to die had a quality life.

With advances in medical sciences, more sophisticated technology and increased evidence-based practice, we can see a greater integration of palliative care into all diseases now as well as in the future. The commencement of palliation at any point along the disease trajectory and symptom management play an important role in achieving an enhanced quality of life. The chapters in this book highlight the multidimensional nature of palliative practice encompassing not only knowledge of the disease state, but an understanding of the role government policy, the economy, family, the interdisciplinary team, support services, existential issues such as spirituality contribute to the provision of optimal palliative care for all. The diversity of topics in this book is also a reflection of the multidimensional nature of palliative care. It represents the contributors vision of how palliative care should be implemented and what are the challenges for the future.

This book has also been designed to provide comprehensive information on key contemporary issues associated with palliation. The reader will find viewpoints that are challenging and sometimes discerning, but at the same time motivating and thought-provoking in the care of people in palliation. This book is divided into three sections. Section 1 examines contemporary practice; Section 2 looks at the challenges in practice; Section 3 discusses the models of care. This contemporary and innovative book is scholar, accessible, reality based and practical. It is an excellent resource for students, practising clinicians and academics for understanding the issues of quality of care in the area of palliation. By reading the book, reflecting on the issues, challenges and opportunities ahead, we hope it will create within the reader a passion to take on, explore and further develop their palliative care practice. This will enable future generations of people requiring palliation to be the recipients of the best possible care available that meets their needs, when they are at their most vulnerable. It is also through this passion that clinical practice, research and teaching of future palliative care practitioners will be improved.We extend our sincere appreciation to the contributors for the work, shared interest and concern with the issues and challenges of palliation. This book would not be possible without them. Many thanks to Ana

Pantar from InTech Open Access Publisher for inviting us to be editors of this book ; special appreciation to Martina Durovic for her encouragement and superb support during this whole process. Finally, we are indebted to our respective husbands, Ron Chang and Robert Johnson for their continuous patience, understanding and support while we worked on this project.

Professor Esther Chang and Dr Amanda Johnson
University of Western Sydney
Australia

Part 1

Contemporary Practice

1

Cross-Cultural Issues in Academic Palliative Medicine

Mira Florea
Faculty of Medicine, University of Medicine and Pharmacy "Iuliu Hatieganu", Cluj-Napoca, Romania

1. Introduction

1.1 The influence of cultural diversity in palliative medicine

The definition of culture, as an integrated pattern of learned beliefs and behaviors that include thoughts, styles of communicating, ways of interacting, values, practices, and customs has evolved, over time, but the underlying understanding is that culture is the lens through which people give the world meaning and which shapes their beliefs and behaviors. Culture is a system of shared ideas, concepts, rules and meanings that underlies the way we live – and approach death. Cultural diversity refers to more than ethnic diversity; age, gender, sexual preference, capabilities, education, place of residence, and occupation also contribute to diversity of culture. [Lickiss, 2003]. Cultures change or evolve over time and this affects many areas. In palliative medicine attitudes and practices regarding care of the incurable patient, of the dying (and dead) have changed, from unspeakable neglect common to the multiple contemporary patterns.[Kellehear , 2001]. The role of culture is significant in palliative care, and how it is conceptualized and applied has enormous consequences for patients, families and health care providers. It influences communication patterns, decision-making styles, responses to symptoms, treatment choices, and emotional expression at end of life [Valente, 2004; Werth et al, 2002]. Studies show that when cultural differences are inadequately addressed, inferior care occurs, affecting trust, and leading to patient dissatisfaction, nonadherence. [Betancourt & Green, 2010; Bruera et al., 2001; Ward et al., 2004]. The progress in palliative medicine requires balancing clinical art with science while paying due attention to cross-cultural differences that influence patients' and physicians' attitudes toward health care matters. The importance of cultural sensitivity for oncologists is now increasingly recognized and teaching and training in cultural competence are mandatory. [Betancourt & Green, 2010; Biasco & Surbone 2009].

1.2 Cross-cultural medical education and the need of cultural competence in the modern medical school

In the medical encounter of the multicultural universities, there is interaction between the culture of the medical students, the culture of the patients, and the medical culture that surrounds them. Physicians increasingly encounter patients of diverse racial, ethnic, linguistic, and religious backgrounds, making effective cross-cultural communication skills essential. They should be sensitive to the diverse patients' health values that may be based on multiple cultures which they belong to (race, ethnicity. religion, gender, socioeconomic status, occupation, disability etc). The need for training in cultural competence is currently a requirement for medical schools. [Chun et al. 2010; Rodriguez et al. 2011]. Cultural competence refers to an ability to interact effectively with people of different cultures. It comprises four components: (a) awareness of one's own cultural worldview, (b) attitude towards cultural differences, (c) knowledge of different cultural practices and worldviews, and (d) cross-cultural skills.[Molinuevo & Torrubia, 2011]. Developing cultural competence results in an ability to understand, communicate with, and effectively interact with people across cultures.[Martin & Vaughn , 2007].

Cultural competency is something beyond the somewhat rigid categories of knowledge, skills, and attitudes: the continuous critical refinement and fostering of a type of thinking and knowing—a critical consciousness—of self, others, and the world. [Kumagai & Lypson, 2009]. As the european countries population and their universities become more diverse, racially and ethnically, demographic differences between physicians and patients increase, and the medical profession itself becomes more diverse, cross-cultural medical training takes on greater significance.[Rosen , 2004] .Cross-cultural education become important in preparing medical students in order to meet the health needs of the growing, diverse population. It has emerged because socio cultural factors are critical to the medical encounter.There are some medical universities which have been incorporated cross-cultural curricula into undergraduate medical education. [Betancourt, 2003; Betancourt, 2005; Davis & Smith, 2009].

The goal of these curricula is to prepare students to care for patients from diverse social and cultural backgrounds, and to recognize and appropriately address racial, cultural, and gender biases in health care delivery. Despite all changes, academic medical curriculums seldom prepare students for the realities of caring for patients with chronic progressive life threatening illnesses. An imbalance has been created in medical education which led to public concerns about poor communication and a perception that doctors lack care. [Taran, 2010]. The increasing attention to palliative medicine education has created major opportunities for improving education about care of the chronic progressive illnesses and for addressing multicultural issues in medical education. [Shanmugasundaram et al., 2009]. Medical schools offer some formal teaching about palliative and end-of-life care, but there is evidence that training is inadequate. [Lloyd-Williams & Macleod, 2004].

1.3 Motivating factors for cross-cultural medical education in palliative medicine

There are some motivating factors for cross-cultural medical education as folows:

- perception of chronic ,progressive illness, disease, causal factors, and treatment varies by culture
- diverse belief systems exist related to health, healing, and wellness
- culture influences attitudes toward health-care providers and motivations for seeking health care
- individual preferences and culture affect traditional and nontraditional approaches to health-care delivery and decision making

- communications between patient and health-care providers need to be clear and convey respect for individual beliefs and differences
- health-care providers in the delivery system are increasingly from culturally diverse and underrepresented minority groups
- patients have personal experiences of biases within health-care systems perceived as a reaction to their culture, ethnicity or religion

1.4 Spiritual dimensions of the health care in palliative medicine

Religious beliefs and practices are part of culture. Patients desire conversations with their health-care providers about spiritual and religious concerns. Physicians should ask about customs and practices, listen, explain and correct for their own cultural biases A good caring relationship is the greatest insurance against, and antidote for, the inevitable cultural mistakes.[Williams et al., 2011].

The advances of modern medicine increased life expectancy and this generated complex issues of the chronic progressive diseases' management. Increasing attention is being paid to the spiritual dimensions of the health care. The avoidance of the spiritual needs assessment in clinical practice and in the academic medical education may constitute a negligence and an important ethical issue. [Florea et al., 2008].

Palliative medicine and one of its core element, the spiritual care, provides a holistic patient-centered care applying a novel philosophy on living with incurable diseases and on death. Physicians, medical trainers mostly those using high medical technology and their students need special skills to communicate with patients and families. The compassionate care of the whole person-body, mind and spirit-has long been an ideal of medical education and practice. Many studies highlight the role that spirituality, culture, and end-of-life issues play in the future of medical education. [Azad, 2002; Betancourt, 2003; Betancourt 2006; Rosen et al. 2004].

Spirituality and religion, while often indistinguishable from culture, are beginning to be addressed in medical education, introducing palliative medicine module in medical schools curicula. A large segment of people claims belief in a higher being, and studies indicate that patients who have some religious commitment benefit in terms of stress reduction, recovery from illness, reduction of depression, and adjustment to disability. [Koenig et al., 2000 ; Lo et al., 2002; Williams et al., 2011 ; Wright, 2004] .

This evidence has provided the impetus among medical educators to include spirituality and health in undergraduate medical school curricula in order to increase sensitivity awareness about spiritual issues and to teach students communication techniques about different patients' spiritual beliefs, as they may affect their health and health care. Greater understanding of the diverse social, cultural, and spiritual contexts in which patients seek health care will facilitate more-favorable health outcomes and the cross-cultural medical education will have the potential to positively influence disparities in health. [Azad et al,.2002]. Some medical universities expand their students' and residents' education by integrating spirituality and medicine in the curriculum. Some of the europen and american medical schools, as our university, have been introduced courses in palliative medicine, including spiritual needs assessment and support, and many international hospitals have spiritual care initiatives.

Our university's undergraduate and postgraduate curriculum offer training in palliative care in a patient-centered model, including spiritual care and cultural diversity issues. Students are skilled in the understanding of human relationships, cultural sensitivity awareness in order to be able to integrate the personal meanings of values for both themselves and their patients, achieving a required cultural competence.

1.5 Obstacles to the inclusion of multicultural health content in the curricula of medical schools

To achieve the competence necessary to provide culturally appropriate education and culturally appropriate health care is a learning process that requires time, effort, practice, and introspection.

There are a number of obstacles to the inclusion of multicultural health content in the curricula of medical schools:

- difficulties in introducing new materials and experiences into an already overcrowded curriculum,
- lack of specialized teaching and learning resource materials,
- insufficient numbers of faculty prepared to teach the subject.

2. Methodology

The purposes of this study was to explore medical students' skills in cultural competence, their cultural sensitivity awareness, using 32 oncological outpatients with different cultural backgrounds, included in palliative care programs.

2.1 Recruitment process

2.1.1 Criteria for patients

Criteria for patients were a diagnosis of cancer and registration with a palliative care programme. The patient and family member had to be aged over 18 years, without obvious cognitive impairment as judged by referring health professionals. They had three different ethnicity (Romanian, Hungarian, German) and different religions (Orthodox, Catholic, Lutheran).

Patients designated the family member most involved in decision making regarding their illness (often but not necessarily the immediate carer) and from both of them formal consent was obtained.

2.1.2 Criteria for students

32 international students in the sixth year of their medical studies, from our university, were selected. They were from different cultural backgrounds: eight from United States, eight from Asia (two Chinese, four Indians, two Pakistani) eight from Africa (six Tunisian, two Moroccan) and eight from european countries (France, Germany, United Kingdom, Bosnia, Portugal).

Students attended the palliative medicine module as elective and all performed at least one summer practice in palliative care settings of their home countries.

The palliative medicine program included a number of six hours devoted to cultural sensitivity training. Methods that were used to integrate culturally sensitive topics into the curricula were: lectures, PBL (problem -based learning) cases with patients selected from three diferent romanian ethnic groups, creative teaching methods using simulated patients with diverse cultural backgrounds and small-group discussions.

All the students responded positively to our request to take part in an interview about palliative care, including spiritual care, even though most had before very limited knowledge of the subject.

2.2 Data collection and analysis

Students used a semistructured interview (one-to-one interview) (average one hour) with patients, focused on four basic dimensions in palliative medicine that vary culturally.

The four dimensions focused in the patients' interview were:

- communication of "bad news", eliciting detailed descriptions of patients' perceptions of their experiences of disclosure about the illness
- spiritual needs assessment: difficult subjects approach, recognizing symptoms and behaviors which may be related to spiritual pain and the relationship between pain and spiritual/psychological healing.
- locus of decision making
- attitudes toward advance directives and end-of-life care.

Semi structured interviews were selected because they are flexible, interactive, allow for deeper understanding of issues, and a greater exploration of cultural diversity issues. They are also dynamic and responsive to the language and concepts of individuals.

The students were divided into four focus groups. The focus groups were multi-cultural and included international medical students of different cultures to give a more diverse mix, palliative care professionals and medical teaching staff. Focus group discussions were effective in eliciting data on the cultural diversity of the patients and of the future physicians and in generating broad overviews of issues of concern to the cultural patient group.

A second interview was conducted with the same 32 international students in the sixth year of their medical studies, from our university, before and after they participated to palliative medicine module and group discussions.

All the students' interviews were personal meetings with teaching staff in palliative medicine that lasted about an hour and they took the form of a free and open discussion facilitated by a guiding questionnaire that had been drawn up in advance.

Some guidelines aimed at:

a. communication skills in different cultural environment :active listening,; common cultural variations regarding physician-patient communication; assess patients' knowledge of disease and prognosis; breaking bad news; strategies regarding ethnic, racial, and religious differences; common cultural variations regarding medical decision making; dealing with dificult questions ; eliciting and responding to patients' fears ; assessing spiritual needs as part of the initial assessment and ongoing care

b. student perception of palliative medicine module
c. student perception of cultural diversity, cultural sensitivity, cross-cultural issues integration in palliative medicine module

3. Results

3.1 Findings from patients' interviews

3.1.1 In the communication process with their patients, students appreciated:

- what are the patient's needs, with specific focus on information needs, views of patients in palliative care and family members regarding their experiences of disclosure and information sharing during the course of the illness
- how to identify common concerns or issues that might be used by students to shape and develop plans with respect to communication, with particular sensitivity to ethnic and cultural differences.

Patients and their relatives'need for sensitivity and respect for individual wishes in the communication process emerged as a central theme in the interviews. While this was especially important at the time of the initial disclosure, it recurred at all the different stages of information provision during the illness and affected the way in which content was perceived. The content needs most important to patients and families was related to prognosis and hope. Open communication regarding all aspects of the illness and its progress was reported as desirable by almost all participants, regardless of cultural backgrounds.

Almost all *patients,* 87% said they wanted to know the diagnosis of their illness. With four exceptions (in patients who shared information only in later stages) they thought it is important that information was fully shared with their families during all of the illness. A perception of insufficient information was reported to add stress, frustration, and uncertainty.

Of the respondents, 90% of the family members thought it was important for the patient to know the diagnosis. Three family members had requested that the patient must be not fully informed.

Students expressed different opinion: Bosnian, Indians, Pakistani and Chinese students expressed evasiveness regarding complete disclosure of the diagnosis to the cancer patients. They motivated their evasiveness with four reasons for nondisclosure:

- Bosnian culture believes that open discussion of serious illness may provoke unnecessary depression or anxiety in the patient
- Indians culture specifically views discussion of serious illness and death as disrespectful or impolite
- Chinese culture believes that direct disclosure may eliminate hope;
- Pakistani culture believes that speaking aloud about a condition, even in a hypothetic sense, makes death or terminal illness real because of the power of the spoken word.

In many Asian cultures, it is perceived as unnecessarily, cruel to directly inform a patient of a cancer diagnosis. Emotional reaction to news of serious illness is also considered directly harmful to health. Indians, Pakistani, Chinese and Bosnian students preferred to act like "going around" the diagnosis and being indirect about serious illness in contrast to the emphasis on "truth telling" of the American students, whose directness they described as hurtful. Asian students' strategies commonly employed to minimize direct disclosure include using terminology that obscures the seriousness of a condition or communicating diagnostic and treatment information only to the patient's family members. Students agreed that, in certain cultures, while communication about serious illness and death may not be overt, information may be conveyed with subtlety. Facial expressions, voice tone, and other nonverbal cues may convey the seriousness of a patient's status without the necessity for explicit statements.

Most patients, 91%, wanted to know their prognosis, and family members respected their wish to know or not, although some would have wanted to protect the patient from details regarding prognosis.

All the students agreed to inform completely the patients and their relatives about prognosis in order to increase adherence to palliative care. They viewed information as a mechanism that enhanced decision making and keeping some control. Most patients wanted their family member present when they met health carers, although a small number expressed a desire to be the first to know or to control how much or when the family member should be told.

3.1.2 Spiritual needs assessment was a real challenge for the students

They used their spiritual-assessment skills (e.g., compassion, presence, and active listening) in understanding how spirituality affects health and appreciating the spiritual needs of patients from diverse cultural and spiritual backgrounds. Students identified as spiritual needs of their patients:

- to have the time to express true feelings without being judged,
- to speak of important relationships,
- to have hope,
- to deal with unresolved issues, to prepare for death.

They recognized spiritual pain as loss of meaning, loss of hope, loss of identity due to lost roles, lost activity, lost independence. Its characteristics identified by the medical students were: constant and chronic pain, insomnia, withdrawal or isolation, conflict with family members, friends or medical staff, anxiety, fear, mistrust of family, friends, physicians, hospice staff, depression, hopelessness, feeling of failure with life.

Despite most of the students considered themselves to be not religious or slightly religious and the heterogeneity in self-reported faith traditions: Christian (n = 7), Hindu (n = 4), atheist (n = 5), Catholic

(n = 6), Jewish (n = 2), Muslim (n = 8) they recognized the appropriate conditions which recommend clergy involvement. The specific situations identified to make referrals to chaplains as part of the interdisciplinary team were:

- when spiritual issues seem particularly significant in the patient's suffering,
- when spiritual/religious beliefs seem of particular help and support for the patient,

- when addressing the spiritual needs of a patient exceeds the physician's comfort level,
- when specific community spiritual resources are needed,
- when physician or nurse suspect spiritual issues which the patient denies,
- when the patient's family seems to be experiencing spiritual pain,
- when the medical staff (doctors, nurses, students) seems to be experiencing spiritual pain or is in need of support - multiple deaths, issues of injustice, particular attachment to a dying patient.

In the feedback gathered from patients, the majority of the participants (95%) felt their symptoms management needs and spiritual needs had been addressed and viewed their interaction with the students involved in palliative care positively. According to patients' responses, the majority wanted their doctor to be interested in their spiritual care.

3.1.3 Locus of decision making

With regard to decision making, american students emphasised on patient autonomy which contrasted with preferences for more family-based, physician-based, or shared physician- and family-based decision making among Indians and Tunisian students'opinion. Pakistani students shared that in their culture, physicians may be adopted into the family unit and addressed as parent, aunt, uncle, or sibling.

European students emphasised that in their culture patients prefer that physicians, because of their expert knowledge, make independent decisions to reduce the burden on patients and their families.

In group discussions, the students discussed choices regarding strategies for managing disease, approaches to symptom relief, or partnership in facing profound existential issues and facilitating personal growth. Decision making involved ethical principles (understood in the light of cultural sensitivity), with considerations of autonomy, justice, beneficence, and maleficence.

3.1.4 Attitudes toward advance directives and end-of-life care

Concerning the advance directive completion, this had lower rates among romanian patients of specific ethnic backgrounds, which may reflect distrust of the health care system, current health care disparities, cultural perspectives on death and suffering.

Chinese students emphasised that in their culture, people are less likely to sign their own do-not-resuscitate (DNR) orders because of its negative emotional impact on health.

By paying attention to the patient's values, spirituality, and relationship dynamics, students elicited cultural preferences. They actively developped rapport with ethnically diverse patients simply by demonstrating an interest in their cultural heritage.

3.2 Findings from students' interviews

3.2.1 Initial students' feedback, before palliative medicine module attendance

They discussed their self-perceived learning needs in dealing with patients with advanced diseases and different cultural backgrounds. Of the respondents 81 % students considered that they were not prepared for all the skills/competencies needed to approach cultural diversity issues in palliative care. We identified many common themes and concerns emerged from students' interviews, including:

- lack of knowledge about palliative care and lack of understanding about spiritual care,
- confusion as to the difference between spiritual and religious needs,
- concern about how healthcare and social services would relate to spiritual care, finding a way to develop spiritual care and successfully integrate it into the general health and social services systems.

3.2.2 Interviews after students completed this module

They shared their educational and training experiences and made suggestions about cultural diversity issues in palliative care management and its influence in learning environment. Most students respondents (96%) thought that general communication skills, e.g. communicating with patients and patients' relatives, counselling skills such as dealing with difficult questions, eliciting and responding to patients' and relatives' fears, breaking bad news, crosscultural issues were well covered in the paliative medicine module and group discussion.

Focused was on:

- communication issues, including disclosure and consent;
- modes of decision making: how or when is the patient or family involved
- concepts of disease, meaning of pain and other symptoms;
- agree priorities with patients with different cultural backgrounds
- fulfil patients' needs for information about treatment
- attitudes to medication (especially opioid drugs and sedatives) and to nutrition
- ways of conceptualising death and dying in relation to the rest of life
- understand issues which surround euthanasia
- spiritual matters, as well as religious issues, including rituals.
- customs surrounding death, burial or cremation, and bereavement
- supporting a bereaved person, preparing family for bereavement.

According to students' responses after palliative medicine training the approach of spiritual care has had a positive and meaningful impact. Students identified two important facilitators of spiritual care: having time, unencumbered by competing clinical demands and effective communication with the patients and their family members. There were also identified the implications for medical care of the spiritual and religious issues:

- if the patient religion forbid any specific parts of medical care (transfusion, surgical therapies),
- barriers to patient-physician communication posed by religion/spirituality complex issues,
- the patient refuse to discuss spiritual or religious implications of his health care.

Students'evaluation before and after this module demonstrated improvement in students' abilities to assess patients' palliative care needs and spiritual needs and negotiate issues regarding complex treatments. They appreciated the interactive nature of palliative medicine program and described it as relevant, balanced, and practical. Students were interested in finding out about new ways to enhance the lives quality of the patients and families in distress and they wanted better understand the challenges facing the development of palliative care. More attention may need to be directed towards the learning environment. The majority of respondents medical students showed that the patient's culture is an important issue when providing care (with 95 % of indicating "moderately important" or "very important"). In the interviews the students also explored educational issues in palliative medicine. They considered the attendance to palliative medicine module as an improved clinical experience and an opportunity for cultural sensitivity and cultural competence achievements. Medical students achieved interviewing skills, abilities to work in a multidisciplinary team, to pay attention to complementary treatments and ethical aspects of cross-cultural issues. Some critical attributes of good communication they identified as important: playing it straight, staying the course, giving time, showing you care, making it clear, and pacing information. They affect the quality of the relationship between health professionals and patients and their families and should be emphasised in the teaching of communication skills. Communication of prognosis to patients with cancer is a sensitive issue and therefore patients' needs for information should be individually assessed. Most students, 91% considered that poorly handled cross-cultural issues may have negative clinical consequences, including longer office visits, patient noncompliance, delays obtaining informed consent, ordering of unnecessary tests, and lower quality of care. A significant proportion of the respondents, 82% thought that they had developed some attributes fully through their work experience in palliative medicine module and group discussions and these were opportunities to consolidate what they had learned in the previous years. The teaching staff involved in this activities appreciated the open-mindedness attitudes, which made students especially receptive to our educational programme.

4. Discussions

The diversity of the cultural and racial orientations of the people means that those who provide health and social services increasingly interact with others of diverse cultural, social, racial, linguistic, and religious backgrounds.[*Green et al,* 2008]. The public is better informed and it has a better understanding of the complexity management of the chronic, life-threatening diseases. [Florea et al, 2008]. Given rapidly changing global demographic dynamics and the evidence regarding health outcomes attributable to cultural competence education, it is time to consider the approach to preparing medical students to reduce health disparities and care for ethnoculturally and socially diverse patients.

In an effort to provide health care professionals with the knowledge and skills to effectively care for diverse populations, an educational movement in "cross-cultural care" has emerged. This field has received a new emphasis during the past 10 years as a result of statements made by the American Medical Association (AMA) and the Accreditation Council for Graduate Medical Education, among others, that crosscultural training is necessary for the effective practice of medicine in this globalizing world.[Weissman, 2005]

The issue of cultural competence training is an evolving element of medical education curricula which must answer to the following questions:

- How can medical curricula be developed so that content is relevant and applicable to the workplace and graduates acquire the personal characteristics and skills required for medical practice?
- What are the obstacles to providing undergraduates with well-managed work experience, adequate exposure to the real world of medical practice and the necessary opportunities to apply knowledge and acquire essential skills, attitudes and personal attributes?

Tomorrow's physicians must be adequately trained to provide optimal care to patients from ethnic, social, spiritual and religious backgrounds different from their own. [Nelda &Valmi, 2011].

Cultural competence translate into improved health outcomes and reduction of disparities in health or health care. [Betancourt , 2006]. Improving student–patient communication is an important component of improving the quality of care generally, and addressing differences in quality of care that are associated with patients' race, ethnicity, or culture more specifically. Many students are unfamiliar with common cultural variations regarding physician-patient communication, medical decision making, and attitudes about formal documents such as code status guidelines and advance directives. End-of-life discussions are particularly challenging because of their emotional and interpersonal intensity. [Far, 2002; Kuin et al 2006; Mueller et al, 2001].

Introducing palliative medicine modules in undergraduate medical education is an important opportunity to enhance students with cultural sensitivity awareness and cultural competence. Despite recent progress and educational efforts, there are attitudinal barriers still thwart the successful integration of palliative care into general medical education. Medical students and residents are uncomfortable facing death and dying. The prevailing medical culture continues to view death as a medical failure. Palliative care, despite its growing scientific base, is often perceived as low-tech or ''soft.'' Many trainees do not view palliative care skills as core clinical competencies. They learn to prescribe antihypertensive and hypolipemiants drugs but they fail to master the use of opioids. These attitudes may contribute to practice patterns that tend to devalue the provision of palliative care even though the public increasingly asserts the importance of humane medical care at the end of life.

Previous efforts in cultural competence have aimed to teach about the attitudes, values, beliefs, and behavior of certain groups. There is no "manual" of how to care for patients from different racial, ethnic, or cultural groups; instead, a more effective approach is to learn about how social, cultural, or economic factors influence patients' health values, beliefs, and behaviors. [Gundersen, 2000; Hibnall & Brooks 2001; Hudson, 2006; Koenig, 2000].

In our study, group discussions were focused on the issues that arise most commonly due to cultural differences, cultural sensitivity. International students' curiosity, empathy, and respect, as well as an understanding of the romanian multiethnic patient's social context, motivated their interest in achieving cultural competence. We approached the concepts of cultural competence and"transnational competence" in medical education, which are not new concepts and have been argued previously, resulting in greater adoption of these principles among medical educators.[Gregg & Saha, 2006].

These principles have now become the blueprint for teaching medical students throughout the country, although adoption of this approach is slow but steady. [Koehn & Swick , 2006]. Training under this approach may be especially helpful in the care of patients who come from cultures different from the culture of the clinician. [Betancourt & Green, 2010]. Cultural competence aims to bridge the "cultural distance" that exists between medical providers and their patients.

Medical students and tomorrow's physicians need a practical set of tools and skills that will enable them to provide quality care to patients everywhere, from anywhere, with whatever differences in background that may exist.

The field of cultural competence aims to assure that health care providers are prepared to provide quality care to diverse populations. There are evidence highlighting the fact that the failure of health care providers to acknowledge, understand, and manage sociocultural variations in the health beliefs and behaviors of their patients may impede effective communication and better patient care. [Betancourt & Green, 2010]. The diversity of the cultural and racial orientations of the people means that those who provide health and social services increasingly interact with others of diverse cultural, social, racial, linguistic, and religious backgrounds. Transnational competence in medical education offers a comprehensive set of core skills derived from international relations, cross-cultural psychology, and intercultural communication that are also applicable for medical education. [Koehn & Swick, 2006].

There is an effort to change the medical education systems. Moderate gains in cultural sensitivity training, such as inclusion of the topic in curricular objectives and content were made. These changes are part of an increased institutional commitment in some medical schools to improve students' abilities to provide culturally sensitive clinical care when they become practicing physicians. Gaps continue to exist in teaching this important skill. To achieve cultural competence, an organized and systematic approach of the objective development, curriculum planning, learning methods, and program evaluation is needed. [Betancourt & Green, 2010; Lie et al., 2006].

In some medical schools informal teaching of culturally sensitive topics have occurred. It is possible that medical students and faculties from different cultural backgrounds learn from each other using students' mobilities and teaching staff's professional mobilities and share their beliefs and attitudes with respect to health practices on an informal basis. Exposure to patients from other cultural backgrounds in practice, as our international students did, might bring culturally sensitive issues to the individual learner. Cultural competency involves an understanding and acceptance of cultural practices and is more than simply being able to speak the same language. Communicating effectively across cultures is a critical factor in providing quality health care to diverse populations. Becoming culturally competent is an ongoing process and a lifelong commitment.

Neglecting cultural issues in palliative medicine should be a possible source of tension in family and of confusion to health professionals. Sensitivity to the cultural nuances of communication (the breaking of bad news), family dynamics, decision making, interpersonal tensions and suffering may add value to attempts to care. Cultural gaps between health professionals and patients are expressed in many ways (from treatment preferences to concepts of spirituality). Bridging the gaps may require long time to be accomplished. This must begin in medical students' training.

As an effort to provide physicians training with the knowledge and skills to address cross-cultural challenges in the clinical encounter, curricula in "cultural competence" have emerged and been integrated into medical education. Cultural competence is a developmental process at both the student and university levels. With appropriate support, students can enhance their cultural awareness, knowledge and skills over time. Cultural strengths exist within our university and they will be better tapped in the training process of our 2800 international medical students, from 50 countries. A process of cultural competence assessment will be developped and students will benefit by heightening awareness, influencing attitudes toward practice, and motivating the development of knowledge and skills. This process also benefits the university by informing planning, policy-making, resource allocation and training/professional development activities. A growing literature delineates the impact of sociocultural factors, race, ethnicity and ethical issues on palliative care. [Florea et al., 2008; Shanmugasundaram et al., 2009; Williams et al., 2011].

Sociocultural differences between patient and physician influence communications and clinical decision making. Medical students and physicians aren't shielded from diversity, as patients present varied perspectives, values, beliefs, and behaviors regarding health and well-being. These include variations in patient recognition of symptoms, thresholds for seeking care, ability to communicate symptoms to a provider who understands their meaning, ability to understand the prescribed management strategy, expectations of care (including preferences for or against diagnostic and therapeutic procedures), and adherence to medical interventions and medications. Evidence suggests that provider-patient communication is directly linked to patient satisfaction and adherence and subsequently to health outcomes. [Betancourt, 2003]. Thus, when sociocultural differences between patient and provider aren't appreciated, explored, understood, or communicated in the medical encounter, patient dissatisfaction, poor adherence, and poorer health outcomes result.

The cultural competence, transnational competence approach will promote advances in preparing medical students to reduce health disparities among patients with multiple and diverse backgrounds, health conditions, and health care beliefs and practices. In palliative care this consistently directs attention to the policy and social factors, as well as the individual considerations, that can alleviate suffering and enhance health in a globalizing world.

Palliative and end-of-life care for a patient born and living in an Anglo-Saxon country may be different from that of a patient in a Latin or Islamic country, as patients' relationships with individual physicians and with institutions, preferences and practices of truth telling, attitudes toward screening, prevention and clinical trials, decision-making styles, and end-of-life choices are all subject to cultural variability. Additional research on how cultural diversity influences patients' and families' preferences in regard to palliative care is needed to meet the needs of different communities and individual patients.[Biasco & Surbone 2009].

Our study, like others, [Chun etal.,2010; Thompson et al, 2010] suggests that specific education, rather than individual experience of crosscultural interactions, which may not always be positive, is needed to improve the cultural competence of tomorrow's physicians and future palliative care professionals. The introduction of humanism, medical ethics and multiculturalism into medical education involves linking the professional training of students with human values, an orientation of education and practice towards addressing human needs and interests. [Kumagai & Lypson, 2009]. We need research to identify, assess, and plan the care of all patients who are sick enough to die, and we need education that keeps alive our humanity and sense of vocation. This is an enormous challenge on the market of healthcare models, but one that will be useful to the chronic, life-threatening ill patients. [Florea et al, 2008].

5. Conclusions

The chapter describes the experiences of international medical students involved in palliative care programme, addressing cross-cultural issues, cultural sensitivity awareness. It draws attention to the complex relationships between different patients' and students' cultural background and palliative care issues and to the need of cultural competence in medical education.

Six-year international students at our medical school appreciated the level to which cultural competence instruction in palliative medicine occurred.

Our sudy also revealed that it is not only the patient's culture that matters; the students' and tomorrow's physicians' culture is equally important. Teaching about palliative care from a crosscultural perspective was favorably received by students and positively influenced students' attitudes.

Palliative medicine training is a complex opportunity of cross-cultural medical education which must be approached and this will increase the cultural competence and standards of the academic medical education. Our findings indicate that multicultural medical education in palliative medicine is an important area for future research and curricular reform.

6. References

Azad N., Power B., Dollin J., Chery S. (2002). Cultural sensitivity training in Canadian medical schools. *Acad.Med.*; 77: 222-228.

Betancourt J. R. (2003). Cross-cultural Medical Education: Conceptual Approaches and Frameworks for Evaluation. *Acad. Med.* 78:560–569.

Betancourt J. R., Green AR, Carrillo JE, Park ER. (2005).Cultural competence and health care disparities: key perspectives and trends. *Health Aff (Millwood).*; 24:499–505.

Betancourt J. R. (2006). Cultural Competence and Medical Education: Many Names, Many Perspectives, One Goal. *Acad Med.* Vol. 81, No. 6 ; :499–501

Betancourt J. R., Green A. R. (2010). *Commentary: Linking Cultural Competence Training to Improved Health Outcomes: Perspectives From the Field. Academic Medicine:* Vol 85 - Issue 4: 583-585

Biasco G., Surbone A. (2009).Cultural Challenges in Caring for Our Patients in Advanced Stages of Cancer. *Journal of Clinical Oncology,* Vol 27, No 1 :157-158 Bruera, E., Sweeney, C., Calder, K., Palmer, L., & Benisch-Tolley, S. (2001). Patient preferences versus physician perceptions of treatment decisions in cancer care. *Journal of Clinical Oncology, 19*(1), 2883-2885

Chun M. B. J., Yamada A.M., Huh J., Hew C., Tasaka S. (2010). Using the Cross-Cultural Care Survey toAssess Cultural Competency in GraduateMedical Education. *J Grad Med* Ed, Vol. 2, No. 1, *96-101;* DOI: 10.4300/JGME-D-09-00100.1

Curlin F. A., Vance J. L., Chin M. H., Lantos J. D. (2002). To Die, to Sleep: US Physicians' Religious and Other Objections to Physician-Assisted Suicide, Terminal Sedation, and Withdrawal of Life Support. *Academic Medicine*; 77(3):193-197

Davis B. H., Smith M. K. (2009). Infusing Cultural Competence Training into the Curriculum: Describing the Development of Culturally Sensitive Training on Dementia Communication. *The Kaohsiung Journal of Medical Sciences, Vol 25; 9: 503-509*

Florea M., Perju-Dumbrava L., Crisan M., Talu S., Miclutia I., Gherman M. (2008). A paliative approach to aids in the antiretroviral therapy era and the impact on medical ethics.*Romanian Journal of Bioethics*, 6 (4): 47-54 *Green AR, Betancourt JR. Carrillo J. (*2008). Integrating Social Factors into Cross-cultural Medical Education. *American Journal of Hospice and Palliative Medicine*, Vol. 25, No. 2, 112-120.

Gregg, J. Saha, S.(2006). Losing Culture on the Way to Competence: The Use and Misuse of Culture in Medical Education. Academic Medicine, Vol 81; 6 : 542-547

Koehn P., Swick H. (2006). Medical Education for a Changing World: Moving Beyond Cultural Competence into Transnational Competence *Academic Medicine*: Vol. 81; 6 : 548-556

Gundersen L. (2000). Faith and healing. *Ann Intern Med* ; 132: 169-72

Hibnall J. T., Brooks C. A. (2001). Religion in the clinic: the role of physician beliefs. *South Med J*; 94: 374-9. Hudson P L, Kristjanson J, Ashby M. (2006).Desire for hastened death in patients with advanced disease and the evidence base of clinical guidelines: a systematic review. *Palliative Medicine*;Vol. 20, No. 7, 693-701

Kuin A., Deliens L., Zuylen L. van, Courtens A. M,. Vernooij-Dassen M. J, Linden B. van der, and Wal G. van der (2006). Spiritual issues in palliative care consultations in the Netherlands. *Palliative Medicine*, September 1; 20(6): 585 – 592

Kellehear A. (2001). The changing face of dying in Australia. *Med J Aust* ; 175: 508-510

Koenig H.G. (2000). Religion, spirituality, and medicine: application to clinical practice. *J Am Med Assoc*; 284: 1708.

Kumagai A.K., Lypson M.L.(2009). Beyond cultural competence: critical consciousness, social justice, and multicultural education. *Acad Med.*; 84(6):782–787

Lickiss J. N. (2003). Approaching death in multicultural Australia. *Med J Aust*; 1796 Suppl): S14-S16

Lie D., Boker J., Cleveland E. (2006). Using the Tool for Assessing Cultural Competence Training (TACCT) to measure faculty and medical student perceptions of cultural competence instruction in the first three years of the curriculum. *Acad Med.*;81:557–64.

Lo B. (2002). Discussing religious and spiritual issues at the end of life. *JAMA*, 287(6), 749-754.

Martin M., Vaughn B. (2007). "Strategic Diversity & Inclusion Management" magazine,. *DTUI Publications Division: San Francisco, CA: 31-36*

Lloyd-Williams M., M. Macleod R. (2004). A systematic review of teaching and learning in palliative care within the medical undergraduate curriculum. *Medical Teacher*, Vol. 26, No. 8: 683-690 (doi: 10.1080/01421590400019575)

Molinuevo B., Torrubia R. (2011). Validation of the Catalan Version of the Communication Skills Attitude Scale (CSAS) in a Cohort of South European Medical and Nursing Students. *Education for Health* 11 (online),: 499. http://www.educationforhealth.net

Mueller, P.S., Plevak, D.J. & Rummans, T.A (2001). Religious involvement, spirituality and medicine: Implications for clinical practice. *Mayo Clin Proc.*;76, 1225-1235.

Nelda C. M,Valmi D. S. (2011). Cross-Cultural Validation and Psychometric Evaluation of the Spanish Brief Religious Coping Scale (S-BRCS). *J Transcult Nurs. 22: 248-256, doi:10.1177/1043659611404426*

Rodriguez F., Cohen A., Betancourt J.R., Green A.R.(2011). Evaluation of medical student self-rated preparedness to care for limited english proficiency patients. BMC Med Educ. 11: 26. doi: 10.1186/1472-6920-11-26

Rosen J., Spatz E.S.; Gaaserud A. M. J., Abramovitch H. , Weinreb B., Wenger N. S., Margolis C. Z. (2004). A new approach to developing cross-cultural communication skills. *Medical Teacher*, vol 26, nr 2, 126-132

Shanmugasundaram S., O'Connor M., Sellick K. (2009). A multicultural perspective on conducting palliative care research in an Indian population in Australia. *International Journal of Palliative Nursing,* Vol. 15, 9; 25: 440 - 445

Taran S. (2010). An Examination of the Factors Contributing to Poor Communication Outside the Physician-Patient Sphere. *MJM*;13(1):86-91

Thompson BM, Haidet P, Casanova R, Vivo RP, Gomez AG, Brown AF, Richter RA, Crandall SJ. (2010). Medical students' perceptions of their teachers' and their own cultural competency: implications for education. *J Gen Intern Med.* 25(Suppl 2):S 91–94.

Valente, S. M. (2004). End of life and ethnicity. *Journal for Nurses in Staff Development, 20*(6), 285-293.

Ward, E., Jemal, A., Cokkinides, V., Singh, G. K., Cardinez, C., Ghafoor, A., et al.(2004). Cancer disparities by race/ethnicity and socioeconomic status; 54(6):369]. *CA -- A Cancer Journal for Clinicians, 54*(2), 78. Weissman JS, Betancourt JR, Campbell EG, et al.(2005). Resident physician's preparedness to provide cross-cultural care. *JAMA.*;294: 1058–67.

Werth, J. L., Jr., Blevins, D., Toussaint, K. L., & Durham, M. R. (2002). The influence ofcultural diversity on end-of-life care and decisions. *American Behavioral Scientist, 46*(2), 204-219.

Williams J. A., Meltzer D., Arora V., Chung G. and Curlin F. A. (2011). Attention to Inpatients' Religious and Spiritual Concerns: Predictors and Association with Patient Satisfaction. *J.Gen.Intern Med,* DOI: 10.1007/s11606-011-1781-y.

Wright M. (2004). Hospice care and models of spirituality. *Eur J Palliat Care*;11:75-78

2

Teaching Palliative Care in a Free Clinic: A Brazilian Experience

Thais Pinheiro, Pablo Blasco, Maria Auxiliadora Benedetto,
Marcelo Levites, Auro Del Giglio and Cauê Monaco
Brazilian Society of Family Medicine (SOBRAMFA),
Brazil

1. Introduction

There is no curricular palliative care teaching in Brazil. Brazilian's doctors are not training to deal with terminally ill patients.

We believe that we can teach some important skills using palliative care. Some essential topics that students can finish medical training in Brazil, without any formal contact. We can provide different approach in communication's skills by teaching in a palliative care setting.

In our group, Brazilian Society of Family Medicine (SOBRAMFA), we diced to create a palliative care setting. Our main objective was to observe students and residents and try to identify how this experience can influence their medical training.

The ideas presented here are the final result of a qualitative analysis about the students and residents' experience. We used the stories related by them to exemplify what they learned.

2. An overview of palliative care

Palliative Medicine is an ancient practice. Some centuries ago the only thing that doctors could do was palliative care (Melo,2003).

Palliative comes from *palliare,* a Latin term that means to cover, to decrease difficulties, exactly what medicine was.

An example that shows us how the intention to care and relive people of suffering can be transformed in science is this description from Ambroise Paré, a barber-surgeon from France in 18th century. It was accepted practice at that time to pour boiling elder oil on an amputated limb to cauterize it and keep away "bad humors". As a military barber-surgeon operating in the Apennine Alps, Paré saw hundreds of patients a day. One night, in the thick of battle, he ran out of elder oil and had to devise a salve of egg, oil of rose, and turpentine. The salve he applied was soothing and causes his patients no pain. The next morning, half the patients treated with elder oil were dead and the other half in agony while all his patients treated with the salve were resting peacefully and healing well. When he saw his new treatment worked more effectively and caused less pain to his patients, Paré would not change his methods (Helliwell,1999).

In the beginning of 20th century William Osler, a famous doctor at that time, was the first scientist that wrote about palliative care. The patients and doctors use to correlate suffering with the end of lifetime and Osler tried to change this idea (Irigoyen,2002).

Osler was a general practitioner, he was considered the smartest, the best one in his time;. His diagnostic ability was fabulous. The title of his biography written by Reid is "The great doctor". It's amazing that in a time where there weren't efficient therapeutics like today, Osler became a healer. It seems that his secret was to know people, not just diseases. He could understand human suffering and he respected that. He tried to understand more than physical and chemical diseases consequences, to be able to share feelings and spiritual thoughts. He was an optimist and had a big compassion. His relationship with patients was a kind of religious thing. Osler blessed them and they got better. He used few drugs and didn't believe in many therapeutic methods. But he believed in human being. He always treated patients well and transmitted security to them. He believed in "bed medicine" (Relman,1989).

Cecily Saunders in 1960 developed the principles of modern hospice and palliative care. She heard patients and learned with them their real necessities deciding to dedicate her life to care of terminally ill patients. Saunders started a "hospice" called Saint Christopher's Hospice, in London (Figueredo,2003; Melvin,2001; South-Paul et al, 2004). She emphasized excellence in pain and symptom management; care of the whole person including their physical, emotional, social and spiritual needs; and the need for research in this newly developing field of medicine.

She used to say to her patients "You are important because you are unique. You will be important to us until the last moment of your life, and we will make everything we can, not just that you die in peace, but that you live until your death moment" (South-Paul et al, 2004).

Nowadays, this philosophy is present in a lot of countries and in many palliative care services.

In 1968, Dr Elizabeth Kuebler-Ross, a psychiatrist working closely with terminally ill people in the United States, published her seminal work, *On Death and Dying*. This book, for the first time, described the psychological crisis of the terminally ill person in terms of defined stages -denial, anger, bargaining, depression, and acceptance. This book has since become essential reading for clinicians who care for the terminally ill. She was the first to show the needs of dying, stressing the need for personal autonomy, death with dignity, and the benefit of death at home versus in a health care facility (Melvin,2001; South-Paul et al, 2004).

2.1 Palliative education setting

Human suffering and death are real facts in daily doctors' activity. In spite of that, we still observe a big lack of professionals that are properly trained and prepared to deal with this subject (Blasco, 1997).

Death is a phenomenon that disrupts medical practice. It is not uncommon that doctors don't consider death as a real possibility. Death is not some unhappy fact that comes and makes the doctor's brilliant acting more difficult. Nowadays we can find doctors that use high-level technology but, in some way, give up their incurable patients, with whom their technical knowledge doesn't work. They are doctors for "new cars", "runners for short running". They are unable to remain comfortable in situations where purely biomedical technical skills are not enough (Blasco, 1997).

Experts agree that experimentally based and developmentally appropriate ethics education is needed during medical training to prepare medical students to provide excellent end-of-life care (Ahmedzai, 1982; Billings & Block , 1997;Caralis &Hammond , 1992; Lloyd-Williams & MacLeod, 2004).

In U.S. a survey had demonstrated that the majority of medical schools do not provide palliative care knowledge during graduation. The researchers suggested the implementation of palliative guideline in medical curriculum (Aalst-Cohen et al, 2008)

2.2 Suffering and death: Palliative care

Palliative Medicine is the study and management of patients with illness in which cure is no longer possible and an end point of death is expected within a finite period of time. The focus is on the control of symptoms and maximizing patient' self-defined quality of life (Melvin,2001; Rakel,1995). The complex goal of relief suffering can't be one-dimensional but must include the four human dimensions of human experience: physical (pain, dyspnea, cough, constipation, delirium), emotional (anxiety, depression, grief), social (financial concerns, unfinished business) and spiritual (guilt, sadness, worthlessness). To provide this complete assistance the palliative care is usually made by an interdisciplinary team (Melvin,2001; South-Paul et al, 2004).

According to World Health Organization, palliative care is an approach that improves the quality of life of patients and their families facing the problem associated with life-threatening illness, through the prevention and relief of suffering by means of early identification and impeccable assessment and treatment of pain and other problems, physical, psychosocial and spiritual. Palliative care provides relief from pain and other distressing symptoms; affirms life and regards dying as a normal process; intends neither to hasten or postpone death; integrates the psychological and spiritual aspects of patient care; offers a support system to help patients live as actively as possible until death;offers a support system to help the family cope during the patients illness and in their own bereavement; uses a team approach to address the needs of patients and their families, including bereavement counseling, if indicated; will enhance quality of life, and may also positively influence the course of illness; is applicable early in the course of illness, in conjunction with other therapies that are intended to prolong life, such as chemotherapy or radiation therapy, and includes those investigations needed to better understand and manage distressing clinical complications

2.3 Family medicine and palliative care

The reason to have a family doctor in a palliative care service becomes clear if we understand the principles of family medicine.

Family Medicine's focus and action fields are: primary care, medical education and leadership. Trained in a specialty that is focused on person, the family physician is a person's specialist (Blasco et al,2003).

Irygoyen says that the Family Medicine participation on palliative care occurs because both specialties focus on continuity care, prevention and family dynamics study.

Family Medicine's philosophy promotes doctors that have as a professional objective to improve health and quality of life of their patients in a broader sense. The doctor-patient relationship doesn't end with some incurable and deathly disease, even with the patient's death, as the relationship with the family goes on after that (Irigoyen,2002).

To provide this kind of care to patients with cancer, a palliative care outpatient clinic started on March 2004 after an agreement between the oncology department of ABC Medical School in Santo André (Brazil) and the Brazilian Society of Family Medicine (SOBRAMFA).

This ambulatory gives medical assistance to patients that the oncologists consider out of traditional therapeutic possibilities. The objective is to training doctors in skills necessary to provide this kind of assistance.

3. Methodology

Students and residents consult terminally ill in a free clinic that provides medical assistance to patients who are referred by oncologists. In the setting the learners are orientated to the principles of palliative care, narrative medicine and have required readings related to these issues. A reflective writing session, in which patients´ stories and doctors' and students' feelings and concerns are shared in a narrative perspective, closes the ambulatory day.

A structure interview was used after nine months of work to express the doctors' reflection clearly.

About the palliative care ambulatory:

- What was the most important aspect for you?
- In which way did this ambulatory experience contribute to your training as a future doctor?
- Did you have any negative experiences?
- Which was your best experience?
- Please write down a patient's story that has drawn your attention.

3.1 Objectives

Identify the educational impact of palliative medicine in family medicine training.

3.2 Setting

In 2004 the Brazilian Society of Family Medicine (SOBRAMFA), in partnership with the oncology department of ABC Medical School, created a Palliative Care Ambulatory Clinic (PCAC). The PCAC is a free clinic that provides medical assistance to patients who are referred by oncologists. The clinic takes place once a week and is staffed by family physicians, residents, and medical students.

Family members are usually present at the encounters, but both patients and relatives have the opportunity to talk individually to members of the team.

At the end of each day, a reflective environment is created. So, students, residents and faculty take part in a reflective writing session in which the patients´ stories, doctors' and students' feelings and concerns are shared in a narrative perspective.

Our study analyzes a period from March to November 2004, were we had 37 patients (22 men; 15 women) and 24 of them had died.

3.3 Analisys

We decided to look at the educational impact of the PCAC using a qualitative method of thematic analysis. The research had the approval of SOBRAMFA's Ethics Committee.

Data was collected from three sources: a journal composed by the preceptors who acted as participant observers, a questionnaire given to the residents and students at the end of their rotation, and the reflective papers written by students and residents.

The teachers that participated in the PCAC, individually, did an analysis of this material and list some topics. After five discussion meetings they decided by tree different topics: keep the focus on the patient, learning to deal with families and from fear to comfort.

4. Findings

4.1 Keep the focus on the patient

Palliative care patients usually have a lot of symptoms,either caused by cancer, like pain and fatigue, or non related to it, like headache or hypertension.

The learners had chances to diagnose and treat some symptoms or diseases that were not so visible in the first contact.

It is important to note that every family doctor during his/her professional life will likely need to offer palliative care to his/her patients, and this doctor has to be able to do so.

4.1.1 What bothers the patient?

"Mr. J comes to palliative care ambulatory because of a liver cancer (without confirmation diagnosis). It was all we knew about him, besides that he hadn't had a good treatment response. After some conversation he told us that what was really bothering him was a sinusitis that nobody had treated before. So we gave him some general orientations and focused treatment on his respiratory problem. His cancer was under control, and after our intervention he had an improvement in his respiratory symptoms. In the following visits he would breathe deeply several times to show us how better he felt."

4.1.2 Can we always do something for our patients?

"One of the most significant patients was Mr. J, a middle aged man who had a larynx tumor, tracheotomy, cachexia, radiotherapy complications and a lot of pain even with morphine in high doses. At first sight he looked like an untreatable patient, and many doctors and family members had

abandoned him. When we listened to his needs, we realized the possibility to improve analgesics to better pain control using amitriptylin and carbamazepine, which worked well. The orientations to offer food in small quantity several times during the day, about intestinal habit and wound care made possible a better pain control and a more comfortable end of life. The family members felt more comfortable too and realized they could do something for the patient's comfort. There is no doubt those doctors' care and family love made the difference for the patient who never missed one consultation not even in the last days of his life."

About the ambulatory context one of the doctors wrote: "Any time the team is trying to release suffering and make something to the patient with the family help. Even if nothing more can be done clinically, we can help the patient feel that he has not been abandoned and that somebody still cares about him".

4.1.3 How do I take all these medications, Doc?

"In his first consultation Mr. J, 65 years old, with a larynx cancer (already treated), hypertension and hypothyroidism after radiotherapy, brought a bag with his medications. We discovered that he couldn't read which makes it difficult for him to know how to use all that. A colorful table and the identification of the medication was enough to him to learn how to do it."

4.2 Learning to deal with families

The families have an active participation in this end of life stage and need orientation about nutrition, hygiene, sadness, suffering and death.

The residents and students could understand the importance of setting opportunities for family members to talk about patients' feelings and about their own feelings and difficulties.

"It is necessary to spend additional time with family members. As a result of that special attention, they can provide better care to the patient at home." Residents and students noticed that even when patients had difficulty visiting the office, the family would still come.

Some family members would express their gratitude through letters, calls, or even visiting the clinic after the patient's death. Occasionally, they came back because they had a need to share experiences and feelings from the patient's final moments.

4.2.1 Receiving news

"It is obvious that the relationship depends on the family and patient. It is interesting to note that the family, perhaps, because of this intense participation in the patient care, feels comfortable to continue to visit us after the patient dies. In these months we had the opportunity to receive some calls, letters or ambulatory visits were the family express their gratitude and inform us about how the patient died. Difficult moments where we can noticed that we were poor prepared and trained during the medical school to deal with ours and patient's families' emotions and feelings."

"Mrs. L, 65 years old, had a huge stomach adenocarcinoma that provoked massive ascites. She was not having dyspnea that day, but her two daughters were worried about her ascites and told us that the procedure made to reverse that was not very efficient. They had a paper with a well-done description from medication and the time to take each one. They had come to us to relieve their mother's pain. We explained to them how to use morphine and other symptomatic medication, diuretics to eliminate the ascites, and gave them a cellular phone number to call if they needed. After that, the patient got better for a few days, but the ascites relapsed. She went to the hospital where they did another procedure and after that she got really worse and died some hours later. Next week, during our clinical discussion time, the receptionist told us that the Mrs. L daughters were there to talk to us. They had come to tell what had happened in their mother's last moments and thanked for what we had done for their mother."

4.2.2 What can I give him to eat?

"The families have a lot of doubt about nutrition, even in patients without tubes. We saw a son that wouldn't let his mother eats ice cream because he thoughts that she could get cold and wives that didn't offer a typical Brazilian food twice a week because it is very spicy. We had noticed with time that it is very important to tell family members what they can give to the patient and how to do it. Patients felt better because they had something like a "medical authorization" to eat what they wanted."

4.3 From fear to comfort

The first contact with a terminal disease was usually frightening for our residents and students. "I think I will be useless here." "During usual training we are taught to solve medical problems. Subjects such as pain, suffering, and death are almost ignored, as if they don't represent important elements of daily medical practice."

"I panic just thinking that I won't know how to behave." Such reactions denote the lack of preparation to approach the usual issues related to terminal patients.

Nevertheless, step by step, trainees acquired more and more ability to deal with the issues they considered difficult. They realized that by listening to the patients and relatives it is possible to detect their real needs. "I could see that my patient did not want to be seen as a special person whose death is inexorable but as a patient like any other. He became calm when I listened to him with attention and was very satisfied with the prescription of the medicines." "Often, the solutions are simpler than we can imagine." "For me, this is something new. I saw the whole team trying to do their best to alleviate suffering and get the family involved in the care. I realized that, even if healing is no longer possible, we can help patients feel they are not alone because there is somebody with them, very interested in helping them."

4.3.1 Do I have cancer, Doctor? Will you help me?

"In the beginning I thought that this first question would be frequent, but because of the advanced disease's stage most of the patients knew what was going on.

The second question is the most common question in the ambulatory setting. Sometimes patients think we are their last hope, someone that can improve their condition. This question is very hard to answer, because we will try our best to each one, even knowing that, almost ever, we will be unable to do something clinically for them.

We have a strange feeling like "I don't know if I want to return to the room and finish the consultation". Maybe because of those feelings the discussion with all the team is more important in this place. It's not just the clinical decision but how to communicate with the patient that matters. "Remember that is always useful to repeat information to the patient and family and try to find little solutions that can make a big difference to the patient's comfort. It helps to learn how to face consultations in a different way, with other kinds of expectations."

5. Discussion

The PCAC provided a unique training apprenticeship for medical students and residents. They learned specific issues, like pain control, and had the opportunity to discuss about aspects of caring for dying patients.

Medical students usually do not learn how to deal with feelings that emerge when they are with a dying patient. On the contrary, they are told to keep a certain distance from the patient and their relatives (Hennezel & Leloup, 2000).

Realizing that this kind of attitude is not helpful, the trainees were receptive to the new approaches that we presented. They were able to face death, pain, and suffering as natural as possible. Events that are part of human life, without losing a respectful attitude.

Students learned that when doctors act with goodwill, humility, compassion, and honesty, patients and their families always benefit (Taylor et al, 2003). Residents learned that family physicians need skills in palliative care since they frequently encounter dying patients. They realized that family members play an important role in a patient's end of life period and must also receive support.

The outcomes described were, in some way, consequence of the application of a narrative approach at the PCAC. By listening to terminal patients with empathy and compassion, we can make them feel that they are not alone, a frequent sentiment in this kind of patients. When they meet an attentive listener and have the opportunity to organize the chaos in their life and to find a meaning in which their illness becomes a teaching condition for all involved.

The students learned that when, apparently,there is nothing to do, we can still listen. The journal writing (De Benedetto et al,2007) were effective in promoting reflection and it is an excellent tool for dealing with chaos stories. Writing in prose or poetry to express feelings that we have difficulty dealing with can have healing effects.

The medical educators noted a necessity of the importance to teach palliative care and are trying to improve this in medical school. There are evidences showing that the lack of palliative care training can be negative to doctors and patients. For example, an ineffective doctor-patient communication can affect the patient's satisfaction (Torke et al,2004).

The barriers for an adequate care are from three types: no specific training, personal attitudes against death and political disinterest (Irigoyen,2002). So, this kind of initiative can help in this improvement in medical education.

6. Conclusion

The students' experiences were essential to promote reflection about difficult themes and to break barriers that prevent them from dealing properly with terminal patients. Our learners had the opportunity to learned how to manage terminal patients in a holistic way.

The technical knowledge provided in Palliative Care Ambulatory Clinic alliedto the creation of an ambiance propitious to reflection, made it, in an educational way, a unique setting to a continuum learning. The idea that palliation is a failure of treatment was quickly abolished.

This activity should be maintained and expanded to other didactic Palliative Care settings as hospice, hospital and home care.

The results of these preliminary evaluation became a stimulus for expanding the Palliative Care Program in Brazil.

7. References

Ahmedzai S. (1982) Dying in hospital: the residents' viewpoint. *British Medical Journal* , Vol 285, pp 712–4.

Blasco, P. G. (1997). *O medico de familia hoje* (1ªed), São Paulo.

Blasco, P.B., Janaudis, M.A.& Leoto, RF at al(2003.) *Principios de Medicina de Familia* (1ªed), São Paulo.

Billings JA & Block S. (1997) Palliative care in undergraduate medical education. *JAMA*,Vol 278,pp 733–8.

Caralis AV & Hammond JS. (1992)Attitudes of medical students, housestaff,and faulty physicians towards euthanasia and termination of lifesustaining treatment. *Critical Care Medicine*,Vol 20,pp 683–90.

De Benedetto MAC, Castro AG &Carvalho E. et al. (2007). From suffering to transcendence: narratives in palliative care. *Can Fam Physician*, Vol53, pp1277-9.

Figueredo, M. T. A. (2003).Educação em cuidados paliativos: uma experiência brasileira,.*O mundo da saúde*, Vol 27, No 1,pp165-9.

Helliwell, AJ.(1999) *A* sabe, a chat, and a bloodletting: two bits. The evolution and inevitability of family practice. *Canadian Family Physician*, 1999. Vol 45, pp 859-61

Hennezel M& Leloup, J. (2000) *A Arte de Morrer*,Petrópolis.

Irigoyen, M. (2002).*El paciente terminal: Manejo del dolor y Cuidados Paliativos em Medicina Familiar.*

Jubelier, SJ, Welch, C & Babar Z. (2001) Competences and concerns in end of life care for medical students and residents. *The West Virginia Medical Journal* ,Vol 97, pp118-21.

Lloyd-Williams M & MacLeod R.(2004) A systematic review of teaching and learning in palliative care within the medical undergraduate curriculum. *Med Teach*,Vol 26,pp 683–90.

Melo, A.G.C.(2003). Os cuidados paliativos no Brasil. *O Mundo da Saúde*, Vol 27, No1,pp58-62.

Melvin, A.T. (2001); The Primary Care Physician and Palliative Care. *Palliative Care*, Vol 28, No2:pp 239-45.

Rakel, R.E.(1995). *Text book of Family Medicine.*(6 edição) , Philadelphia.

Relman AS. (1989). The Johns Hopkins Centennial. *New England J Medicine*, Vol 320, pp1411.

South-Paul, J.E.,Matheny, S. C. &Lewis, E.L. (2004).*Current Diagnosis e Treatment in Family Medicine.*

Taylor,L, Hammond J & Carlos R. (2003). A student initiated elective on end of life care: a unique perspective..*Journal of Palliative Medicine,* Vol 1, pp86-90

Torke, A.M.,Quest, T.M.& Branch, W.T. (2004).A Workshop to Teach Medical Students Communication Skills and Clinical Knowledge About End-of-Life Care..*Journal of General Internal Medicine,* Maio, Vol 19, pp540-44.

Van Aalst-Cohen,E.S.,Riggs R. & Byock, I.R.(2008), Palliative Care in Medical School Curricula:A Survey of United States Medical Schools. *Journal of Palliative Medicine,* Vol 11, No 9, pp 1200-02

3

Are Anxiety and Depressive Symptoms Related to Physical Symptoms? A Prospective Study of Patients with Advanced Chronic Disease

María Ignacia del Río, Alejandra Palma, Laura Tupper, Luis Villaroel,
Pilar Bonati, María Margarita Reyes and Flavio Nervi
Department of Medicine, Program in Palliative Medicine and Continuos Care,
Pontificia Universidad Católica de Chile,
Chile

1. Introduction

Access to increasingly sophisticated medical care over the last century has improved the prevention and treatment of many diseases that had previously been fatal, including pneumonia, tuberculosis, acute and chronic renal failure, some cancers, and myocardial infarction. Despite these important curative advances, insufficient emphasis was initially placed on the importance of relieving symptoms and providing continuing support to patients with limited prognosis of survival. A response to this deficiency was the emergence, in the sixties, of Hospice and Palliative Care movements, which sought to improve the quality of care of terminally ill patients and their families (Saunders, 2004).

The primary goal of palliative care therapy is the optimal relief of multiple physical and psychological symptoms, with careful consideration of the spiritual and social needs of the patients and their families (Billings, 1998; WHO, 2004). To achieve optimal symptomatic relief, it is important not only to assemble a multidisciplinary team that is able to consider all aspects of the patient's situation, but also to ensure that they are able to provide coordinated and interdisciplinary therapeutic assistance to the patient. To achieve this, it is necessary that the members of the team fully understand the relationship between the myriad physical, psychological, spiritual, and social aspects of the individual and his environment.

It is sometimes assumed in clinical practice that symptoms of depression or anxiety can influence the intensity and persistence of certain physical symptoms (Vignaroli et al., 2006). Another common assumption is that physical symptoms can trigger depression or anxiety. However, these assumptions are not firmly supported by scientific data, as a number of international studies that have attempted to explore this relationship have reported contradictory results (Lloyd-Williams et al., 2004a; Chen & Chang, 2004; Teunissen et al., 2007a). There are no national studies to explain the potential link between emotional suffering and the intensity and frequency of physical symptoms other than pain.

Depressive and anxiety symptoms can reflect the existence of a psychiatric pathology. Anxiety and mood disorders occur frequently in patients with advanced chronic disease,

(Teunissen et al., 2007b; Lloyd-Williams et al., 2003; Wilson et al., 2007; Durkin et al., 2003; Meyer et al., 2003; Noorani & Montagnini, 2007) with the observed prevalence fluctuating between 17 and 46% for the former disorder, (Teunissen et al, 2007a) and between 5% and 26% in the latter (Hotopf et al., 2002). Regardless of the frequency of these disorders and their relevance to diagnosis and treatment, they are frequently under diagnosed (Vignaroli et al., 2006; Durkin et al., 2003; Palma et al., 2008; Breitbart, 1995). This low level of detection may be related to the as-yet-incomplete incorporation of mental health professionals into medical teams, as well as to insufficient medical training in the detection, assessment, and treatment of psychiatric disorders.

The Hospital Anxiety and Depression Scale (HADS) is one of the more commonly used tools to screen for anxiety and depression in hospitalized patients. Although this scale has proven to be a reliable and valid instrument for assessing anxiety and depression in patients with physical illness (Bjelland et al., 2002), its length makes it difficult to apply in terminally ill patients, who require continuing assessment of multiple additional symptoms. The Edmonton Symptom Assessment System (Bruera et al., 1991; Dudgeon et al., 1999; Chang et al., 2000) (ESAS) is a concise, valid, and internationally used tool in palliative care Chang et al., 2000), which uses self-report scales to evaluate objectively the multiple symptoms observed in this group of patients. A particular advantage of the ESAS is that it is a simple and quickly administered tool that requires very little effort and concentration from the patient. Nevertheless, the anxiety and depressive components of this scale in Spanish have not been validated for the detection of depression and anxiety.

The main goal of this study is to determine if anxiety or depressive symptoms shows a positive correlation with the intensity and frequency of physical symptoms in hospitalized patients with advanced chronic diseases. Additionally it seeks to compare the ESAS and HADS as screening tools for anxiety and depressive symptoms in this population.

2. Material and methods

This study was conducted in the internal medicine wards of the Clinical Hospital of the Pontificia Universidad Católica de Chile during seven months, and Sotero del Río Hospital during four months. It was approved by the ethics committee of both hospitals.

During the study period, 2280 patients were hospitalized in the internal medicine wards of both hospitals. Of these, 150 patients met the initial criteria for inclusion by being diagnosed with chronic disease at an advanced stage, including: (1) advanced cancer, including haematological neoplasia or solid metastasis not responding to medical treatment; (2) pulmonary obstructive lung disease with a functional class NYHA III-IV and/or requiring additional oxygen on a permanent basis; (3) chronic liver failure categorized as Child C in its basal condition; or (4) heart failure with functional class NYHA III/IV in its basal condition. The main exclusion criteria was the presence of delirium, assessed with the Confusion Assessment Method. Of this group, 124 did not present with delirium and were admitted to our study.

On each service, the patients admitted each day were evaluated according to these criteria by systematic review of their medical charts, lab tests and clinical status. Patients with no evidence of delirium were asked to sign an informed consent form. Social, demographic and clinical data were registered: age, sex, health insurance, educational level, date of diagnosis of the underlying disease, cause of hospitalization, co-morbidities and basal Karnofsky score.

2.1 Patient assessment

We used ESAS scale to evaluate the presence and intensity of physical symptoms reported by each patient. Symptoms of anxiety and depression was evaluated using HADS and ESAS scales, both of which have been validated and translated into Spanish (Vignaroli et al., 2006; Bjelland et al., 2002; Bruera et al., 1991; Dudgeon et al., 1999; Chang et al., 2000; Herrero et al., 2003; Walker et al., 2007; Quintana et al., 2003; Tejero et al., 1986).

The ESAS scale evaluates the symptoms that occur most frequently in advanced chronic disease, including: pain, fatigue, nausea, depression, anxiety, somnolence, dyspnea, insomnia, and reduction of one's global sense of wellness. Each symptom is assessed using a self-reporting scale where 0 mean absence of symptom and 10 indicates the presence of the symptom at its maximum possible intensity. Symptoms of anxiety and depression were considered to be present when the intensity of the symptom was 1 or more. The HADS scale consists of two 7-item subscales, one for depression and one for anxiety. Each item is rated on a 4-point scale, scored from 0 to 3. In 1983, the authors of the scale, Zigmond and Snaith, proposed that a score greater than 11 indicates a clinical problem and a score from 8 to 10 indicates that the status of the symptom is uncertain, while a score of 7 or less indicates the absence of the symptom(25).

All researchers participating in the study had been previously trained in the proper application of the scales used. A separate investigator was assigned to audit the correct registration of findings in each of the cases included in the protocol. In order to avoid registration errors, two additional researchers coded and tabulated the information in an electronic database.

2.2 Statistical analysis

The numerical variables of the study were presented as mean with standard deviation, or, in a small number of cases, as the median. Categorical variables were presented as number of cases and percent. We used the nonparametric Mann-Whitney test to compare numerical variables between groups, and the chi-square or exact Fisher tests to compare percentages.

To determine the validity of the ESAS as a diagnostic test, using the HADS as the gold standard, we analyzed both sensitivity and specificity. The grade of agreement between ESAS and HADS was determined by the Kappa test. P values not greater than 0.05 were considered significant. All statistical analyses were carried out using SPSS 16.0 software.

3. Results

To evaluate the relationship between physical symptoms and symptoms of anxiety or depression, profiles of depressed and non-depressed patients and anxious and non-anxious patients were compared in terms of the number and intensity of symptoms.

Of 124 patients who met the inclusion criteria of the study, 5 were too emotionally disturbed to answer the HADS, and were excluded to receive psychological assistance. Of the remaining 119 patients, most were female (58%), with an average age of 66.9 years (range 35–95), and a mean basal Karnofsky score of 70 (range 30–100). Regarding their admission diagnosis 55 patients had cancer and 61 were diagnosed with non-oncological diseases.

Variables	N	%	Median (range)
Total participants	119	-	-
Age (years)	-	-	66.9 (35-95)
Sex (M/F) (n,%)	49 / 70	48 / 52	-
Married or communal	72	60.7	-
Single	16	13.4	-
Separated or widow	31	25.9	-
With Religion	102	85.7	-
Working	29	24.4	-
Stopped Work	28	23.5	-
Retired	56	47.1	-
Karnofsky	-	-	69.8 (30-100)
With Cancer	55	47.4	-
1. Digestive	14	25.5	-
2. Blood	11	20.0	-
3. Lung	13	10.9	-
4. Breast/Gynological	02	3.6	-
5. Other	15	27.3	-
Wihtout Cancer	61	52.6	-
1. Chronic Liver Failure Child C	17	27.9	-
2. Chronic Cardiac Failure CF IV	24	39.3	-
3. Pulmonary Obstructive Lung Disease	20	32.8	-

Table 1. Clinical characteristics and social demographics of the study cohort

We found a high prevalence of physical symptoms, fatigue being the most common (78.9%), followed by insomnia (78.7%), anorexia (76.2%), and somnolence (71.3%). At least 60% of patients reported their symptoms were of moderate to severe intensity (between 4 and 10 points on the self-report scale).

Symptoms	Frequency (%)	Mild (%)	Moderate (%)	Severe (%)
Pain	61.8	22.8	26.8	12.2
Fatigue	78.9	21.1	42.3	15.4
Nausea	17.1	8.9	5.7	2.4
Drowsiness	71.3	23.0	36.1	12.3
Dyspnea	60.7	18.0	31.1	11.5
Anorexia	76.2	18.9	30.3	27.0
Depression	68.3	26.8	24.4	17.1
Anxiety	71.3	23.8	34.4	13.1

The symptoms were catalogued as mild-moderate-severe in accordance with ESAS scoring: Mild 1-3 / Moderate: 4-7 / Severe: 8-10.

Table 2. Frequency and intensity of symptoms

According to HADS scoring, 13.6% of the patients presented with depression and 32.5% with anxiety. Using a cutoff score of 2, for ESAS, 67.5% of patients experienced anxiety and 60.2% reported depressed mood.

There was no significant difference in age, religious or marital status between patients with significant psychological distress, in the form of depression or anxiety according to HADS, and those who exhibited no psychological distress (Table III). However, significant statistical differences were found in gender, employment status and Karnofsky index. We observed that patients with psychological distress tended to be female, unemployed (87.2% of the subjects with psychological distress were not working), and having a lower basal Karnofsky index of 65, compared to 75 observed in the second group with no psychological distress (p = 0.027).

	Significant Psychological Distress*						
	Present			Absent			
	N	(%)	Median	N	(%)	Median	P
Age	-	-	63.23	-	-	66.94	.154
Men	10	25	-	39	49.4	-	.014
Women	30	75	-	40	50.6	-	
With religion	36	92.3	-	66	88	-	.477
Without religion	3	7.7	-	9	12	-	
Single	3	7.9	-	12	16.2	-	.365
With a partner	23	60.5	-	45	60.8	-	
Separate or Widow	12	31.6	-	17	23	-	
Working	5	12.8	-	24	32.4	-	.006
Not working**	34	87.2	-	50	67.6	-	
Karnofsky	-	-	65.43	-	-	74.93	.027

** Presence of depression or anxiety matching HADS store.*
*** Unemployed, not working, retire or pension*

Table 3. Analysis with respect to socio-demographic characteristics. for medical reason.

3.1 Comparison of assessment tools for depression and anxiety

Using HADS as a gold standard, ESAS was tested as a screening tool to detect depression and anxiety (Table IV). Using a cutoff score of 2 or more, we obtained a sensitivity of 87,5% for depression and 86.8% for anxiety and negative predictive values of 95.7% for depression and 86.8% for anxiety. These parameters dramatically decreased when a cutoff score of 5 was used, obtaining sensitivity of 68% for depression and 63% for anxiety.

	ESAS Depression		ESAS Anxiety	
Cutoff Point	2 (%)	5 (%)	2 (%)	5 (%)
Sensitivity	87.5	68.8	86.8	63.2
Specificity	44.1	71.6	41.8	74.7
Predictive value (+)	19.7	27.5	41.8	54.5
Predictive value (-)	95.7	93.6	86.8	80.8
Kappa	.129	.247	.224	.364
P	.016	.002	.002	.000

Table 4. Sensitivity, specificity and predictive values of the ESAS as a diagnostic test using the HADS as the gold standard

3.2 Analysis based on physical symptom profiles

Patients with anxiety had higher incidence of physical symptoms and greater severity of several symptoms compared with controls. As shown in Table V, the presence of anxiety was associated with a greater incidence of pain (p = .006), insomnia (p = .002), fatigue (p = .380), and nausea (p = .009). Likewise, as shown in Table VI, the presence of anxiety was associated with greater severity of pain (p= .001), fatigue (p= .003), anorexia (p= .022), insomnia (p= .001) and nausea (p= .009). Patients with anxiety also reported a greater loss of the sensation of global well-being (p= .004).

Patients with depression also had a higher incidence of physical symptoms and greater severity of several symptoms relative to healthy controls. As shown in Table V, depressed patients had a higher frequency of anorexia (p = .014), fatigue (p = .021), and insomnia (p = .021) than controls. These symptoms (p == .014, p = .023, p = .044, respectively), in addition to nausea (p = .017), were more severe in the depressed group (Table VI). The sensation of well-being did not differ between depressed and control individuals (p > .05).

	Frequency of Symptoms (%)					
	Anxiety			Depression		
	Yes (N:38)	No (N:80)	P	Yes (N:16)	No (N: 102)	P
Pain	78.9	52.5	.006*	81.3	57.8	.074
Fatigue	89.5	72.5	.038*	100	74.5	.021*
Nausea	28.9	10.0	.009*	37.5	12.7	.023*
Drowsy	71.1	69.6	.874	75	69.3	.774
Dyspnea	63.2	57.5	.559	62.5	58.8	.781
Anorexia	84.2	71.3	.127	100	71.6	.014*
Insomnia	94.7	70.0	.002*	100	74.5	.021*
Global Well Being	97.4	75.9	.004*	100	80.2	.070

Table 5. Frequency of symptoms: comparative analysis in patients with and without depression or anxiety

	Depression			Anxiety		
	Yes (N:16)	No (N: 102)	P	Yes (N:38)	No (N:80)	P
Pain	4.00 ± 3.25	2.66 ± 3.03	.075	4.26 ± 3.38	2.16 ± 2.69	.001*
Fatigue	5.63 ± 2.73	3.67 ± 2.99	.023*	5.18 ± 3.27	3.34 ±2.72	.003*
Nausea	1.06 ± 1.88	.51 ± 1.71	.017*	1.13 ± 2.43	.33 ± 1.21	.009*
Drowsiness	4.06 ± 3.36	3.35 ± 3.0	.427	3.87 ± 3.37	3.24 ± 2.88	.362
Dyspnea	4.06 ± 3.44	2.92 ± 3.21	.261	3.95 ± 3.71	2.66 ± 2.94	.092
Anorexia	6.50 ± 3.03	4.13 ± 3.66	.014*	5.58 ± 3.58	3.91 ± 3.60	.022*
Insomnia	6.06 ± 2.43	4.17 ± 3.54	.044*	5.92 ± 3.11	3.71 ± 3.42	.001*

(Mean± Standard Deviation of scores of the ESAS Depression and anxiety in accord with the HADS scale (≥ 11); Mann-Whitney Test)

Table 6. Presence of depression and anxiety, and intensity of physical symptoms.

4. Conclusion

The high levels of anxiety (32.5%) and depression (32.5%) we found in this study are consistent with those reported in several previous international studies of patients with advanced chronic disease (Teunissen et al., 2007a; Lloyd-Williams et al., 2003; Wilson et al., 2007; Durkin et al., 2003; Meyer et al., 2003; Noorani & Montagnini, 2007; Hotopf et al., 2002). From these results, we conclude that in patients with anxiety and depressive symptoms there is a strong association between the frequency and intensity of physical symptoms and the presence of psychological symptoms. Additionally our results suggests that the ESAS can be a useful screening tool to improve the clinical detection of anxious or depressive syndromes in terminal patients.

We found that psychological disturbance was associated with significantly more frequent and intense physical symptoms. The explanation for this correlation might be that physical symptoms play an etiologic role in triggering psychological disturbance, or, conversely, that anxiety and depression tend to increase the perceived intensity of a symptom already experienced by the patient. Although our results do not allow us to decide between these alternative theories, they do indicate that, in the presence of intense and frequent physical symptoms, the probability of finding psychological disturbance is significantly higher. This finding underlines the importance of performing a comprehensive and multidisciplinary assessment of all terminally ill patients.

Although multiple studies have sought the connection between depressed mood and physical symptoms, few have focused on the role of anxiety in this context. Chen and Chang (Chen & Chang, 2004) compared the physical symptom profiles of depressed and non-depressed patients and found, as we did, that the former group presented with a significantly larger number of symptoms. They observed a higher prevalence of insomnia, pain, anorexia, and fatigue in patients who were classified by HADS as being depressed. Our results confirm these, although, in the case of pain, the differences between depressed and non-depressed patients were not statistically significant. A study by Lloyd-Williams et al. also showed a close association between physical symptoms and depression in palliative patients (Lloyd-Williams et al., 2004a). However, the results we and others have reported lie in contrast to a Dutch report (Teunissen, 2007a). In that study, whose design was very similar to ours, no association was found between depressed or anxious mood and the presence of physical symptoms. We believe the different results may be due to cultural differences between Chilean and Dutch patients, as well as to national differences in Karnofsky score (average 65 and 50 in the Chilean and Dutch population, respectively). It should also be noted that the previous study included fewer subjects than did the current one, potentially lending less validity to their data.

The usefulness of the ESAS as a screening test in anxiety and depression is derived mainly from its sensitivity and negative predictive value. To comprehensively evaluate the usefulness of a screening test, sensitivity, specificity, and negative and positive predictive values must be evaluated. It is essential that both the sensitivity, which measures the ability of a particular tool to detect disease when it is present, and the negative predictive value, the probability that an individual with a negative test is healthy, be as higher as possible. Because a screening test is not intended to diagnose, it is less important that it has high specificity, which measures the probability of detecting the absence of disease when there is none, because, after subjects with potential disease are identified, their assessment should always be confirmed and complemented by an adequate diagnostic procedure (in this case psychiatric interview based on DSM-IV).

When we used a cutoff score of 2, the ESAS had high sensitivity and negative predictive value for both anxiety and depression, each exceeding 86%. When the cutoff score was raised to 5, the performance dropped considerably. Thus, in agreement with the results of a previous American study (Vignaroli et al., 2006) that also used the HADS as the gold standard, our data suggests that the ideal ESAS cutoff point to achieve an acceptable level of sensitivity and specificity when screening depression and anxiety in terminal patients is 2.

Lloyd Williams et al. (2004b) found that the sensitivity and specificity of posing the simple question: are you depressed? to patients in palliative care was 74% and 55%, respectively. In addition to HADS, other tools have been designed to detect psychiatric syndromes, such as the Beck questionnaire, the Edinburgh Depression Scale, and the Schedule for Affective Disorders and Schizophrenia (SADS). However, because of their length, none of these instruments is practically applicable in clinical settings requiring daily simultaneous assessment and management of physical symptoms whose high frequency and intensity has been documented by this study and others (Chen & Chang, 2004; S Teunissen et al., 2007a; 2007b; Oi-Ling et al., 2005). For this reason, we propose ESAS as a useful and sensitive tool that can help physicians to identify, and refer to psychiatric evaluation, those patients for whom advanced disease is accompanied by symptoms of depression or anxiety.

In conclusion, in a sample of hospitalized patients with advanced chronic disease, we found that high levels of anxiety and depression were correlated with a higher frequency and intensity of physical symptoms. We found that for ESAS the ideal cutoff point to detect depressive mood and anxiety was a score of 2, which allowed ESAS to serve as a useful screening tool in this clinical context.

5. Acknowledgements

This study was supported by International Association for Hospice & Palliative Care (IAHPC).

6. References

Billings, A. What is palliative care? J Palliat Med 1998;1: 73-81.

Bjelland, I., Dahl, A., Tangen Haug, T., Neckelmann, D. The Validity of the Hospital Anxiety and Depression Scale. An updated literature review. J Psychosom Res 2002; 52: 69-77

Breitbart W. Identifying patients at risk for and treatment of major psychiatric complications of cancer. Support Care Cancer1995; 3: 45-60

Bruera, E., Kuehn, N., Miller, M., Selmser, P., Macmillan, K. The Edmonton Symptom Assessment System (ESAS): Asimple method for the assessment of palliative care patients. J Palliat Care 1991; 7: 6-9

Chang, V., Hwang, S., Feuermen, M. Validation of the Edmonton Symptom Assessment Scale. Cancer 2000; 88: 2164-2171

Chen, M., Chang, H. Physical symptom profiles of depressed and nondepressed patients with cancer. Palliat Med 2004; 18: 712-718

Dudgeon, D., Harlos, M., Clinch, J. The Edmonton Symptom Assesment Scale (ESAS) as an audit. Tool.J Palliat Care 1999; 15: 14-19

Durkin, I., Kearney, M., O`Siorain, L. Psychiatric disorder in a palliative care unit. Palliat Med 2003; 17: 212-218

Herrero, M.J., Blanch, J, Peri, J.M , Pablo, Pintor, L., Bulbena, A. A validation study of the hospital anxiety and depression scale (HADS) in a Spanish population. Gen HospPsychiatry 2003; 25: 277–283.

Hotopf, M., Chidgey, J., Addington-Hall, J. and Lan Ly, K. Depression in advanced disease: a systematic review Part 1. Prevalence and case finding.Palliat Med 2002; 16: 81-97

Lloyd-Williams, M., Spiller, J., Ward, J. Which depression screening tools should be used in palliative care? Palliat Med 2003; 17: 40-43

Lloyd-Williams, M., Dennis, M., Taylor, F. A prospective study to determine the association between physical symptoms and depression in patients with advanced cancer. Palliat Med 2004; 18: 558-563

Lloyd-Williams, M., Dennis, M., Taylor, F. A prospective study to compare three depression screening tools in patients who are terminally ill.Gen Hosp Psychiatry 2004; 26: 384–389

Meyer, H., Sinott, C., Seed, P. Depressive symptoms in advanced cancer. Part 2.Depression over time; the role of the palliative care professional.Palliat Med2003; 17: 604-607

Noorani, N., Montagnini, M. Recognizing depression in palliative care patients. J Palliat Med2007; 10: 458-464

Oi-Ling, K., Man-Wah, D. Kam-Hung, D. Symptom Distress as rated by advanced cancer patients, caregivers and physicians in the last week of life. Palliat Med 2005; 19: 228-233

Palma A, del Río I, Bonati P, Tupper L, Villarroel L, Olivares P, Nervi F. Frequency and assessment of symptoms in hospitalized patient with advanced chronic diseases: is there concordance among patients and doctors? Rev Med Chil 2008; 136:561-9.

Payne, A., Barry, S., Creedon, B., et al. Sensitivity and specificity of a two-question screening tool for depression in a specialist palliative care unit. Palliat Med 2007; 21:193-198

Quintana JM, Padierna A, Esteban C, Arostegui I, Bilbao A, Ruiz I Evaluation of the psychometric characteristics of the Spanish version of the Hospital Anxiety and Depression Scale. Acta Psychiatr Scand 2003;107: 216-221.

Saunders, C. Foreword In: Doyle, D., Hanks, G., Cherny, N. &Calman, K., editors. Oxford Textbook of Palliative Medicine.Third ed. Oxford University Press; 2004.

Smith, E., Gomm, SA, Dickens, CM Assessing the independent contribution to quality of life from anxiety and depression in patients with advanced cancer. Palliat Med 2003; 17: 509-513

Tejero A, Guimera E., Farré JM, Peri JM. Uso Clínico del HADS (Hospital Anxiety and Depression Scale) en población psiquiátrica: un estudio de sensibilidad, fiabilidad y validez. Revista del departamento Psiquiatría la Facultad Med Barcelona 1986; 12: 233-238

Teunissen, S., Graeff, A., Voest, E., Haes, J. Are anxiety and depressed mood related to physical symptom burden? A study in hospitalized advanced cancer patients. Palliat Med 2007; 21: 341-346

Teunissen SCCM, Wesker W, de Haes JCJM, Voest EE, de Graeff A. Symptom prevalence in patients with incurable cancer: a systematic review. J Pain Symptom Manage 2007; 34: 94-104

Vignaroli, E., Pace, E., Willey, J., Palmer, J., Zhang, T., Bruera, E. The Edmonton Symptom Assessment System as a screening tool for depression and anxiety. J PalliatMed 2006; 9: 296-303.

Walker, J., Postma, K., McHugh G., et al. Performance of the Hospital Anxiety and Depression Scale as a screening tool for mayor depressive disorder in cancer patients. J Psychosom Res 2007; 63: 83-91.

Wilson, K., Chochinov, H., Graham, M., Allard, P. et al Depression and anxiety disorders in palliative cancer care. J Pain Symptom Manage 2007; 33: 118-129.

World Health Organization. Palliative Care Symptom Management and end-of-life care. Interim guidelines for first-level facility health workers. 2004. Available from World Wide Web: http://www.who.int

Zigmond AS, Snaith RP. The Hospital Anxiety and depression Scale. ActaPsychiatrScand 1983; 67: 361-370.

4

Designing for the Experience of Pain

Elizabeth Lewis
Sydney,
Australia

1. Introduction

Pain management within a palliative care context offers many opportunities for designers to innovatively push boundaries as they provide new perspectives on experiences. Additionally, the designer's ability to remain grounded in the needs of the care environment is dependent on their ability to draw on the experiences of others. This paper discusses the importance of experience and the way it can be explored as a key problem-solving tool. Experiential research aims to guide the design process and subsequent solutions towards products and systems that are deeply rooted in the needs of pain sufferers.

Breakthroughs in science and technology have led to the development and implementation of innovative concepts, which have shaped and improved the lives of pain sufferers. Innovations such as Transdermal Patches, TeleMedCare Health Monitor and NeuroTherm radiofrequency nerve ablation systems have been nurtured, guided and bought to realisation as physical products by diverse and skilled professionals in the field of science, medicine, engineering and design.

As the realm of pain management in palliative care becomes both broader in its capabilities and highly specific in application, designers are asking the question, "How do we design for a pain sufferer if we have not experienced that for which we are designing?" There are various tools and strategies available to designers to ensure innovative solutions are formulated, but the initial problem must still be defined. Similarly, the solution must reflect the values and cultural beliefs of the community.

In order for products and systems to maintain innovation, the design process may involve experiential research. There are difficulties associated with this, primarily due to cost and timing but also communication barriers, cultural differences and availability of resources. If this key research activity is not undertaken, there is potential for pain management products to be disengaged from daily experience. The importance and placement of experiential research within the design process and the greater development of pain management products will be discussed in this paper.

2. Concepts

2.1 The role of experience in shaping our understanding

Our perception of the environment we encounter will be affected consciously to some degree by everything we have learned about it up until now (Hughes, 2000). These perceptions are driven by a culmination of experience, knowledge, memory, reflection and analysis. It is through experience that we are able to analyse the present and imagine for the future.

Experience may define to a large extent of who we are, what we do and what we have done (Bate and Robert, 2007); however it is not necessarily understood very well. Subsequently, it may be questionable as to why the study of experience is important in our understanding and development of services, systems, and processes and in the subject of this paper, design. As researchers and developers of community resources, designers could develop for behaviour which is observable or attitudes which are measurable (Bate and Robert, 2007), however our behaviours, attitudes, logic, memories, opinions, actions and reactions are interpreted through personal and social significance gained through experience (Suri, 2002). By addressing the core experience or couplings of experience, designers are able to build relationships of phenomena and strongly address the needs of the user.

Bate and Robert (2007) describe the elements of experience on page 41 as

- Reflection and awareness (awareness of self, others and the environment in a conscious and subconscious manner)
- Sensation (kinaesthetic)
- Perceptions
- Thought
- Memory
- Imagination
- Emotions and expressions
- Desire
- Actions and conduct

Within each experience, the levels and impact of these elements may be minimal or maximal. During an experience, it may be unlikely that individuals are identifying, recording and reflecting upon such elements. The challenge for researchers is guiding individuals in their reflection of such elements in a meaningful manner, which will allow insightful contribution to the design process.

The design profession requires experience, as it will lead to a change in perspective from which the problem is defined. Hubbell (1994, p61) describes this process: "Experiential analysis is a form of research that encourages the researcher to use a variety of alternate techniques as a means of learning about a particular socio-political phenomenon." Through the experience, the designer comes face to face with the problem. Examination of the elements allows for problems to be identified, prejudices to be overcome, the ability to reflect on that which is not normally acknowledged and the time to formulate solutions that directly relate to the context. This allows the initial design process to be led by the context and those within it as opposed to user testing a prototype several stages down the track.

Experience design can be applicable to any field in which creative process and cross-pollination of ideas results in a designable scenario. Chapman (2005) explores the potential for experience and states, "The most important concept to grasp is that all experiences are important and that we can learn from them, whether they are traditional, physical, offline experiences or whether they are digital, online or technological experiences."

Experiential research offers the greatest opportunity for all areas of the context to be explored, for all disciplines to offer perspectives and for the focus of product development to be driven by the key user groups. This form of investigation is crucial within the early stages of design development, prior to attachment of ideas, materials and technologies.

Although several areas of discourse would benefit from the inclusion of experiential research during investigative design phase, the following discussion is formulated around the palliative care environment.

2.2 The palliative environment as a design setting

Australians are becoming increasingly aware of the cost and financial expenditure of healthcare, especially as the aging workforce moves towards retirement. The Australian Government budget estimates that there are approximately two million Australians aged over 70 years, with this figure expected to double by 2029. The Minister for Health and Aging acknowledged that each year more than 20,000 Australians receive some form of specialist palliative care and more than 500,000 patients, carers and families are affected (Elliot and Roxon, 2010).

In 2010, the Australian government dedicated a further $14.3 million to fund projects for improved palliative care services, research, training and information (Elliot and Roxon, 2010). Acknowledgment of the current need for investment in palliative care to create a health care system that has service sustainability provides incentive for the growing numbers of professionals looking at ways of contributing to this field.

As a service industry, the health care sector draws on the products and resources that have been developed and produced by the private sector. The private sector is therefore most likely see the greatest development and generation of consumer products, systems and services that will cater for the growing palliative market. It is important that the priorities of communities and individuals will be recognised in the commercialisation process of the private sector with the additional investment of time and funds by governments globally. It is on this level that experiential research and data that is collected will become most valuable to the developing body, with innovations reflecting the insights gained through this alternative, experience-centred perspective.

Products, systems and environments are rarely experienced without some kind of service affiliation (Suri, 2002). Suri (2002, p162) illustrates this trait through the example of the overall quality of interaction with a telephone or a hotel having as much to do with the characteristics of the service encountered as with the design of the physical elements interacted with. Service industries are commonly associated with corporations that are customer service focused such as hospitality franchises, information technology and telecommunications companies, whereby the customer experience is a crucial element of the company's evaluation of performance.

For example, telecommunications companies are able to provide the customer with the physical artefact of a mobile phone, which has been designed to be ergonomic, aesthetically pleasing, and inclusive of emerging telecommunications technology. Once connected to a service provider, the capabilities of the phone extend well beyond the physical elements to a realm of digital interaction. Throughout the use, the customer will evaluate both the physical artefact itself and the corresponding service. At times, the individual may not be able to differentiate between the two and might mistake poor performance as either physically or service related. Subsequently, this affects the experience that the customer has of both the phone and the service.

Within healthcare environments, patients are not referred to as customers. Healthcare does, however, provide services, expectations and discussions like any service industry. Receiving institutionalised care for a period of time, patients are more likely to evaluate the more complex elements of experience. Berry (2006) comments on this idea by stating 'few service experiences are more important, variable, complex and personal than being hospitalised and patients are likely to be eager for any evidence of the hospital's competence and caring'. Although this statement comments on the environment of a hospital, this idea may be applied to any notion of care that is provided to patients and generates care experiences.

Australian attitudes and behaviours in responding to death and the environment in which this occurs are derived for the most part from our English heritage (Kellehear, 2002). As the dying population within Australia (i.e the proportion of the population within their final years) becomes multicultural, perspectives on the ideal palliative care services and the way in which they meet personal identity and social needs will challenge these environments, those who provide care and the subsequent device and systems designed to be used in administering care.

It is also acknowledged that the needs of palliative care patients are becoming more complex as many patients may not suffer of one life threatening disease but a culmination of several physical and psychological aliments (Dale et al, 2009). This in turn changes the predictability of a patient's journey and experience as they enter the palliative phase.

Although it has been identified as a service industry, there are also unique qualities that separate palliative care from general healthcare. The role of this form of care-giving is to provide a support framework for the patient and provide a central, long-term care system for health professionals and family members as trust and friendship are built over the period (Ersek and Wilson, 2003). It is a multidisciplinary, holistic approach to care that encompasses physical, emotional and spiritual needs (Noell, 1995). The palliative approach is particularly unique as the care focus becomes concerned with alleviating symptoms such as pain as opposed to treating the illness directly.

Furthermore, in extending the care environment to the physical environment, it is important to acknowledge that devices, objects and systems impact all levels of care. Noell (1995), states that communities should be seeking to "highlight the quality of the human experience and shift medical services and dehumanising equipment into the background", and that "a physical environment for older people must be designed to celebrate life". Medical devices, services and equipment are important, and in some cases crucial, to the care of patients. Noell (1995) has also brought to the attention of developers the need to be exploring the innovation of emotionally rich interactions (Djadjadiningrat et al, 2002). Through a greater understanding of both the emotional and physical requirements, designers are provided with the opportunity to alter the experience of palliative care and interaction through innovation.

Such interactions may become the driving force for problem identification as the designer moves towards creating for the experience as opposed to the development of a product. Bate and Robert, (2007) use the example of seeing not a glass half empty or a glass half full, but questioning as to why it is a glass at all. Through this questioning phase, designers are able to generate ideas for the experience of drinking water as opposed to producing a glass, thus opening a greater spectrum of possibility. In the realm of medical design, the complexity of the product most often extends beyond the simplicity of a glass. Nanotechnology, remote telecommunication and interactive materials are only skimming the surface in the depth of technologies employed within healthcare.

Due to technological development, there is a greater emphasis on a carer's ability to be technologically competent and proficient. New technologies allow carers to perform their role efficiently, effectively and accurately, however there is concern that the care provided is governed by the physicality of an object (Locsin, 2005). This notion is also applicable for palliative patients, as their quality of life is greatly affected, and can be restricted, by the functionality of medical devices.

Beyond technical aspects, our perception of products and our response to them is not solely an outcome of cognitive processing but also an emotional response. There is a particular manner in which humans feel and perceive the tactile and aesthetic nature of a product (Suri, 2002). Consumers will often consider the way in which a product reflects their current lifestyle whilst also aspiring to a projected lifestyle. Issues of aesthetics, functionality and past experience will guide the consumer in making informed choices that determine future experiences.

Suri (2002, p163) further develops this through the example of purchasing a briefcase, Individuals may consider the aesthetic and practical issues involved with using a briefcase such as capacity and features that may be needed as well the message that the bag portrays within the community. Terms such as 'serious', 'professional', 'arty' or 'hip' may be used as a way of individuals classifying the emotional and physical characteristics of the briefcase based on their understanding of the objects meaning. Through this example it becomes clear that prior to making a purchase, it is possible for individuals to build a relationship with an object based on both past and projected future experiences.

Additionally, emotional responses play a role in consumers' expectations and affordances offered to a product. Djadjadiningrat el al (2002) discuss' the role of applying respect within the foundations of a products sensibility. Through the comparison of a vending machine with a sales assistant, Djadjadiningrat el al (2002), encourage not only designers and the product development team but also most importantly consumers to question acceptable and desirable interactions of use within innate products.

When considering the same perspective in a pain management device, the provision given to individual experience, cultural context, communication barriers, emotional requirements and changing physical condition is very different. The considerations of size, shape and materiality are still equally important however the choices are limited to functionality.

The following section of this paper explores the role of the subcutaneous syringe driver in managing pain for palliative patients. This product was chosen as a case study as the experiences and functionality of the product are complex and multiple, therefore allowing for a detailed analysis. This case study will demonstrate the importance of acknowledging experience in development of new syringe driver models in the future.

2.3 Pain management: palliative care principle

The goals of palliative care as outlined by The Therapeutic Guidelines - Palliative Care - of Australia (2005) are;

- To provide relief from pain and other distressing symptoms
- Affirms life and regards dying as a normal process
- Intends neither to hasten nor postpone death
- Integrates the psychological, emotional, spiritual and social aspects of care for the patient, the family and close carers in a culturally sensitive manner
- Offers a support system to help patients live their lives as actively as possible
- Offers a support system to help the family and carers cope during the patient's illness and the patient's death.

The Therapeutic Guidelines – Palliative Care – of Australia (2005) acknowledges that there are potential problems in providing palliative care within Australian communities. The inability to provide high quality care is often due to relatively low staffing levels (both nurses and other members of the palliative team) and the possibility of having limited access to outside expertise due to funding restrictions and the consequent lack of resources.

The first goal of palliative care, to provide relief from pain and other distressing symptoms, involves multiple and varied experiences which in turn affect the subsequent mentioned goals. Through a greater understanding of the pain experience, it is felt that improved systems, products and environments may result which in turn will improve the overall palliative experience.

The International Association defines pain for the Study of Pain as 'an unpleasant sensory and emotional experience associated with actual or potential tissue damage, or described in terms of such damage." (The Therapeutic Guidelines - Palliative Care - of Australia, 2005)

Pain has the ability to affect a patient's physical response and condition in conjunction with affecting their psychological mood. It is acknowledged that pain is a personal experience whereby the experience and perception of pain is influenced by a patient's state of mind. If pain is a subjective experience, then the care environment should in turn recognise and treat the pain as described and reflected by the patient (Wilson, 2007).

As discussed earlier, the palliative patient is more often suffering from numerous diseases which will affect their ability to describe, analyse and reflect on their acceptance and experience of pain. Furthermore, two patients may be suffering from similar sensation of pain, but their experience of the pain may be different.

This creates barriers to effective pain management and makes the task of gathering experiential data all the more difficult. In Section 2 this paper, possible strategies will be explored that may be employed in order to gain a greater understanding of the experience of pain for not only designers but also for the health care industry and for the greater product development team.

3. Frameworks

3.1 The use of narratives in analysing experience

As an individual moves into the palliative phase, the power to communicate emotions, thoughts, and medical needs is extended beyond the patient to those that surround and care for them. The following description has been given by a chaplain after holding a discussion with a patient"…terminally ill or extremely distressed, in pain suffering extreme handicap, or suffering from something that makes life hard for them to bear, they feel that they are completely useless. They feel that they have nothing to give and that the person with them is giving everything and they are receiving; whereas in fact, they are giving out an enormous amount without even knowing it. In fact I found that very ill people generate a tremendous spiritual energy and for the most part they are quite unaware of it. When you tell them that they are giving you back something of immense importance, they can't understand what you are saying. But it is tremendously real." (Jenkins, 1997)

As humans, we tell stories often and in a variety of manners whether verbal or written, through motion and sound, collections of images and the use of props. Story telling offers the opportunity for individuals to culminate their interpretations, emotions and responses in a way that is personal. Through an audience or a story told to ones' self, the narrative is a natural way of recounting an experience in a structured form (Moen (2006). Through the narrative, a sequence of events is recalled and individual thoughts are captured. Stories may include elements that are not always easily identifiable or directly relevant and offer much greater value than that of a structured interview.

The narrative research approach has been growing in use as researchers have become aware of the possibilities and opportunities that it can offer as a way of learning about context, interaction, culture and perception. Although storytellers may alter, opinionate, exaggerate and hypothesise, the story itself offers a vivid reflection on the experience being described (Bate & Robert (2007). Through rich descriptions, the mind of the listener is able to wander, reflect, interpret and imagine the event, with the hope of building a foundation of the experiential narratives.

The palliative environment is rooted in the relationships that are built over time. These relationships are founded on trust and friendship that will have built through discussions and stories as patients and carers describe the experiences of entering end of life care. Over the past 25 years there has been an increase in published stories of both carers and patients facing the prospect and the stage of being within palliative care (Bingley et al, 2008). As identified earlier, the palliative experience is difficult to explore and analyse first hand, resulting in research that may be quantitative and statistics based. Stories offer an insight into the complex experiences of end of life care as recounted by the environment and act as a key research tool to designers in the development of pain management tools.

The validility of stories and narratives can be questioned and analysed. Bingley et al (2008) identify key narrative analysis methods that can be implemented for the review of research.

These methods explore the analysis of stories in terms of life grid timelines, through the structure and the form, through a holistic approach of stories or a sequence of stories and through biographical analysis whereby the same biography is presented by a variety of individuals. These techniques allow for narratives to be interpreted and translated by researchers and allow for the greatest amount of value to be sought.

Researchers may explore the narratives in such analytical ways as listed above, however designers often iterate between design research, practise and process whereby the analysis of the narrative is incorporated within design responses. The experiences of patients and carers as collected through narratives offer designers the opportunity to co-design with the environment. As the sequence of narratives expands, designers are able to pose solutions and responses to the environment with the hope of further narratives developing.

The palliative environment offers both unique and challenging obstacles in the drawing of narratives as a reference material. Traditionally user studies in the design field are based on an object centric perspective (Redstrom, 2005) whereby designers are able to explore a context through existing products and rituals of use. Although this process will lead to innovative progression in product development, the integration and use of narratives aims to redirect development towards rituals of experience, thus encapsulates a much larger spectrum of ideas.

Palliative Care Australia, in collaboration with patients and carers, produced a collection of stories in 2007 written by those that have followed the palliative journey. This initiative not only performs as a research base but also allowed individuals the opportunity to share, educate and heal through the act of writing.

Gai Gibson shared the story of her husband Greg who was diagnosed with lung cancer. Gai recounted the successes and trails of the palliative environment as she and her family experienced it. Phrases such as "We tried going to day procedures on the first occasion but they didn't even have a bed to lie on, just a very hard recliner chair", conjure images in the mind of a sparse room, the hard square recliner chair, the difficulties of mobility for the ill, the anxiety for Greg as he would need to lie for a long period of time and the overwhelming feelings that Greg and Gai must have felt when entering into a foreign medical environment. Although the story has been interpreted and assumptions have been made in relation to the physical and emotional aspects of this narrative, this interpretation has been made by the researchers linking similar personal experience. Researchers may make further analyses of the stories and develop critical links, for example is the hard recliner chair similar to that of a dentist chair. This will lead to identification of where design subjects overlap.

Further into the story, Gai states "For what was once a simple trip into town we now needed to take a seemingly endless list of supplies, including oxygen cylinders; an oxygen conserving device; wheelchair; Roho cushion; mask as well as nasal prongs; morphine nasal spray; Ventolin and mobile phone in case of breakdown, A doctor's appointment at 11:00am required as to make a start at 7:30am – the care was constant." This statement allows for empathy to be generated between the reader and Gai. Gai's reflection may spark previous experience for parents that have had sick children, or those that have had to take an elderly relative out for a day. It is these connections that we draw between the experiences of others and those that are personal that act a foundation for problem analysis.

The design profession is posed with the task of making this trip easier, by simplifying objects, by making the oxygen cylinder lighter or more compact, by simply reducing the number of tasks needed to get from the home to the doctor. Designers may turn to inspiration from children's prams, luggage design and compact storage systems to draw design qualities and innovations that may add value to this environment. Innovations in commercial markets can be utilised and adapted for use in the medical field.

These narratives build a collection of experiences in which the designer can begin to map the areas of concern. It provides the designer with the ability to follow a progression of experience by first entering into the context, learning about the context as it exists, hypothesise about the ideal experience and responding with a concept. Although technologies, resources, manufacturing and materials manipulate the product development process, budgets and timelines, this particular progression allows the practises of medicine and design to inspire and co-create.

3.2 Experience based co-design

Co-design or co-creation of products, is a term that is often associated with marketing infrastructure whereby the customer is given the opportunity to yield some form ownership over the design process. This tool is often seen as a way of improving customer satisfaction within products whilst also allowing variance and personalisation of products in a large market. In corporations such as motoring, telecommunications and fast moving consumer goods, the majority of participation is generated through the use of multimedia and multi channel process whereby customers can contribute remotely to the questions or ideas posed by developers and manufacturers (Pini, 2009). When comparing this to the medical service industry, the process of generation and collaboration should occur differently based on the introduction of experience.

As analysed earlier, the generation of narratives allows for the co-design and generation of ideas to occur at the root level of experience. This is particularly important, as the range of range of products that may be utilised in the treatment of pain is much narrower than that of other fields. The design process for medical devices may also be considerably longer and complex, resulting in fewer developments and options available to patients at any one point in time.

Through the collaboration of the palliative environment with designers, engineers, scientists and manufacturers, it is hoped that the resulting products will be able to provide for the market more effectively and efficiently. It is also hoped that as the collaborations take place, a database of experiences, inspirations and ideas will culminate and therefore the process will develop more rapidly.

The translation and communication of ideas within the collaborative framework may occur through the generation of storyboards, mind-maps, analogies, props, photographs, short films, personas, touch points, brainstorming and sketching (Makela, 2006).

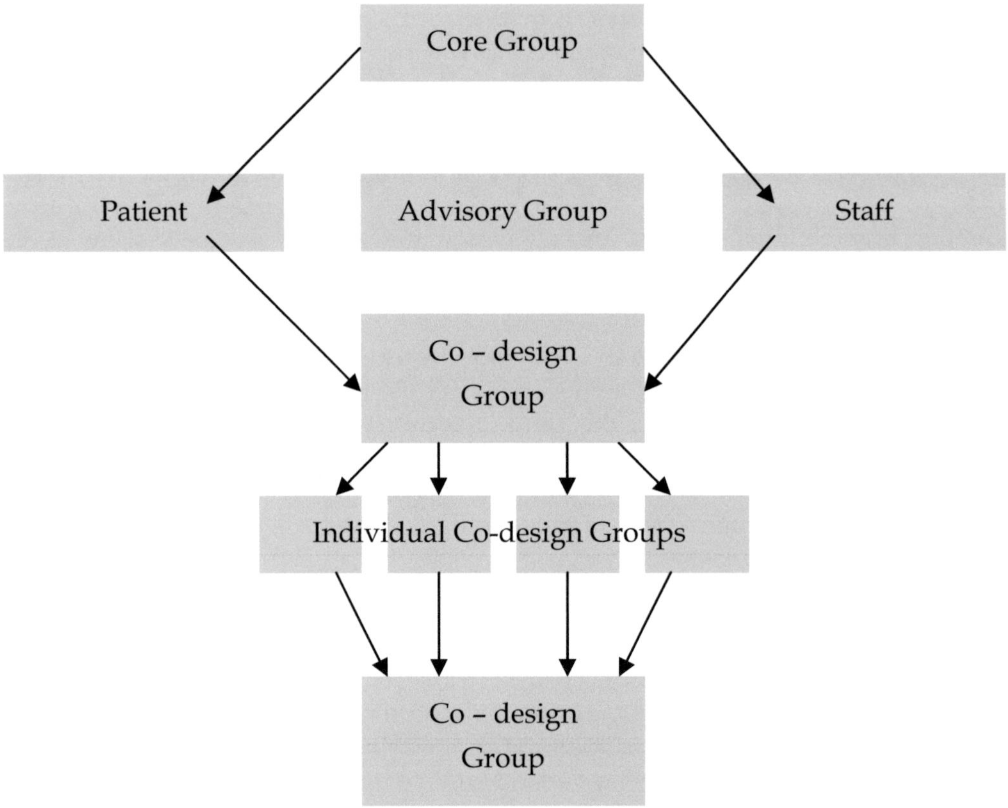

Fig. 1. The experience based co- design process abstract from *Bringing User Experience to Healthcare Improvement* by Bate and Robert (2006) on page 120.

Bate and Robert (2007) identified key groups in the experience based design process. Through this process the leadership is shared between patients and staff as they distinguish the common needs and requirements for the co development process. The identification of a core group turns attention towards the needs of all those that come into contact with the environment as opposed to a purely patient led or user led process.

Figure 1 has been drawn from Bate and Robert's study *Bringing User Experience to Healthcare Improvement* (2007 p120). This process map offers a visual indication as to the various groups that encompass the co-design process. It is important to acknowledge the specialised skills of the development team such as designers and engineers. Although the aim of co-design is to allow collaboration and a continuous feedback cycle, there is knowledge and skills that designers possess and also draw upon from external sources in order to best lead the design process.

Figure 2 illustrates the way in which the co-design and design process may flow in an experience design situation. The design process may be fluid, stagnant, structured or disjointed in its progression, dependent on designer's style and discipline. Throughout, the designer must retain direction to ensure that paths of exploration can be executed within a design solution.

The design process may involve a cycle of progressions, and the core group, patients and carers may be drawn upon at several stages along the process. Although the figure demonstrates a somewhat structured direction, the designer may move backward and forward amongst the collaborators as ideas are explored, questioned and reviewed.

The designer's priority during the co-design process is to act as an agent for those within the palliative framework. The final design solution(s) will represent the partnership between patients, carers and specialists, in a resolved product that can be presented and communicated to manufacturers, government bodies, specialist developers and investors within the private sector. By drawing on experiences, interactions, feedback and inspiration, the product solution will quantify the needs of palliative care.

The subcutaneous syringe driver is a pain management tool that is utilised within palliative care. This particular product has been the focus of review within Australia since the primary model was withdrawn from the Australian market in 2007. The operation and interaction of syringe drivers requires numerous processes and effects several members of the palliative care team. The experiential design model will be applied to the syringe driver in the form of a case study to explore the relationship between experience, product design and the palliative framework.

4. Practise and process

4.1 Case study - syringe driver

A syringe driver is a power driven device for pushing the plunger of a syringe forward at an accurately controlled rate. Syringe drivers are used within palliative care environments as a primary way of conducting pain management for patients who suffer from chronic pain through the implementation of pharmacology.

The medication is administered through the subcutaneous route and diminishes the need for constant injections whilst allowing adequate pain medication levels. Nurses are able to mix together 3- 4 drugs in a syringe and set the device for 24 hours. This elevates stress and anxiety for the patient, as they are able to perform daily rituals such as eating and sleeping without the worry of having to engage with a device for pain management.

There are several models of syringe drivers available on the Australian market and many of these are utilised daily within hospitals, nursing homes, hospices and homes around the country. The primary model, the Graseby MS26, has been withdrawn from the Australian market for purchase but will remain operable within Australia until November 2012. As a result, the Australian government has sourced replacement models that meet the Australian Therapeutic Guidelines and all practise standards and has communicated these suggested models to palliative networks around the country. Although an opportunity for critique and revitalisation of such devices has arisen, barriers such as timing, financial, resource availability, private sector investment and added medical value, has resulted in the provision of replacement as opposed to regeneration. Image 1 presents the functions and key features of the primary model, the Graseby MS26.

The following discussion explores the implementation of experience-based models in the reflection and redefinition of medical processes and service.

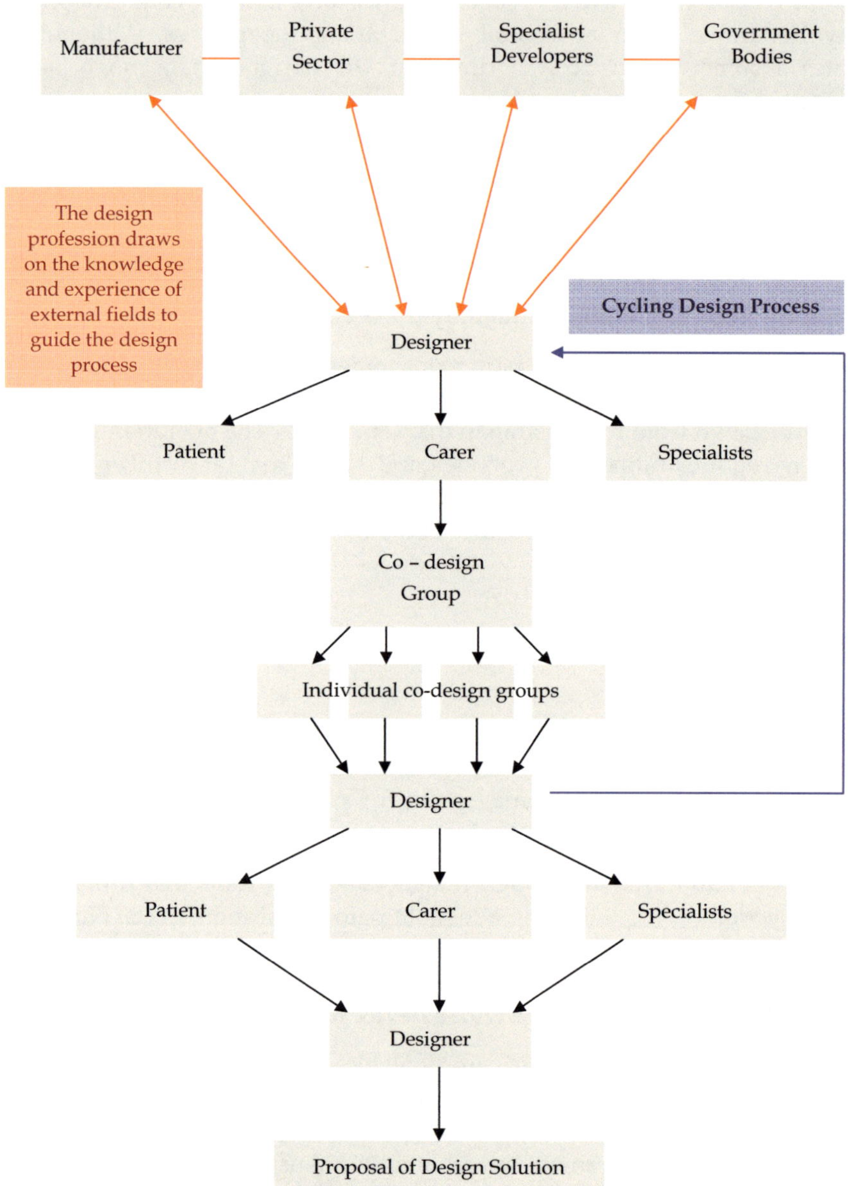

Fig. 2. The experiential design process model.

4.2 From object to user to experience

Over time designers have been exploring the relationship between objects and humans, either through aesthetics, function, materiality, experience, rituals, technology and the natural environment. Different design movements have explored fundamental design principles and have contributed to the design approach both practised and taught amongst the design community.

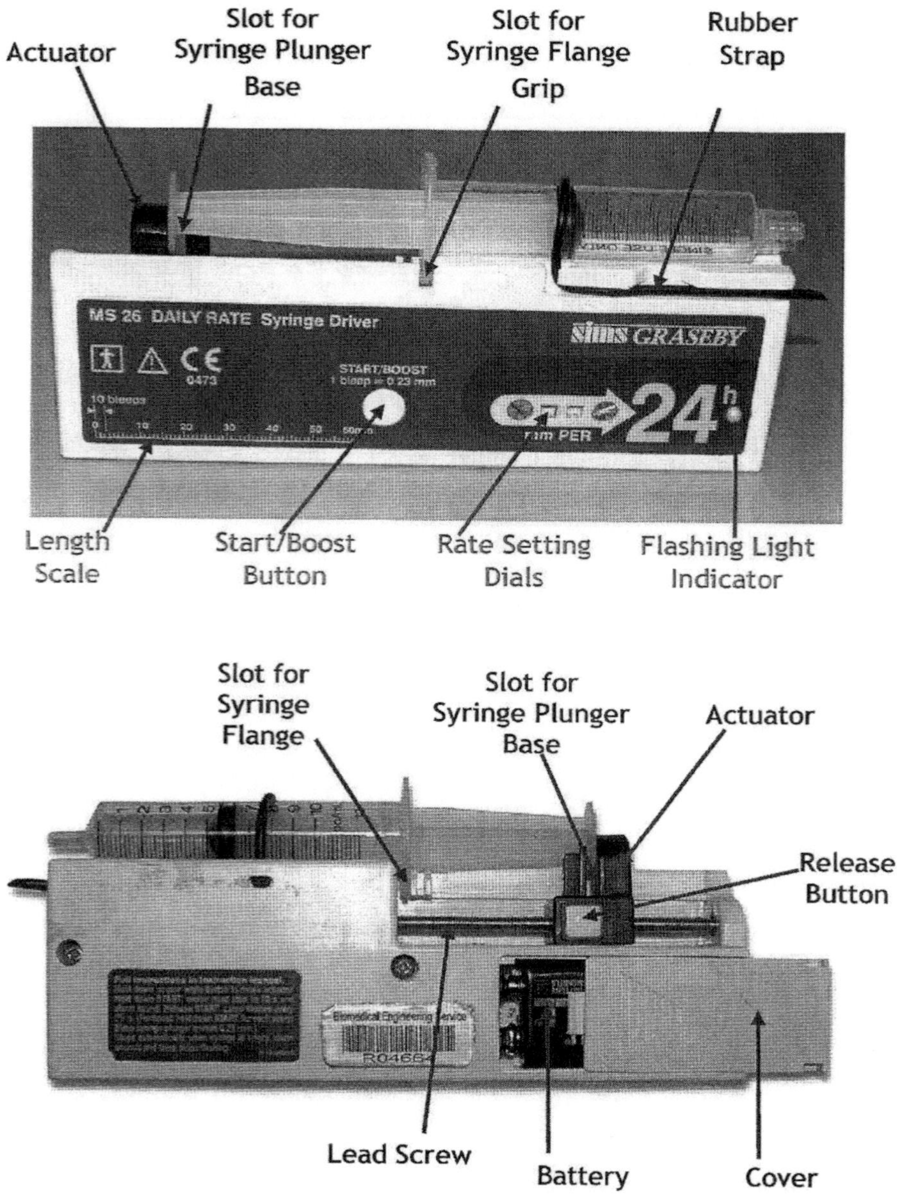

Image 1. Key Functions and Features of the Graseby MS26 (Ballarat Health Services, 2004).

The exploration of syringe driver practise and review would commonly begin with an analysis of current rituals, processes, engagement, satisfactions and disappointments centred on the object and its intended user. The explorative phase occurs on the premise that there is an active product in which to review, that the relationship built between object and user is centred on the capabilities of the object and the way in which the object fits to the user needs and desires. This form of exploration is demonstrated in Figure 3. By placing the syringe at the centre of interaction, users such as patients, carers and specialists must engage with the syringe driver to carry out daily rituals and behaviours.

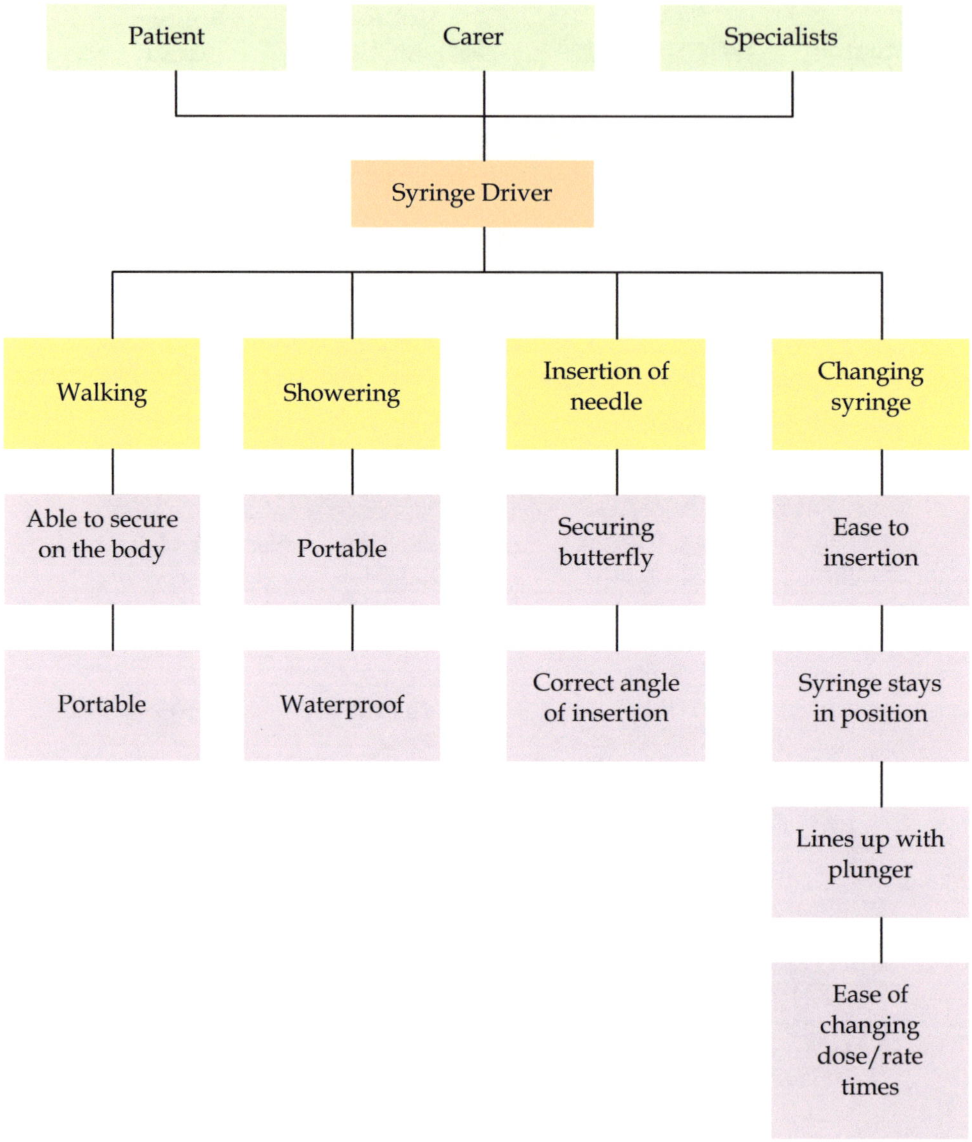

Fig. 3. *Object to User* Product Analysis Approach.

The flowchart maps the relationship between the intended user and the object. As the user engages with the product through daily rituals, the design process is informed about desired or required functions, form, bodily interactions and processes. The designer may then create a checklist or formulate a design hierarchy for evaluation. For example, a designer observed a carer changing the syringe. During the observation, the designer noticed that the carer was having difficulty keeping the syringe in place once secured back into the driver. The designer was drawn to the functional problem that the nurse was experiencing at the time. The nurse's comment on the situation was "I know that when I walk away, the patient will pick the driver up and the end of the syringe will no longer be sitting in the ridge. Maybe I'll put a piece of sticky tape over the top." This observation prompted the designer to make note of form and placement of syringe and may lead to innovative forms, material choices and mechanisms that would influence experiences.

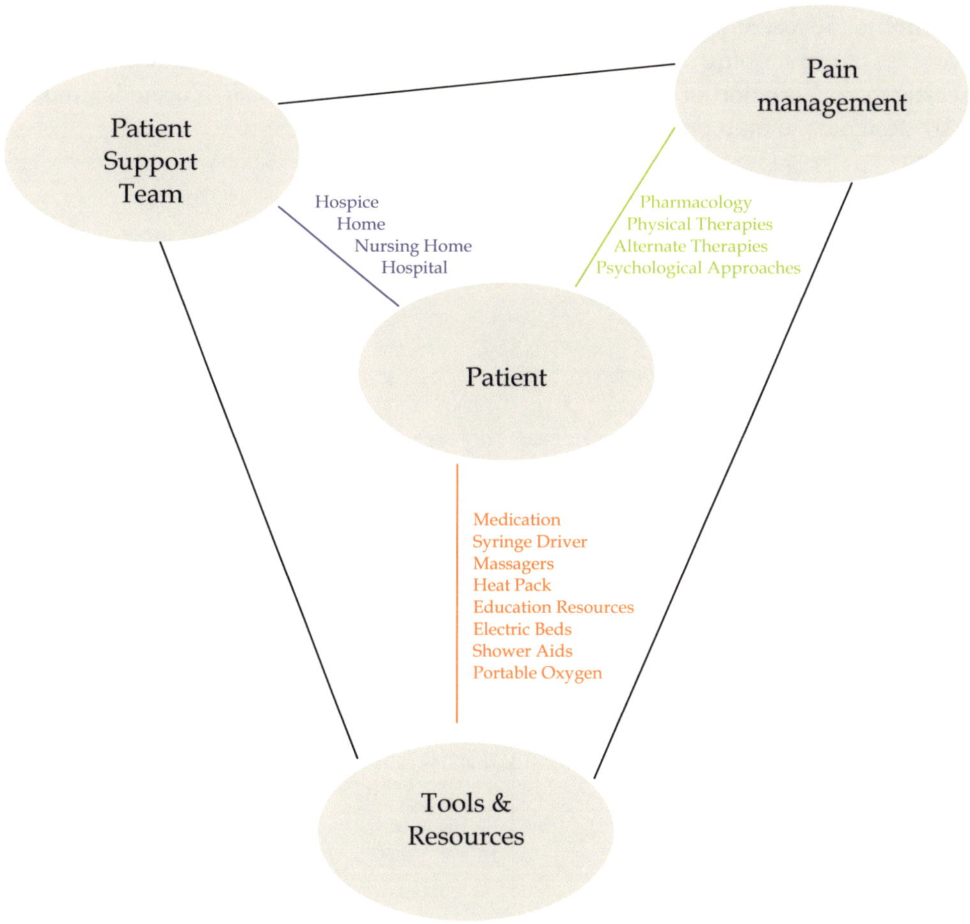

Fig. 4. Patient Centred Care Approach.

Through alteration of the model to reflect a patient centred care philosophy, the dynamic between the palliative frameworks will offer a holistic and broadened experience. In this model, the framework is turned towards the service offered and provided by the support team, pain management and the tools and resources. Pathways of exploration become clear as interactions and experiences become apparent. The syringe driver falls within the relationship between the patient and tools and resources but may also be expanded as experiences between the syringe driver and other factors crystallises.

In figure 5, examples of relationships between the syringe driver and the support framework have been identified. It through the relationships that experience can be evaluated and determined. The experience of use of the syringe driver may be very different in the home where the carer may be emotionally exhausted, stressed and anxious in comparison to a hospice where there are several trained carers available. The expansion of design possibility may also be questioned. New relationships between the syringe driver and physical therapies may challenge designers to reconsider the purpose and intent of such a device. Materiality and form may offer a new form of therapy, for example textures that reflect different levels of pain or form that can be squeezed and moulded as pain increases. This process of questioning and reflection aims to redirect understanding and open the area of investigation. Variation of experience can be identified within such a model and drawn upon by designers to map points of direction and research.

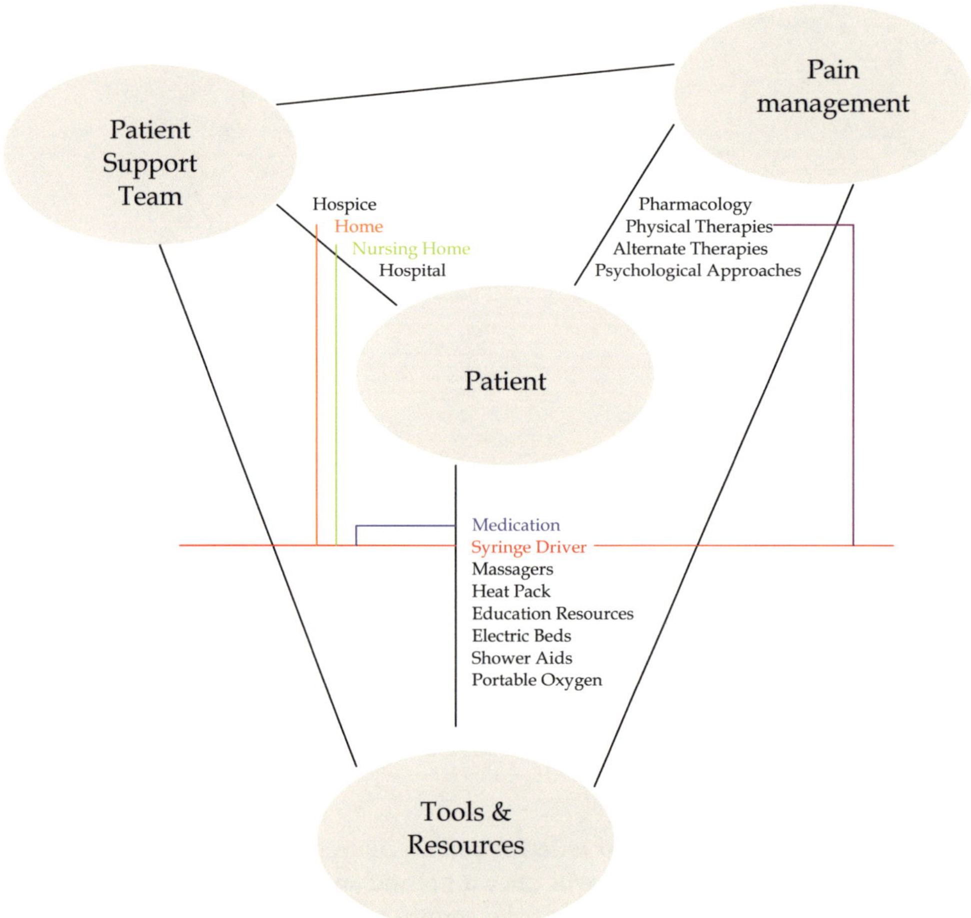

Fig. 5. Relationships formed1 with a palliative framework.

The frameworks illustrated reposition the palliative environment towards a service centred provider. Through mapping relationships, new research possibilities become evident. This process is primarily object centred and explores relationships and needs that pre-exist. Touch points within an experience may redefine the elements that contribute to the current syringe driver design and identify new points of exploration through narratives and feedback.

Through a flow chart of touch points the designer is able to reconstruct the experience prior to syringe driver use, identify the patients understanding of pain management and reconsider the positioning of the syringe driver within the experience. The flowchart shown in Figure 6 illustrates the touch points that may be encountered from the initial phone call to the palliative team to the first home visit by the community nurse. Alongside each touch points are concerns, questions or points of interest that the patient or carer may be experiencing during the process.

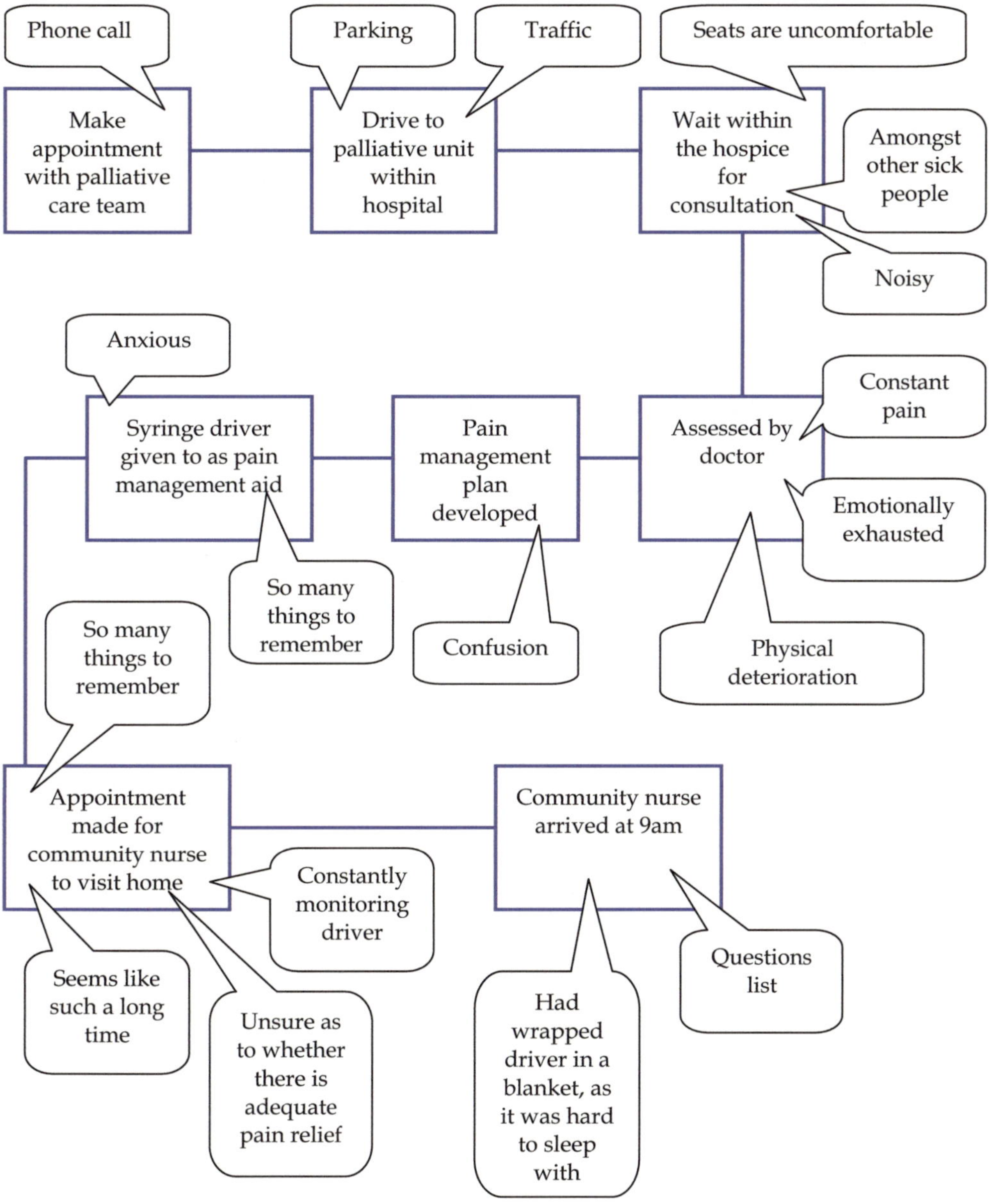

Fig. 6. Patient experiences map.

The patient experience map exposes elements that contribute to the patient's evaluation of the palliative service. The syringe driver that the patient engaged with may have posed difficulties and frustrations. When grouped with surrounding experiential factors such as the noise in the waiting room, uncomfortable chairs, being overwhelmed with information and suffering from sever pain, it may be evaluated that if design changes were made to the syringe driver to improve ease of use, the experiential analysis may still be poor. Through the map it becomes clear to the development team that the first of interaction, the phone call, is where the service to the patient begins.

As health services develop, integrated systems and technologies may aid in reducing poor touch points. The realm of digital health service aids, online training and support will help to reduce the pressure and stress placed on carers and patients. The design of products such as the syringe driver must reflect the way in which we interact with common service providers and the rising needs and expectations of the community. Whilst reflecting on the patient experience of a syringe driver, the development team may question the core ideals of the product, which is to provide consistent pain relief through pharmacology. By returning to the primary need, designers may begin to pose opportunities and new directions through questioning and evaluation. For example, is it necessary to use a syringe? Can we redesign the syringe to reduce the size? Can we design a syringe that is flexible? Can we design the whole device so that it is flexible?

4.3 Evaluation of experience and its role in shaping our understanding

The syringe driver case study demonstrated a strategy for the integration of experiential research within the design process. The experience of pain and its management is personal and unique to each individual. By drawing upon the experiences of others, the development team, particularly designers, is able to consider the complex needs of the patient. Through sketches, mind maps, touch points, photographs and videos the designer is able to respond in an interactive manner to the experiences presented. The ideal integration for experience is to provide a product to a patient that fulfils all the functions of a syringe driver but offers an emotional response. Future products should delight and surprise patients, they should be compassionate and understanding, trustworthy and honest. It is through innovative design concepts and strategies that products can endeavour to reflect human values.

4.4 Conclusion

The dynamic relationship between patient and carer is the centre of palliative care. It is a relationship that develops from a medical stem and matures into a connection based on emotions, spirituality, experiences and trust. Design is concerned with the development of physical forms and systems that acts as a response to the needs and experiences of this form of relationship. Design does not take the lead but rather acts as an aid. It aims redefine the development process, to demonstrate to the environment the possibilities and opportunities and if executed correctly, design should be deeply embedded in the experiences of the patient.

5. References

Bate, P & Robert, G. (2007). *Bringing User Experience to Healthcare Improvement,* Radcliffe Publishing, ISBN-13:9781846191763, United Kingdom

Berry, L et al. *(2006)*. Service Clues and Customer Assessment of the Service Experience: Lessons from Marketing, *Academy of Management Perspectives,* Vol.20, No.4, pp. 43-57

Bingley et al. (2008). Developing Narrative Research in Supportive and Palliative Care: the Focus on Illness Narratives, *Palliative Medicine,* Vol.22, pp 653-658

Chapman, J. (2005). *Emotionally Durable Design,* Earthscan, ISBN 1-84407-181-2, United Kingdom

Djadjadiningrat, T et al. (2006). Beauty in Usability: Forget Ease of Use!, In: *Pleasure with Products: Beyond Usability,* Green, S and Jordan, P, pp.9-17, Taylor and Francis, ISBN 0-415237041, Cornwall

Elliot, J & Roxon, N. (2010). Media Release, *Australian Department of Health and Aging,* 01.08.2011, Available from <http://www.health.gov.au/internet/ministers/publishing.nsf/Content/mr-yr10-nr-nr112.htm>

Ersek, M & Wilson, S. (2003). The Challenges and Opportunities in Providing End-Of-Life Care in Nursing Homes, *Journal of Palliative Medicine,* Vol.6, No.1. pp 45-57

Hubbell, L. (1994). Teaching Research Methods: An Experiential and Heterodoxical Approach, *PS:Political Science and Politics,* Vol. 27, No 1

Hughes, R. (2000). The Mechanical Paradise, In: *The Shock of the New,* pp.16-17, Thames & Hudson, ISBN 0-500-27582-3, London

Jenkins, B. (2002). Offering Spiritual Care, In: *Spirituality and Palliative Care, Social and Pastoral Perspectives,* Oxford University Press, Melbourne, pp118-119, 124-125

Kellehear, A. (2001). The Changing Face of Dying in Australia, *Medical Journal of Australia,* viewed 11 March 2009

Locsin, R. (2005). Technological Competency as Caring in Nursing, *Sigma International,* Indianapolis, pp. 86-94

Makela, A. (2006). Collecting Stories on User Experiences to Inspire Design - a Pilot, In: *Pleasure with Products: Beyond Usability,* Green, S and Jordan, P, pp333-343, Taylor and Francis, ISBN 0-415237041, Cornwall

Moen, T. (2006). Reflections on the Narrative Research Approach, *International Journal of Qualitative Methods* Vol. 5, No. 4, pp.1-11

Noell, E. (1995). Design in Nursing Homes: Environment as a Silent Partner in Caregiving, *Generations,* Vol. 19, No. 4, pp. 14

Pini, F. (2009). The Role of Customers in Interactive Co-creation Practises: The Italian Scenario, *Knowledge, Technology and Policy,* Vol. 22, pp. 61-69

Redstrom, J. (2005). Towards User Design? On the Shift from Object to User as the Subject of Design, *Design Studies,* Vol. 27, No. 2, pp. 123-139

Suri, J. (2006). Designing Experience: Whether to Measure Pleasure of Just Tune In?, In: *Pleasure with Products: Beyond Usability,* Green, S and Jordan, P, pp.161-173, Taylor and Francis, ISBN 0-415237041, Cornwall

Wilson, B. (2007). Can Patient Lifestyle Influence the Management of Pain?, *Journal of Clinical Nursing,* No. 18, pp, 399-408

(2007). Greg's Story, as told by his wife Gai Gibson, In: *Aaron McMillan Palliative Care Story Collection,* Palliative Care Australia, pp.14

(2005). Therapeutic Guidelines of Australia - Palliative Care, *Therapeutic Guidelines of Australia*, Department of Health and Aging.

(2004). Clinical Practise Guideline, Syringe Driver – Graseby MS26, *Ballarat Health Services*, 04.04.2009, Available from <http://grpct.grampianspalliativecare.com.au/policy_proceed/syrinvedriver/syringedriver.htm>

5

Predictors in Complicated Grief: Supporting Families in Palliative Care Dealing with Grief

Pilar Barreto-Martín, Marián Pérez-Marín and Patricia Yi
University of Valencia,
Department of Personality,
Assessment and psychological Treatment,
Spain

1. Introduction

The construction of a person's identity is an evolutionary process. Living implies passing through a series of bereavements and this development gives time to the ego for the management of loss. It also permits recovery from the transitory moments of alteration of identity (Grinberg, 1980). As it has been thoroughly documented, in problematic cases, if the management of bereavement fails, serious disturbances in bereavement or pathological formations happen (Gamo & Pazos, 2009).

As it is known, bereavement is the natural result of the loss of any person, thing or value, one has developed an affective link with. As such, it is a natural and human process and not an illness which must be avoided or cured. The expression of bereavement includes reactions which very often appear similar to those which accompany physical, mental or emotional disorders (Payas, 2007).

Different researchers, even using different conceptual models, agree that bereavement is a complex and multidimensional process, influenced by physical, psychological, social and cultural elements (Barreto & Soler, 2007; Corr & Coolican, 2010; Meuser & Marwit, 2001; Kissane, Block & Mckenzie, 1997; Stroebe, Hansson, Schut, & Stroebe, 2008). Thus, research in bereavement has increased in recent years around the world and many efforts toward consensus have been made (Stroebe et al., 2008).

Early studies were systematic reviews of a conceptual nature, symptoms and types of grief (normal versus complicated, chronic, prolonged, delayed, inhibited, absent grief) and their effects on health.

From a conceptual viewpoint, bereavement is the term used to denote the objective situation of having lost a significant one through death. Grief is the term applied to the primarily emotional (affective) reaction to the loss of a loved one through death. Mourning is related to the public display of grief, the social expression or expressive acts of grief that are connected to the beliefs (often religious) and practices of a given society or cultural group (Stroebe et al, 2008).

Moreover, grief is a process of affliction, sorrow, regret and/or pain, challenging the person actively. The emotional experience of dealing with loss is called the grief process and it refers to the need to adapt to a new situation. We also know that bereavement is a common, painful and universal human experience (Bayes, 2001; Bayes, 2006; Corr & Coolican, 2010). We all suffer loss and we feel the anguish that it is involved with it.

Full of basic notions, bereavement is simultaneously universal and individual, benign and malignant. It is helpful and harmful, active and passive, internal and external, a state and a process (Moules, Simonson, Fleiser, Prins & Glasgow, 2007). Bereavement is universal in the sense that it is an unavoidable aspect of life because we are finite beings. It is individual because people develop their own, intimate, personal and unique bereavement. Bereaved persons may development a substantial change in their vision of the world. It can lead to personal growth, and in that sense it is benign and helpful. But it also implies the danger of regressing or becoming paralyzed and in that aspect it is malignant and harmful. Worden is one of the authors who most insist on the active role of the person in the development of bereavement (Worden, 1991/1997). Finally, bereavement is a dynamic process which evolves over time although in the emotionally painful moment the sufferer has the impression that the world is paralyzed.

In the specialized literature we can find a large number of attempts to define it, which illustrates its multidimensionality and its primarily active and adaptive role (Bonnano et al, 1999; Altet &Boatas 2000; Gamo, Del Alamo, & Hernangómez, 2000, Gamo & Pazos, 2009; SECPAL 2002; Barreto & Soler, 2007)

The American Psychiatric Association has also tried to delineate the concept of bereavement. Thus, in the Diagnostic and Statistical Manual of Mental Disorders (APA, 2003) bereavement figures as a reaction to the death of a loved one, an entity which may need clinical attention and which may have symptoms similar to major depression, such as sadness, insomnia and anorexia.

Most of the people immersed in the process of bereavement will recover more or less in a relatively short period of time which usually ranges from two to three years (Limonero, 1996; Neimeyer, 2002; Worden, 1997; Amurrio & Limonero, 1997). However a group of factors referred to by clinicians and investigators, can condition negatively or positively this process, increasing or ameliorating its intensity and duration and, therefore, the suffering (Bonnano & Katlman,2001; Zhang et al, 2006). These aspects are related to the characteristics of the person who died (the affective significance of the loss), the relation maintained with the deceased, the characteristics of the family member, the circumstances of the death, the strategies of coping, social assistance and religion (Parkes, 1988; Herbert et al. 2009; Stroebe et al., 2001b; Sanders, 1999; Wortmann & Part, 2008; Wortman et al., 1999). In the same way, different investigations have shown that mourners in general have a higher rate of morbidity and mortality (Stroebe et al, 2007; Zivin & Christakis, 2007), and that more than 25% of outpatient care requests are related to psychological aspects which have their origin in the loss of a loved one (Bayes, 2006; McChrystal, 2008).

Thus, we need to keep in mind that for some mourners the process of bereavement can become complicated and extended in time (Limonero et al, 2009), bringing additional suffering. When risk factors have been detected in the mourners, it is necessary to offer them effective psychological and/or pharmacological treatment. And for them to accept it.

Given this scenario, good practice requires evaluating the existence of risk factors, the evolution of the manifestations during the process, the collection of family data which facilitate greater precision in the evaluation and the previous psychological alterations exhibited by family members in mourning (Kissane et al, 1997; Barreto et al, 2008; Chiu et al, 2010). All these factors give a personal profile which can detect individuals more prone to complications in the bereavement process and therefore in more need of specialized interventions (Barreto et al., 2008; Limonero et al., 2009; Soler & Barreto, 2003; Kristjanson et al., 2005).

It is also important to point out how social changes imply variations in the community support individuals receive (Gil-Julia et al. 2008) and also, as Rando (1993) refers, in the increased prevalence of complicated bereavements in the current population. This author attributes this increase to some socio-cultural and technological changes prevalent today, which influence types of death, characteristics of personal relations, personality and the resources of mourners. These facts emphasize the relevance of the sociocultural context (Walter, 2000) and the malleability of bereavement as affected by sociocultural variables (Yi et al., 2006).

Currently, grief support to relatives of patients in palliative care is recognized as a fundamental practice within palliative medicine.

Working with the objective of improving psychological care for persons in bereavement, our research group has obtained interesting results in studying the following themes: determination of the degree of implantation of psychological services in palliative care units in Spain for persons in bereavement; the indicators of a complicated bereavement process; and the risk and protective factors which can perturb or facilitate an adaptive development of the bereavement process.

In this chapter, we try to synthesize the results of our research group with those reflected in the literature, all in the light of the authors' clinical experience. Thus, we will discuss the manifestations of grief, its evolution and we will review the existing knowledge about the factors (mainly risk) prior to the loss that may predict subsequent complications in the mourning of family caregivers of patients in palliative care.

2. Manifestations of grief: An overview

According to Bayés (2001, 2006), we can consider three components in the grieving process: (a) a universal reaction to loss, in the sense that it is a facet which appears in all cultures, although its manifestations may be very different. (b) suffering, which may be associated with active behaviors of discomfort and with passive depression-like behavior. (c) possible negative effects on the health of the person who is grieving.

Most people deal with loss without professional help, but some, a minority, risk suffering lasting effects on health and it is essential to know the indicators that warn us about the danger of complicated grief in order to prevent it (Lacasta & Soler, 2004, Barreto & Soler, 2007; Cunill et al., 2010).

Grief indicators include reactions that often are similar to those that are expressions of physical, mental or emotional disorders. It is important to be very careful in the interpretation of certain reactions of grief that may look like as pathological, when they could be natural and appropriate manifestations according to the particular circumstances of the loss (Gil-Julia et al. 2008).

Grief manifestations include a variety of feelings, thoughts and physical and motor aspects. Among the most commonly described feelings are sadness, anger, anxiety, helplessness, shock, yearning, and emancipation. We see a great variety of these manifestations in cognitive, physical and motor areas (Gil-julia et al., 2008, Barreto & Soler, 2007):

Studies show us how these manifestations can change with the passing of time and prevail more in certain moments of the grief process (Maciejewski et al., 2007).

The grieving process goes through different stages although there is a disagreement over what they are and their empirical validity. These stages are highly variable from person to person (Maciejewki et al., 2007). The first descriptions of the grieving process proposed the existence of successive, essentially static stages: disbelief and shock, yearning, angry protests, depressive mood (hopelessness) and recovery or acceptance (Kubler-Ross, 1969/1975/2000), Bowlby 1993, Parkes, 1970). Nowadays, rather than speaking of specific successive stages, it is beginning to be accepted that although the symptoms of grief come and go, there is a gradual movement towards adaptation as time goes by (Hansson and Stroebe, 2007)

An important empirical study of the grieving process (Maciejewski et al, 2007) has shown that these phases are actually found in the normal process. This study also revealed some aspects not previously considered, such as, for example, that acceptance is an indicator that shows up at the moment that we learn about the loved one's death but that its maximum expression occurs after 2 years. This seems to be the time when the person really emotionally accepts the death. On the other hand, the so-called adverse or negative indicators (denial/disbelief, yearning, anger/rage and depression) have their onset peak before 6 months after the death.

Uncomplicated bereavement involves reconciliation: "the process that occurs as the bereaved individual works to integrate the new reality of moving forward in life without the physical presence of the person who died". Reconciliation is achieved through specific tasks that take place during bereavement.

Authors such as Worden (1991/1997) consider it appropriated to speak of tasks in the grieving process, implying that the person is active and can do something. Phases imply certain passivity, something that the grieving person goes through. Thus, Worden includes four grieving tasks: (a) accept the reality of the loss, (b) work on the emotions and pain caused by the loss, (c) adapt to an environment in which the loved one is absent and (d) emotionally relocate the deceased person and more on.

Similarly, Parkes & Weiss (1983) consider three necessary tasks: (a) intellectual recognition and explanation of the loss, (b) emotional acceptance of the loss and (c) assumption of a new identity.

It is difficult to determine the completion of bereavement. Some authors (Moules et al., 2007) think that it really never ends, but it is considered that the most critical process ends when the person is able to retrospectively remember the deceased with serene affection, and this period seems to last between one and two years.

Likewise, the manifestations of grief are modulated by variables such as gender, age, relationship to the deceased, the cycle of family life and the cultural background of the bereaved (Payas, 2008). The main areas to be assessed to understand and prevent the inadequate progression of mourning would be the following: family structure and functioning, the story of the death, individual and family needs, behavioral problems and requests for intervention.

2.1 A general definition of the grief phenomenon

Although it has been widely studied, there is still disagreement about the definition of grieving (Howarth, 2011).

The Diagnostic and Statistical Manual of Mental Disorders (DSM-IV-TR) (APA, 2003) includes bereavement as an additional problems which may need clinical attention and defines it as the reaction to the death of a loved one.

According to the DSM-IV-TR, a bereavement V-code can be used when the focus of treatment is a client's reaction to the death of a loved one. Use code V62.82, not attributable to mental disorder. For them, bereavement or grief is an entity able to receive clinical attention that may cause symptoms similar to major depression, posttraumatic stress, sadness, insomnia and anorexia, with a chronic evolution implying a great deal of suffering and considerable healthcare costs. The manual indicates that during the first two months the bereaved may present depressive symptoms characteristic of a major depressive episode. They may be considered normal if it does not last longer or there is no suspicious of the presence of pathological mourning. On the other hand, the loss of loved ones is among the major psychosocial problems related to primary support group and social environment, classified on axis IV of the multiaxial classification (Barreto et al., 2008; Prigerson & Jacobs, 2001; Stroebe & Schut, 2001; Hansson & Stroebe, 2007; Tomarken et al., 2008).

The international classification of diseases ICD-10 Mental and Behavioural Disorders (OMS-WHO, 1992), in factors that influence health status and contact with health services, in problems associated with the support group, including family circumstances, uses code Z63.4 for normal grief (disappearance or death of a family member), while uses code F43.2 adjustment disorders for grief reactions of any length which are considered abnormal because of their manifestations or content (Gil-Julia et al. 2008).

Since most people come to terms with the death of a loved one and regain their interest and engagement in ongoing life, as we commented earlier, clinicians should be cautious about suggesting that a bereaved person can expect to follow a predictable pathway (Shear & Mulhare, 2008).

Adjustment occurs during a period of acute grief, when confrontation with the painful reality oscillates with defensive exclusion, in the form of numbing, focusing on positive memories, imagined reunion, and other forms of respire in which attention is directed toward neutral or positive thoughts (Shear & Mulhare, 2008).

Acute Grief lasts most of the day, every day for up to 6 months. It is characterized by: a sense of disbelief; difficulty accepting the death; a mix of emotions with painful emotions usually dominant; thoughts and memories of the deceased are prominent and preoccupying; interest and engagement in ongoing life is attenuated and focused on bereavement-related activities (Shear & Mulhare, 2008).

Integrated Grief is primarily a background state; grief occurs intermittently and changes over time. It is characterized by: comprehension of the death; thoughts and memories of the deceased accessible but not preoccupying; interest and engagement in life are re-established; a mix of emotions with positive emotions usually dominant (Shear & Mulhare, 2008).

Its not easy to establish the differences between normal and pathological bereavement or grief (Altet & Botas, 2000; Corr & Coolican, 2010).

2.2 Complicated grief: A brief history of the evolution of the concept

Complicated grief has been defined as a deviation from the normal (in cultural and social terms) grief experience in either length of time, intensity, or both, entailing a chronic and more intense emotional experience or an inhibited response, which either lacks the usual symptoms or in which onset of symptoms is delayed (Stroebe et al., 2007).

Among the terms that have been used in the bereavement literature to describe atypical grief are: complicated grief (CG); traumatic bereavement; childhood traumatic grief; and, lastly, prolonged grief disorder (PGD) (Howarth, 2011).

Complicated grief interferes significantly in the overall functioning of people, compromising their health and as stated by Maddocks (2003), it may last for years or even become chronic (Barreto et al., 2008)

It is difficult to estimate the incidence of complicated grief in the general population. Different authors are interested in this problem and have observed that after the loss of a significant person, speaking of estimated averages, in the general population, two thirds of mourners evolve normally and the rest suffer alterations in their physical health, mental health or both (Olmeda, García Olmos & Basurte, 2002). Jacobs (1999) for example, reports a percentage of 10 to 20% having problems in resolving their grief, Bonanno and Kaltman (2001) noted 10 to 15% of their samples, and Maercker et al (2005) found only 7.4% of people with complicated grief in a sample of older people. Different populations and clinical criteria may account for these discrepancies.

If we estimate that each deceased leaves an average of 5 mourners (Shear et al., 2005) and of these about 15% develop complicated grief, we will have about 300,000 people with complicated grief per year in the USA, for example.

Currently, there is no consensus diagnosis in part because complicated grief is not included in the classification of the DSM-IV-TR. However, certain symptoms that are not characteristic of "normal" bereavement and may be useful in differentiation from major depressive disorder have been included in additional problems that may need clinical care. The first is guilt for things, rather than actions, received or not received by the survivor at the time of death of the loved one. The second is thoughts of death rather than will to live with the feeling that the survivor should have died with the deceased. The third is morbid preoccupation with uselessness. The fourth is pronounced psychomotor slowing. The fifth is pronounced and prolonged functional impairment, and the sixth is hallucinatory experiences other than hearing the voice or see the fleeting image of the deceased.

As noted above, the line between normal grief and complicated grief can be very thin. The findings suggest that if not treated appropriately the condition may cause negative, long-term, mental health consequences. As a result, researchers are making attempts to define complicated grief, understand its relation to various adaptive responses and desired mental health outcomes, and identify efficacious interventions.

Some researchers have proposed specific diagnostic criteria (Forstmaier & Maercker, 2007; Horowitz, Siegel, Holen, Bonanno, Milbrath, & Stinson, 1998; Prigerson and Jacobs, 2001; Prigerson et al, 2008; Stroebe et al, 2008b; Stroebe et al, 2008c; Shimshon et al, 2008; Frances, Pies & Zisook, 2010).

Traditionally, a classification according to type of complication (anticipatory, chronic, delayed and repressive or avoidant grief) (Parkes, 1990) has been used, but there is currently an attempt to refine the boundaries using the indicators that allow for the diagnosis. The most used in research are those of the DSM -IV-TR (APA, 2003). Others have been operationalized in a questionnaire called the Inventory of Complicated Grief (ICG) established by a group of researchers led by Prigerson.

Both criteria set out different aspects of the phenomenon, the DSM includes mainly the possible psychopathology of mourning, while the ICG includes responses to grief, normal in principle, resulting from the processes of bonding and those that refer to coping with stress. It is also important to note that the DSM criteria is established and accepted in this field and the ICG is still under revision.

Fortunately, the group effort of Prigerson (Prigerson et al. 1999; Prigerson & Jacobs, 2001) can reduce the lack of consensus. According to them, the syndrome or disorder of "traumatic grief" brings together distinct manifestations which can be grouped into two different categories referred to, on one hand, as separation distress (intrusive thoughts about the deceased, longing for the deceased, searching for the deceased despite knowing that he is dead and loneliness as a result of the death) and, on the other hand, the symptoms of traumatic distress (lack of goals and/or feelings of futility about the future, subjective feeling of indifference or lack of emotional response, difficulties in accepting the death, feeling that life is empty and/or meaningless, feeling that a part of oneself has died, feeling that the way of seeing and understanding the world has been shattered, take on symptoms and/or harmful behaviors of the deceased and excessive irritability, bitterness and/or anger in relation to the death). In summary, the diagnosis of complicated grief requires the death of a significant person, the simultaneous presence of several of the manifestations in each category with a certain intensity, frequency and duration and, finally, a serious deterioration in the social life, work or other significant activities of the bereaved.

These authors defend "traumatic grief" as a distinct entity from other syndromes listed in the DSM-IV-TR, such as major depressive disorder, adjustment disorder and posttraumatic stress disorder.

In addition to the listed events, clinical experience suggests other indicators of complicated grief: prolonged state of shock, antisocial behavior, escapes (running away), house-museum (full of mementos) or phobic avoidance (complete absence of them) (Soler & Jordá, 1996).

Tracking studies tell of poor long-term prognosis. The percentage of people who develop complicated grief is relatively small but they may have physical or mental disorders for years and even decades.

Another interesting question under discussion concerns the time when complications in the process can be diagnosed, with the least possible error. DSM's proposal is that this moment should not be less than 6 months after the loss. However, Prigerson's group insists, following the results of its research and clinical experience, that complications detected at 6 months are already present 2 months after the loss (Prigerson & Jacobs, 2001).

Prior to the Prigerson's group, another system for the diagnosis of complicated grief had already been proposed by Horowitz et al. (1998). Independently, both groups proposed similar symptoms that tend specifically to characterize complicated grief (for example, yearning, disbelief, loneliness, emptiness, avoidance ...), suggesting a general agreement in principle on the symptoms of complicated grief. However, the study comparing the two systems' diagnoses of complicated grief, by Forstmeier & Maercker (2007), found significant differences regarding prevalence and conditional probability, both being higher with the diagnostic system proposed by Horowitz's group. This same study also concludes that the set of criteria established by Horowitz's group is more inclusive and less strict than that of Prigerson's group and thus leads to a higher prevalence (Gil-Julia et al. 2008).

2.3 Complicated grief: Differential diagnosis

The Prigerson's group developed the first criteria for complicated grief. Later, these criteria were translated and adapted to Spanish (Garcia et al, 2002), which led to minor changes in them. Furthermore, these authors developed a diagnosis of complicated grief distinguishing it from other disorders listed in the DSM-IV-TR, such as posttraumatic stress disorder, major depressive disorder and adjustment disorder.

Shear & Mulhare (2008) analyzed the similarities and differences between Complicated Grief (CG), Major Depression Disorder (MDD), and Posttraumatic stress disorder (PTSD):

- Similarities between MDD and Complicated Grief:

  Sadness, loss of interest; Psychomotor retardation; Guilt; Sleep and appetite disturbances; Difficulty concentrating.

- Similarities between PTSD and Complicated Grief:

  Triggered by a traumatic event; Sense of shock, helplessness; Intrusive images; Avoidance behaviour.

- Differences between MDD and Complicated Grief:

  Major Depression: Pervasive sad mood; Loss of interest or pleasure; Pervasive sense of guilt; Rumination about pervasive failures or misdeeds.

  Complicated Grief: Sadness related to missing the deceased; Interest in memories of the deceased maintained; longing and yearning for contact; pleasurable reveries; Rumination focused on death or issues related to the deceased; Preoccupation with positive thoughts of the deceased; intense yearning and craving for the person who died; Intrusive images of the person dying; Avoidance of situations and people related to reminders of the loss.

- Differences between PTSD and Complicated Grief:

  Posttraumatic Stress Disorder: Triggered by physical threat; Primary emotion is fear; Nightmares are very common; Painful reminders linked to the traumatic event, usually specific to the event.

  Complicated Grief: Triggered by loss of a close attachment; Primary emotion is sadness; Nightmares are rare; Painful reminders more pervasive and unexpected; Yearning and longing for the person who died; Pleasurable reveries.

Adjustment disorders are defined in turn as the onset of emotional or behavioral symptoms that occur within three months of a stressor. The reaction must be disproportionate to the stressor and produce significant impairment in social or occupational functioning. Stressors are normal life experiences (change of address, illness or illness of a family member, work problems, relationship problems, separation, job loss, etc.). The DSM-IV-TR distinguishes various types: with depressed mood, with anxiety, with anxiety and depression; with altered behavior; with emotional and behavioral alteration and nonspecific. Although most tend to subside with the passage of time, some may become chronic.

2.4 Complicated grief: New definition and controversial issues of DSM

Currently, the most important social issue with respect to complicated grief involves its status as a pathological condition, as a mental disorder for inclusion in systems such as the DSM. There is a growing debate about whether Complicated Grief should be included in the DSM-V as a disorder.

Recently, Prigerson, Vanderwerker, and Maciejewski (2008) presented a case for changing the terminology from Complicated Grief (CG) to prolonged grief disorder (PGD). They now use the term Prolonged Grief Disorder (PGD) to refer to the syndrome specific to bereavement.

The change in terminology increases clarity in the definition of the disorder.

In the past the term *traumatic grief* created confusion with *posttraumatic stress disorder* (PTSD), and *pathological grief* had pejorative connotations. The concept *complicated* etymologically refers to "problems of analysis, understanding and explanation" and therefore we have considered it inadequate for its use in the new proposal which characterizes the bereavement specific form of distress. In addition, *complicated grief* can be confused with *complicated bereavement* which is the term used in the DSM-IV to refer to symptoms of major depression secondary to bereavement.

The term *prolonged* best expresses the nature of this disorder. *Prolonged* does not imply that duration is the only indicator of the pathological grief, it refers to a persistent set of specific symptoms of grief identified in bereaved individuals with significant difficulties in adapting to the loss (Prigerson et al., 2008, pp. 166).

In addition to proposing specific diagnostic criteria, the authors present descriptive features, risk factors, outcomes, and differential diagnoses for prolonged grief disorder. Prigerson et al. (2008) have produced a diagnostic algorithm for Prolonged Grief Disorder (POD), a criteria set that specifies that the reaction has to follow the loss of a significant other.

The proposed Prolonged Grief Disorder Criteria for the Fifth Edition of the Diagnostic and Statistical Manual of Mental Disorders (Prigerson et al., 2008, pp. 171) is:

Criterion A: Bereavement: the bereaved person must experience at least one of the following three symptoms daily or to an intense or disruptive degree: (a) intrusive thoughts related to the deceased, (b) intense pangs of separation distress, or (c) distressingly strong yearnings for that which was lost.

Criterion B: Separation Distress: The bereaved person must have five of the following nine symptoms daily or to an intense or disruptive degree: (a) confusion about one's role in life or a diminished sense of self (e.g., feeling that a part of oneself has died); (b) difficulty accepting the loss; (c) avoidance of reminders of the reality of the loss; (d) an inability to trust others since the loss; (e) bitterness or anger related to the loss; (f) difficulty moving on with life (e.g., making new friends, pursuing interests); (g) numbness (absence of emotion) since the loss; (h) feeling that life is unfulfilling, empty, and meaningless since the loss; and (i) feeling stunned, dazed, or shocked by the loss.

Criterion C: Cognitive, Emotional, and Behavioural Symptoms: Duration of at least 6 months from the onset of separation distress.

Criterion D: Duration: and the preceding symptomatic disturbance must cause clinically significant distress or impairment in social, occupational, or other important areas of functioning (e.g., domestic responsibilities), Further requirements stipulate that the disturbance is not due to the physiological effects of a substance or a general medical condition and that the symptoms could not be better accounted for by post-traumatic stress disorder (PTSD), major depression(MDD) and generalized anxiety disorder (GAD).

On the other hand, Rubin et al. (2008) have suggested the inclusion of more features, in the category of complicated grief in the DSM, in order to put the focus on the relationship, and not only on the dysfunction, also taking into account the interpersonal nature of the loss.

Rubin et al. (2008) propose the representation of a wide spectrum of responses within the construct of complicated grief. They are concerned about the exclusion of cases of complications in bereavement, and argue that the category should be relevant enough to include the many forms of difficulties that arise in bereavement. They also raise doubts about the "medicalization" of grief responses and the possibility that a formal diagnosis could hinder the care and support offered by the various cultural expressions of grief and natural healing or complications connected with the loss. While considering the nature of complicated grief and its status in the DSM, it is also important to address the question of subtypes. Prigerson and Jacobs (2001) noted that the concept of complicated grief in the DSM was similar to chronic grief. This left out the other subtypes of different origin (involving absent, delayed, or inhibited grief).

Currently, Prigerson et al. (2008), in their proposed criteria for the inclusion of prolonged grief disorder in the DSM, specify that "the particular symptomatic distress must persist for at least six consecutive months, regardless of when those six months occur in relation to the loss". This includes the subtype of delayed grief distress provided the symptom persists for at least six months.

Authors such as Frances et al. (2010) in relation to some of the current proposals to include complicated grief in the DSM-V, say, "The recently posted draft of DSM5 makes a seemingly small suggestion that would profoundly impact how grief is handled by psychiatry. It would allow the diagnosis of Major Depression even if the person is grieving immediately after the loss of a loved one. Many people now considered to be experiencing a variation of normal grief would instead get a mental disorder label.

Undoubtedly, this would be helpful for some people who would receive much needed treatment earlier than would otherwise be the case. But for many others, an inaccurate and unnecessary psychiatric diagnosis could have many harmful effects. Medicalizing normal grief stigmatizes and reduces the normalcy and dignity of the pain, shortcircuits the expected existential processing of the loss, reduces reliance on the many well established cultural rituals for consoling grief, and would subject many people to unnecessary and potentially harmful medication treatment."

Responding to Frances et al. (2010), Pies y Zisook say, "We stand by our previous review of the most pertinent recent data, which informs us that continuing the bereavement exclusion (BE) for the diagnosis of major depression does more harm than good. The BE ignores much of this recent evidence, and we agree with the DSM committee's pithy but astute rationale for discontinuing the BE—that there is no credible evidence that bereavement-related depression is different (in severity, course, morbidity, comorbidity, consequences, or treatment response) from other, non-bereavement-related instances of major depressive episodes.

Notably, the International Classification of Diseases (ICD-10) also omits the BE. While rates of clinically serious depression may be somewhat higher when ICD-10 (vs DSM-IV) criteria are used, we are not aware of any evidence demonstrating an 'epidemic of psychiatric grief' resulting from the use of ICD depression criteria."

Finally, the latest investigations conducted by Prigerson et al. (2008) and Rubin et al. (2008) argue that complicated grief is a distinct clinical entity and that it overlaps little with other diagnostic categories, such as depression.

Clearly, the development of specific diagnostic criteria for Complicated Grief is a current and important debate and direction for future research.

3. Predictors in complicated grief: A risk factor overview

There are a variety of ways and moments to express grief over the death of a loved one. Sometimes people do not follow the "normal" grief process. They express it in a way that does not seem adaptive and it significantly interferes in their general functioning, forcing them to look for professional help. These reactions have been called abnormal, complicated, neurotic, morbid, distorted, traumatic or pathological grief.

Studies of risk predictors allow us to identify people who might need support after the loss of a loved one. If it is possible to anticipate who may have difficulties in resolving the grief, it also may act as a prevention and an early intervention (if necessary) to optimize and avoid possible unresolved grief.

The study of risk factors regarding complicated grief allows for the detection and later followup of people with risk of suffering complications in the process. This benefits the entire health network in the short, medium and long term. Early identification of those people who need help to deal with their grief could facilitate early psychological or medical support. The study of risk factors has an important role in the development and testing of theoretical explanations of the impact of grief on health.

Supporting a person with complicated grief risk could reduce the time of the process and prevent future pathologies, depression being one of the most common (Stroebe & Shut, 2001).

Clinical experience and scientific studies warn of the existence of factors linked to poor results in the adequate resolution of grief. We know that when there is loneliness or intense sadness in conjugal bereavement, the risk of physical problems and death increases. Similarly, the death of a child is associated with high morbidity of the surviving parents. Moreover, factors such as sudden or multiple death, low perceived social support or scarce material resources have also been associated with increased risk of health problems (Sanders, 1999).

A risk factor is a lifestyle or personal behavior issue, an environmental situation or an innate or inherited characteristic based on epidemiological evidence. It is associated with health conditions and it is considered important to prevent (Stroebe & Schut 2001).

From a clinical health perspective, it is necessary to identify risk factors that determine possible complications in the grief process. It is also important to identify those factors that may protect people who are going to experience a grief process. The efficient and effective clinical intervention has always considered important both the recovery and the promotion of the individual's resources and attention to their deficits (Barreto et al., 2008). However, there is little information from which we can draw definite conclusions. There is a lot of work to do in this field in order to obtain indicators related to protective factors.

In this study we show some information regarding risk factors (Barreto et al., 2008). We group them into three categories: situational, personal and interpersonal.

3.1 Situational factors

Situational factors make reference to issues that affect the course of grief. This group includes the way in which death has occurred, the duration of the disease, the existence of a concurrent crisis, insufficient material resources and stigmatized deaths.

Sudden unexpected death takes place as a result of a natural or caused catastrophe, an accident, suicide or murder. Within this group difficulty may be aggravated in the case of a multiple loss (for example, several members of a family die in an accident or attack) or in certain circumstances in which there is no certainty of loss due to a disappearance or the inability to recognize the body.

Sudden unexpected death produces a state of shock that greatly reduces the capacity to cope so that full functioning takes time to recover. The survivors of this type of death show more rage and physical symptoms than members of a family who lose a loved one after an illness. Unexpected death leaves the mourners with a sense of loss of control and loss of confidence in the world in which they had previously put their faith. It is usual that this type of death has a child or a son or daughter as the protagonist, a theme which we will discuss more later, and that obviously aggravates the situation.

Sanders (1999) considers suicide a risk factor for illness and death of the survivors but underlines the difficulty of studying it since people do not usually speak of it. Stroebe and Schut (2001) note the lack of empirical evidence supporting greater difficulty in bereavement for suicide. Probably this is due to methodological problems since this type of death favors sentiments of guilt and rumination about previous situations and the outcome, making it harder for the survivor to recover.

Intuitively we know that the death of one's wife in an accident while going to work is not the same as if it happens after several months of illness. The existence of a serious health problem can prepare one for the outcome and promotes the proper resolution of grief, especially if one has cared for and is secure in having adequately supported the loved one. On the other hand, if the duration of the disease has been very long (more than 12 months) and has required a lot of care, the recuperation is likely to occur more slowly because of the exhaustion of the survivor and the painful memory of the process.

The existence of concurrent crisis, that is to say, additional stressors during bereavement may cause an overload. It is easy to understand that the simultaneous presence of other problems such as the loss of a job or of financial resources, a change of address, the appearance of a disease or the presence of other sick or disabled family members may require the development of adaptive resources at a time when the mourner may be operating at a disadvantage, a situation which makes him even more vulnerable.

Likewise, scarce material resources complicate the painful existence of the survivor, producing a poor adjustment to the loss. On the other hand, the recovery is strongly associated with the bereaved having a good economic situation (Sanders 1999).

Finally, regarding situational factors, stigmatized death should be mentioned. Abortion, suicide (which has already been mentioned), death caused by AIDS or other socially marked diseases, or the loss of relationships that society rejects entail a more difficult mourning because of social disapproval, the accompanying concealment or exclusion in the planning of care during the illness and of funeral rites (Sanders 1999, Worden 1997).

3.2 Personal factors

Personal factors basically refer to the individual features of survivors that influence the process of recovery from loss. Based on available studies, the most important variables are: age and gender of the bereaved, personality, previous health, religion, early loss of parents, previous unresolved grief and emotional reactions of anger, bitterness and intense guilt.

The age and the health of the bereaved are inversely related. Younger age groups present more physical discomfort (headaches or stomach pain) than psychological discomfort as a result of bereavement (Stroebe and Schut 2001; Oltjenbruns 2001 and Balk and Corr 2001).

When age in the marital context has been studied, it has been found that younger spouses have a higher intensity of grief but after two years there is a significant improvement. Being young it is easier to see a better future with new feelings of hope. On the other hand, elderly widows initially show a less intense grief but two years later their health is more fragile and the perception of grief becomes more negative than in the case of younger widows (Sanders 1989,1999).

Regarding the effect of gender on bereavement's outcome there is no agreement in the results of scientific studies. Some conclude that widows suffer more health problems than widowers, although most researchers say the opposite. Others find no significant differences. Sanders (1999) considers that the available body of knowledge supports the conclusion that men suffer more severe health consequences after the loss of a partner than women, although conclusive reasons have not yet been found regarding the causes of this difference.

It is plausible that people with well-adjusted personalities and feelings of control over their lives manage better the impact of stressful life events. On the contrary, those with poor adjustment, difficulty expressing emotions, inability to handle stress, little sense of control and low frustration tolerance are more likely to have difficulties recovering from a relevant loss.

In the same sense, people with fragile mental and physical health previous to a loss worsen in a stress situation. It is known that grief exacerbates congestive heart failure and essential hypertension. Moreover, Bunch (1972) investigated the phenomenon of suicide in mourners and found that 60% of them were under psychiatric treatment before the bereavement. Obviously it is easier to detect and diagnose premorbid physical problems than psychiatric problems because people find it is easier to talk about them, but it is essential to take them into account in the light of experience. It has also been observed that people who use health services prior to the loss of a loved one are more susceptible to complications in the grieving process.

On the other hand, it is believed that religion can influence bereavement through two mechanisms: as social support because of the integration into a group and as a belief system that helps in the search for meaning in death. However, the results of the studies are contradictory and may be due to methodological issues or different modes of experiencing religious phenomena (Stroebe and Shut 2001).

Also, the early loss of parents and previous unresolved bereavements impede recovery, since the new death can make them emerge to an extent that has not been reached before (Neimeyer et al, 2010) or the difficulties created by them have not been resolved.

Finally, experimenting and expressing emotional reactions of anger, bitterness or intense guilt predicts long-term complications in the adequate resolution of bereavement except in those mourners who have maintained very contentious relationships with the deceased (Bonanno, 2001b).

3.3 Interpersonal factors

Interpersonal factors refer to relevant aspects of the relationship with the deceased and the social network. We emphasize within this category kinship, ambivalent or dependent relationship, lack of social support and the painful memory.

Kinship is an important variable in predicting the risk of complications in mourning. Parents are not prepared to survive a child. When this happens, they say that they feel like a part of themselves has died and the "why" becomes an obsessive rumination. The feeling of loss of control over their lives and the world and of insecurity is very strong. Somatic reactions, the degree of depression, guilt and anger are higher than those experienced in the loss of a spouse or elderly parent. It has also been observed that mothers have higher levels of guilt, anger and isolation than fathers and the support they experienced in the past with their partner is often lost and they find it very hard to show their feelings. The dissolution of marriage, divorce or separation is frequent, estimated to be between 50 and 90% of cases (Rando 1983). This type of loss can take several years for resolution and, sometimes, family structure may be undermined in such a way that stability can never be completely recovered as a result of "survivor guilt" (feeling guilty for being alive).

Other difficult situations are the loss of a sibling in adolescence, of the father or mother at an early age and of the spouse (some already mentioned).

Conflicting or ambivalent relationships with the deceased may cause difficulties in the subsequent resolution of grief. The fact of having oscillated between love and hate make more likely the emergence of self-reproaches and self-deprecation which may hamper the recovery.

When the deceased was practically the only source of gratification, problem solving and considering necessary to live and be happy, outliving the deceased may create very high levels of anxiety or hopelessness. These are clear predictors of difficulty in the resolution of bereavement.

The various authors who have worked in this field generally agree about the disturbing role of the lack of social support. A small family with low cohesion and inability to help its members usually will present problems. On the contrary, having family and friends who listen empathetically, without stifling tears or expressions of frustration, has a positive effect on health and will avoid an important risk factor. One example is the added difficulty that may occur by not doing alternative activities and the presence of small children at home, phenomena explained by the social isolation that both situations produce and the consequent decline of social support.

We must not forget that the "painful memory due to late diagnosis, poor control of symptoms or inadequate relationships with healthcare staff are factors that also hinder the resolution of bereavement.

3.4 Situations for children and adolescents

Although predictive factors discussed are applicable to all age groups, we also consider in this study some specific high-risk situations for children and adolescents.

The first is an unstable environment with a person responsible for alternate care. As far as possible this situation should be avoided and efforts must be made to ensure continuity of care when parents are not in condition to provide it. The second refers to the dependence on the surviving parents and their reaction to the loss (it should not be forgotten that for children a very important kind of learning is the model that adults provide for them). The third is the existence of remarriage and the presence of a negative relationship with the new parent. The fourth is the loss of the mother for girls younger than 11 and the father in adolescent boys. And fifth is the lack of consistency in disciplining the child or adolescent.

4. Predictors in complicated grief: Some ideas about protective factors

We also briefly analyze protective factors grouped into three categories (based on review of scientific literature, our preliminary research results and our clinical experience): coping strategies, protectors deduced from the study of risk factors and, finally, other factors identified from clinical experience.

4.1 Coping strategies

Coping strategies are what we call the different ways or strategies that people use consciously, and very often unconsciously, to reduce, manage and survive the physical, mental and emotional symptoms naturally encountered in bereavement.

In the theory of stress, bereavement is considered a stressor which requires coping directed at the problem and coping directed at emotions in different moments. The first type of coping would be more appropriate in situations that can be modified and the second would be more useful in irreversible situations. Therefore, in the grieving process, these two components have different roles at different points in time, from the anticipation of the loss to the resolution of grief.

Some of the few findings in this field are those of Benight, Flores & Tashiro (2001) who found in a sample of widows with a mean age of 54 that dealing effectively with bereavement significantly predicted psychological and spiritual well-being and perception of health 6 months or more after the death of the spouse. These data refer to general mechanisms, not specific to the process, and at present are not clinically applicable.

On the other hand, spirituality is a well-documented resource for coping. Religious and spiritual beliefs and related behaviors appear to facilitate a positive adjustment to the loss of a loved one.

As it can be seen, there is very little data from which we can draw definitive conclusions. It is quite possible that the theme of bereavement has special difficulties preventing it from being investigated in the same manner as other stressors, and probably the instruments designed to assess coping in other areas are inadequate in this area, as mentioned.

4.2 Protectors deduced from the study of risk factors

Obviously, many risk factors can be considered in reverse as protectors. Consider for instance the case of family support, occupation or the absence of economic difficulties. In the same way, these might act as protectors: feelings of usefulness, the absence of prior pathology, knowledge of the prognosis of the illness adjusted to reality, etcetera. (See Risk Factors).

However, we cannot simply assume that the inverse of a risk factor necessarily implies a protector, so we need to empirically assess its specific role in future studies of predictive indicators.

4.3 Other factors identified from clinical experience

Finally, there is another group of variables found in clinical practice that have proven their efficacy as protectors in other areas in the field of health and which would be very interesting to consider in the present one. We refer to fluency in communication, perceived self-efficacy, feelings of usefulness in the care of the sick, the ability for planning and problem solving, mental flexibility, self-care and the ability to find meaning in the experience.

5. Supporting families to deal with grief: Some ideas about intervention

Bereavement is an adaptive process that restores the balance broken after the loss and can positively contribute to personal growth (Davis & Asliturk, 2011). Most people adjust without professional help, but a minority are at risk of suffering lasting health consequences.

There is no final end of bereavement but we can deduce that it is completed when the intense pain gives way to quiet and affectionate remembrance of the past. The duration of the process is usually one to two years but this will depend, like its intensity, on the importance of the deceased, on socio-cultural factors and on certain circumstances which are predictors of greater difficulty in resolving bereavement (Barreto & Soler, 2007; Barreto et al. 2000).

Following Gamo & Pazos (2009) with regard to mourning it is important to consider that:

- There is an interrelation between personal history, psychopathology and bereavement.
- Evolution towards a pathological bereavement occurs only in a minority of cases.
- Bereavements, whether or not ending in pathology, are important milestones in the biographical history because of their character of permanent loss and because they mark the resumption of the biographical line after the loss.
- The effects of bereavement can be very long, variable in time, reactivated by other bereavements, other losses, and by multiple relationships or biographical circumstances. Those occurring at one moment may affect others occurring later.
- Bereavements in infancy may condition later biographical development and configure aspects of the personality.
- Bereavement marks the succession of the generations, some have transgenerational effects.
- Bereavement is implicated in triggering or it is related to a very diverse set of clinical syndromes.
- The understanding of certain symptoms, behaviors and life situations can be related to bereavement: this repositions for us the meaning of certain symptoms or behaviors that can have identifying, imitative, repetitive or compulsive shades of meaning.
- The impact of grief in life is always a process, the important thing is not only the event, but the situation and its evolution. Because of this, relations after bereavement are decisive: support, substitute relationships, later losses.

Psychological support in caring for bereaved people includes a wide spectrum of activities (Raphael et al., 2001/2001b; Barreto & Soler, 2003; Barreto, Yi & Martínez, 2003; Soler & Barreto, 2003). Bereavement is a normal phenomenon and routine psychotherapeutic or pharmacological interventions are not justified (Raphael et al., 2001b). Grief interventions are indicated only in specific circumstances and connected to different moments of the process. Bereavement interventions can be divided into two phases: before and after the death of the loved one (Barreto & Soler, 2007).

From a health perspective we can carry out preventive actions aimed at facilitating the development of grief and minimizing the risk of complicated grief, such as (Barreto & Soler, 2007):

- Identify the needs and preoccupations of the loved ones
- Provide information that facilitates coping with the situations of terminal illness and death
- Help the family accept the death of the patient
- Identify the risk factors for complicated grief
- Identify the protective factors of adaptive grief

Preventive interventions of a universal nature, namely those aimed at the general population of mourners, show inconsistent and disappointing results, except for intervention in children which must follow an age-specific approach. Selective preventive interventions designed for mourners showing greater vulnerability have modest results but very good results for certain groups such as bereaved parents with perinatal or neonatal losses, elderly with risk of depression and widows at risk and needing social support. Preventive interventions programmed for people with an incipient pathology or with high levels of discomfort at the beginning of bereavement, have proven very useful.

In interventions after the death of the patient certain aspects should be considered important (Barreto & Soler, 2007):

- People are unique in their manner of living and expressing their pain at the death of a loved one.
- Bereavement is not an illness: Most people have a 'normal' bereavement and adapt to the loss and its consequences.
- The processes of both normal and complicated bereavement are slow.
- Intervention in bereavement re-orders relations, which does not mean helping to forget the loved one.
- In the course of the process of bereavement a wide range of emotions may be present. Some only negative, such as sadness, anger, impotence, guilt, anxiety, and fear, but also some positive, such as joy, pride, satisfaction, gratitude, love, and others.

Following Rando (Rando, 1993; Solomon & Rando, 2007) the general objectives of the intervention in bereavement would be:

- Develop relationships which connect the bereaved with the deceased in a new form given the deceased's absence. Here the focus is on the loved one who has been lost.
- Personal adaptation to the loss. Here the focus is on the bereaved, implying their revision of their worldview and on their own identity which has been impacted through the loss (Calderwood, 2011).
- Learning to adapt to the new world without the deceased. The focus is on the external world and how the bereaved lives in it.

Therapeutic interventions aimed at helping people showing complications in the mourning, and maintenance interventions, which seek to rehabilitate mourners increasing their quality of life and helping in any residual disorder, have been shown to be largely effective (Altmaier, 2011; Drenth et al. 2010; Molero & Perez, 2009; Lacasta & Soler, 2006; Lacasta & Garcia, 2011, Lopez et al. 2010; Portillo et al, 2002; SECPAL, 2011).

The use of drugs for the treatment of complicated grief should be approached carefully for two main reasons: first, because empirical research is inconclusive about the effects of drugs on the intensity of grief; and second, because it could create counterproductive addictions (Barreto & Soler, 2007; Raphael et al., 2001/2001b, Worden, 1991/1997; Lacasta & Sastre, 2000).

6. Conclusion

In this chapter, firstly we have tried to present an overview of history and current status of some nuclear components of grief. Recently, researchers are working on the clarification of the concept in relation to other phenomena with similar clinical features, the underlying processes, its different manifestations and its evolution (normal and pathological grief). Current studies also consider interpersonal aspects, including social risk factors, the effectiveness of the intervention and the consequences in grief of social networks.

The loss of a loved one normally has different emotional effects on survivors in function not only of their biography but also of the circumstances. The intensity and duration of the emotional impact will depend greatly on the importance of the loss for the survivor and the unexpectedness of the loss. The clinical presentation of bereavement responds to individual, family, environmental, and cultural variables, although there are common tasks that an individual likely goes through to successfully navigate the grieving. It is very important to know the normal manifestations of bereavement and grieving and to be cautious in their interpretation because otherwise we may make the mistake of considering as pathological, some completely natural and adaptive manifestations of the process.

Sometimes, bereavement does not follow its normal course and there are reactions that clearly interfere with the overall functioning of the person to the point of requiring specialized help. These reactions or states constitute what it has been conventionally called abnormal, chronic, pathological, traumatic, complicated bereavement or grief. The term complicated (or traumatic) grief describes grief that appears to deviate from the norm in duration and symptom intensity. Lately, the concept of prolonged grief disorder is being used. Currently, the focus on complicated grief is not intended to imply that this disorder is the only, because other psychiatric disorders, such as major depression disorder, generalized anxiety disorder, adjustment disorder and posttraumatic stress disorder could be possible as well. So a good and fine differential diagnosis will be of major importance.

The second part of the chapter highlights that we should pay particular attention to possible signs of grief that are not following an adequate course. We show in this work some information regarding risk factors. We group them into three categories: situational, personal and interpersonal. We present as well some information on protective factors that could help people to deal with pain. We briefly comment about protective factors grouped in three categories: coping strategies, protectors deduced from the study of risk factors and, finally, other factors identified from clinical experience.

It is especially important consider the predictors of pathological mourning in order to identify people who are most likely to need support after the loss of a loved one and thus try to prevent a possible complicated grief. However, in situations of pathological mourning, one should accurately assess the specific problem that prevents people from functioning effectively in their daily life, as well as address the aspects related to the loss. The study of risk factors regarding complicated grief allows the detection and later following up of people with risk to suffer complications in the process. This benefits in short, medium and long term to the entire health network. Early identification could make easier an early psychological or medical support, reduce the time process and prevent future pathologies.

Finally, we insist in the fact that routine psychotherapeutic or pharmacological interventions are not justified. Grief interventions are indicated only in specific circumstances. These interventions may be preventive, therapeutic or follow-up interventions, universal or guided to the general population, referred to groups of "high risk" or indicated in the case of bereaved people who displayed continuous and very high levels of symptoms related to loss. It is also important to identify and to treat grief pathologies as early as possible. Finally, follow-up interventions try to increase quality of life and to help the bereaved people to live as best as possible with their problem and decreasing their morbidity and disability.

7. References

Altet, J. & Boatas, F. (2000) Reacciones de duelo. *Informaciones Psiquiátricas,* No.159, pp 17-29.

American Psychiatric Association (APA) (2003) *DSM-IV-TR. Manual diagnóstico y estadístico de los trastornos mentales.* Barcelona: Masson.

Amurrio L, & Limonero JT. (2007) El concepto de duelo en estudiantes universitarios. *Med Paliat,* Vol. 14, No. 1, pp. 14-9.

Altmaier, EM. (2011) Best Practices in Counseling Grief and Loss: Finding Benefit from Trauma. *Journal of Mental Health Counseling,* Vol. 33, No. 1; pp. 33-45.

Balk DE y Corr CA (2001) Bereavement during adolescence: A review of research. En: MS Stroebe RO Hansson W Stroebe y H Schut (Ed.) *Handbook of bereavement research: Consequences, coping, and care* (pp. 199-218). Washington: American Psychological Association.

Barreto MP; Molero M & Pérez MA (2000) Evaluación e intervención psicológica en familias de enfermos oncológicos. In: F Gil (Ed.) Manual de psico-oncología. Madrid, Nova Sidonia.

Barreto, P. & Soler, C. (2003). Psicología y Fin de Vida. *Revista de Psicooncologia,* Vol. 0, No 1, pp. 135-146.

Barreto, MP; Yi, Patricia & Martínez, E. (2003). Apoyo psicológico en la fase final de la vida. *Revista de Psicología UniversitasTarraconensis,* Vol. 25, No.1-2 , pp. 193-209.

Barreto P & Soler MC. (2007) Muerte y Duelo. Madrid: Síntesis.

Barreto, P., Yi, P. & Soler, C. (2008) Predictores de duelo complicado. *Revista de Psicooncologia,* Vol. *5,* No. *2-3,* pp.383-400.

Bayés, R. (2001). *Psicología del sufrimiento y de la muerte.* Martinez Roca: Barcelona.

Bayés, R. (2006). *Afrontando la vida, esperando la muerte.* Madrid: Alianza

Benight, C, Flores, J. & Tashiro, T. (2001) Bereavement coping self-efficacy in cancer widows. *Death studies,* Vol. 25, No 2, pp. 97-125.

Bonanno GA, & Kaltman S. (1999) Toward an integrative perspective on bereavement. *Psychol Bull* , Vol. 125, No. 6, pp. 760-77.

Bonanno GA, & Kaltman S. (2001) The variety of grief experience. *Clin Psychol Rev;* Vol. 21, No. 5, pp. 705-734.

Bonanno GA (2001b) Grief and emotion: A social-funtional perspective. En: MS Stroebe RO Hansson W Stroebe y H Schut (Ed.) Handbook of bereavement research: Consequences, coping, and care (pp. 493-515). Washington: American Psychological Association.

Bowlby J (1993) *El vínculo afectivo. La separación afectiva. La pérdida afectiva.* Barcelona: Paidós. Psicología Profunda.

Calderwood, KA. (2011) Adapting the Transtheoretical Model of Change to the Bereavement Process. *Social Work;* Vol. 56, No. 2, pp. 107-118.

Chiu YW, Huang CT, Yin SM, Huang YC, Chien CH, Chuang HY. (2010) Determinants of complicated grief in caregivers who cared for terminal cancer patients. *Support Care Cancer,* Vol. 18, pp. 1321-1327.

Corr, CA, & Coolican, MB, (2010) Understanding bereavement, grief, and mourning: implications for donation and transplant professionals. *Progress in Transplantation;* Vol. 20, No. 2; pp. 169-177.

Cunill, M., Clavero, P., Gras, M. & Planes, M. (2010) Procesos de pérdida: como prevenir futuras dificultades. *Cuadernos de medicina psicosomática y psiquiatría de enlace,* No 93 / 94, pp. 45-48.

Davis, CG. & Asliturk, E (2011) Toward a Positive Psychology of Coping With Anticipated Events. *Canadian Psychology*, Vol. 52, No. 2; pp. 101-110.

Drenth, C., Herbst, A.G. & Strydom, H., (2010) A complicated grief intervention model. *Health SA Gesondheid*, Vol. 15, No 1, pp. 1-8. Available from http://www.hsag.co.za. Art. #415, 8 pages. DOI: 10.4102/hsag.v15i1.415

Forstmeier S, Maercker A. (2007) Comparison of two diagnostic systems for Complicated Grief. *J Affective Disorders*, Vol. 99, pp. 203-211.

Frances, A., Pies, R. & Zisook, S. (May 2010) DSM5 and the Medicalization of Grief: Two Perspectives. *Psychiatric times*, 13 May 2010, No 10168, pp. 46-47. Available from http://www.psychiatrictimes.com/dsm-5/content/article/10168/1568760.

Gamo, E. & Pazos, P. (2009) El duelo y las etapas de la vida. *Revista de la asociación española de neuropsiquiatría*, Vol. 29, No 104, pp. 455-469.

Gamo, E., De alamo, Hernan Gomez (2000) Problemática clínica del duelo en la asistencia en Salud Mental, *Psiquiatría Pública*, 12 (3), 209

García-García JA, Landa V, Prigerson H, Echeverria M, Grandes G, Mauriz A, & Andollo I. (2002) Adaptación al español del Inventario de Duelo Complicado (IDC). *Medicina Paliativa*, Vol. 9, No. 2, pp. 10-1.

Gil-Juliá, B., Bellver, A. & Ballester, R. (2008) Duelo: evaluación, diagnóstico y tratamiento. *Revista de Psicooncologia*, Vol. 5, No. 2-3, pp. 103-116.

Grimberg, L. (1980) *Identidad y cambio*.Buenos Aires, Paidos.

Hansson, R., & Stroebe, M. (2007). *Bereavement in late life*. Washington DC: American Psychological Association

Hebert RS, Schulz R, Copeland VC, & Arnold RM. (2009) Preparing family caregivers for death and bereavement. Insights from caregivers of terminally ill patients. *J Pain Symptom Manage*; Vol. 37, No. 1, pp. 3-12.

Horowitz MJ, Siegel B, Holen A, Bonanno GA, Milbrath C, Stinson CH. (1998) Diagnostic criteria for complicated grief disorder. *Am J Psychiatry*, Vol. 155, No. 9, pp. 1305-1306.

Howarth, A. (2011) Concepts and Controversies in Grief and Loss. *Journal of Mental Health Counseling*; Vol. 33, No 1; pp. 4-10.

Jacobs SC. (1999) *Traumatic grief: Diagnosis, treatment and prevention*. Philadelphia: Brunner/Mazel,.

Kristjanson LJ, Cousins K, Smith J, & Lewin G. (2005) Evaluation of the Bereavement Risk Index (BRI): A community hospice care protocol. *Int J Palliat Nurs*; Vol 11, No. 12, 610-618.

Kissane D, Bloch S & McKenzie D. (1997) Family coping and bereavement outcome. *Palliative Medicine*, Vol. 11, pp. 191-201.

Kubler-Ross, E. (1969/1975/2000). *Sobre la muerte y los moribundos*. Barcelona: Grigalbo Mondadori.

Lacasta MA & Soler MC. (2004) El duelo: prevención y tratamiento del duelo patológico. Cuidados después de la muerte. In: *Manual SEOM de Cuidados Continuos*. Madrid: Dispublic.

Lacasta, M., & Sastre, P. (2000). El manejo del duelo. In M. Die Trill, & E. López Imedio, *Aspectos psicológicos en cuidados paliativos. La comunicación con el enfermo y la familia* Madrid: Ades Editores.

Lacasta MA & Soler MC. (2006) Instrumentos de evaluación en duelo. In: González Barón M, Ordóñez Gállego A. & Lacasta Reverte MA (Eds.) *Valoración Clínica en el paciente con Cáncer*. Madrid: Editorial Médica Panamericana.

Lacasta Reverte MA & García Rodríguez ED (July 2011) *El duelo en cuidados paliativos.* SECPAL. Guías Medicas. Available from: http://www.secpal.com

Limonero JT. (1996) El fenómeno de la muerte en la investigación de las emociones. *Rev Psicol Gen Aplic;* Vol. 49: pp. 249-265.

Limonero, J, Lacaste, M., García, J.A., Maté, J. & Prigerson, HG. (2009) Adaptación al castellano del inventario de duelo complicado. *Medicina paliativa,* Vol. 16: N.o 5; pp. 291-297.

López de Ayala García; C., Galea Martín; T & Campos Méndez, R. (2010) *Guía Clínica. Seguimiento del duelo en Cuidados Paliativos.* Observatorio Regional de Cuidados Paliativos de Extremadura.

Maciejewski PK, Zhang B, Block SD, & Prigerson HG. (2007) An empirical examination of the stage theory of grief. *JAMA,* Vol. 297, No. 7, pp. 716-723.

Maddocks I (2003) Grief and bereavement. *Med J Aust,* Vol. 179 , No. suppl 6, pp. s6-s7.

Maercker A, Fortmeieer S, Enzler A, & Ehlert U. (2005) *Complicated grief as a stress response syndrome: results from the Zurich older age study.* Paper presented at the 7th International conference on grief and bereavement in contemporary society, London,.

McChrystal J. (2008) The psychological impact of bereavement on insecurely attached adults in a primary care setting. *Couns Psychother Res* ; Vol. 8, No. 4, 231-238.

Meuser T & Marwit S (2001) A comprehensive, stage-sensitive model of grief in dementia caregiving. *The Gerontologist,* 41 (5), 658

Molero, M. & Pérez, M. (2009) El duelo, la familia, el trauma y el EMDR: Análisis de un caso clínico. *Mosaico-Revista de la Federación española de asociaciones de terapia familiar,* Vol.42, pp. 28-35.

Moules, N. J., Simonson, K., Fleiser, A. R., Prins, M., & Glasgow, B. (2007). The Soul of Sorrow Work: Grief and Therapeutic Interventions With Families. *J Fam Nurs* , Vol. 13, No. 1, pp. 117-141

Neimeyer RA. (2002) *Aprender de la pérdida.*Barcelona: Paidós.

Neimeyer, R., Burke, L., Mackay, M., Van Dyke Stringer, J. (2010) Grief Therapy and the Reconstruction of Meaning: From Principles to Practice. *Journal of Contemporany Psychothery,* Vol. 40, pp. 73–83.

Olmeda, MS, García, A. & Basurte, I. (2002) Rasgos de personalidad en duelo complicado. *Psiquiatría.com,* Vol. 5, No 5, 1-12.

Oltjenbruns KA (2001). Developmental Context of childhood: Grief and regrief phenomena. En: MS Stroebe, RO Hansson, W Stroebe y H Schut (Ed.) *Handbook of bereavement research: Consequences, coping, and care* (pp. 169-197). Washington: American Psychological Association.

Organización Mundial de la Salud, CIE. (1992) *Clasificación internacional de las enfermedades: Trastornos mentales y del comportamiento.* 10ª ed. Zaragoza: Meditor.

Parkes CM. (1970) Seeking and finding a lost object: Evidence of recent studies of the reaction to bereavement. *Social science & medicine;,* Vol. 4, No. 2, pp. 187-201.

Parkes CM. (1988) Research: bereavement. *Omega,* Vol. 18, No. 4, pp. 365-377.

Parkes CM. (1990) Risk Factors In Bereavement: Implications for the prevention and treatment of pathologic grief. *Psychiatr Ann;* Vol. 20, No. 6, pp. 308-313.

Parkes CM & Weiss RS (1983) *Recovery from bereavement.* New York: Basic Books.

Payás A. (2007) Intervención grupal en duelo. In: Camps C, Sánchez PT, (eds). *Duelo en Oncología.* Madrid: Sociedad Española de Oncología Médica.

Payás, A. (2008) Funciones psicológicas y tratamiento de las rumiaciones obsesivas en el duelo. *Revista de la asociación española de neuropsiquiatría,* Vol. 28, No 102, pp. 307-323.

Portillo, M., Martín, M.J. & Alberto, M. (2002) Adherencia al tratamiento del duelo patológico. *Cuadernos de medicina psicosomática y psiquiatría de enlace,* No 62 / 63, pp. 13-18.

Prigerson, H.G.; Shear, M.K.; Jacobs, S.C.; Reynolds III, C.F.; Maciejewski, P.K.; Davidson, J.R.T.; Rosenheck, R.A.; Pilkonis, P.A.; Wortman, C.B.; Williams, J.B.W.; Widiger, T.A.; Frank, E.; Kupfer, D.J. y Zisook, S. (1999). Consensus criteria for traumatic grief. A preliminary empirical test. *British Journal of Psychiatry,* Vol. *174,* pp. 67-73.

Prigerson, H.G. & Jacobs, S.C. (2001). Traumatic grief as a distinct disorder: A rationale, consensus criteria, and a preliminary empirical test. In: M.S. Stroebe, R.O. Hansson, W. Stroebe & H. Schut (Eds.), *Handbook of bereavement research: Consequences, coping, and care* (pp. 613-645). Washington: American Psychological Association.

Prigerson, H. G., & Jacobs, S. (2001). Traumatic grief as a distinct disorder: A rationale, consensus criteria, and a preliminary empirical test. In M.S. Stroebe, R.O. Hansson, W. Stroebe, & H. Schut (Eds.), *Handbook of bereavement research: Consequences, coping, and caring* Washington, DC: American Psychological Association.

Prigerson, H. G., Vanderwerker, L. C, & Maciejewski, P. K. (2008). A case for inclusion of prolonged grief disorder in DSM-V. In M.S. Stroebe, R.O. Hansson, H. Schut, & W. Stroebe (Eds.), *Handbook of bereavement research and practice: Advances in theory and intervention* Washington, DC: American Psychological Association.

Rando TA (1983) An investigation of grief adaptation in parents whose children have died from cancer. *Journal of Pediatric Psychology,* Vol. 8, pp. 3-20.

Rando, T. (1993) *Treatment of complicated mourning.* Champaign, IL: Research Press

Raphael B, Middleton W, Martinek N, Misso V. (2001) Counselling and therapy of the bereaved. In: M.S. Stroebe, R.O. Hansson, W. Stroebe y H. Schut, eds. *Handbook of bereavement research: Consequences, coping, and care.* Washington: American Psychological Association.

Raphael, Minkov, and Dobson (2001b). Psychotherapeutic and pharmacological intervention for bereaved persons. In: M.S. Stroebe, R.O. Hansson, W. Stroebe y H. Schut, eds. *Handbook of bereavement research: Consequences, coping, and care.* Washington: American Psychological Association.

Rubin, S., Malkinson, R., & Witztum, E. (2008). Clinical aspects of a DSM Complicated Grief Diagnosis: Challenges, dilemmas, and opportunities. In M. S. Stroebe, R. O. Hansson, H. Schut & W. Stroebe (Eds) *Handbook of Bereavement Research and Practice: Advances in Theory and Intervention* (pp 187 - 206). Washington, DC: American Psychological Association Press.

Sanders CM (1999) Risk factors in bereavement outcome. In: MS Stroebe, W Stroebe y RO Hansson (Ed.) *Handbook of bereavement: Theory, research, and intervention* (pp. 255-267). Cambridge: Cambridge University Press.

Secpal (2002) *Guía de cuidados paliativos.* Madrid: Secpal.

Shear, M.K., Frank, E., Houck, P.R., & Reynolds, CF. (2005). Treatment of complicated grief: A randomized controlled trial. *JAMA,* Vol. 293, pp. 2601-2608.

Shear, MK. & Mulhare, E. (2008) Complicated Grief. *Psychiatric annals,* Vol. 38, No. 10, pp. 662-670.

Shimshon, S., Malkinson, R. & Witztum, E. (2008). Clinical aspects of a DSM complicated grief diagnosis: challenges, dilemmas and opportunities. In M.S. Stroebe, R.O. Hansson, H. Schut, & W. Stroebe (Eds.), *Handbook of bereavement research and practice: Advances in theory and intervention* Washington, DC: American Psychological Association.

Sociedad Española de Cuidados Paliativos (SECPAL). (July 2011) *Guía de duelo para familiares.* Sociedad Española de Cuidados Paliativos. Available from http://www.iconcologia.net/catala/hospitalet/imatges /model_guiadol.pdf.

Soler, M. C. & Jorda, E. (1996). El duelo: manejo y prevención de complicaciones. *Medicina Paliativa, Vol 3/2,pp.* 66-75.

Soler, C. & Barreto, MP. (2003). Intervención Psicológica en el duelo. *Revista de Psicología UniversitasTarraconensis, Vol.* 25, No. 1-2, pp. 218-233.

Solomon, R. & Rando, T. (2007) Utilization of EMDR in the Treatment of Grief and Mourning. *Journal of EMDR Practice and Research,* Vol.1, No 2, pp. 109-117.

Stroebe W & Schut H (2001) Risks factors in bereavement outcome: a methodological and empirical review. In: Stroebe M et al. (Ed.) *Handbook of bereavement research: consequences, coping and care.* Washington: American Psychological Association,

Stroebe, M.S., Hansson, R.O., Stroebe, W. & Schut, H. (eds.) (2001b) *Handbook of bereavement research: Consequences, coping, and care.* Washington: American Psychological Association.

Stroebe, M.S., Schut, H & Stroebe, W. (2007) Health outcomes of bereavement. The Lancet, Vol. 370, No. 9603, pp. 1960-1973.

Stroebe, M.S., Hansson, R.O., Schut, H.A.W. & Stroebe, W. (Eds.) (2008) *Handbook of bereavement research and practice: Advances in Theory and Intervention.* Washington: APA.

Stroebe, M.S., Hansson, R.O., Stroebe, W. & Schut, H. (2008b) Bereavement research: contemporary perspectives. In M.S. Stroebe, R.O. Hansson, H. Schut, & W. Stroebe (Eds.), *Handbook of bereavement research and practice: Advances in theory and intervention* Washington, DC: American Psychological Association.

Stroebe, M.S., Hansson, R.O., Stroebe, W. & Schut, H. (2008c) Bereavement research: 21st century prospects. In M.S. Stroebe, R.O. Hansson, H. Schut, & W. Stroebe (Eds.), *Handbook of bereavement research and practice: Advances in theory and intervention* Washington, DC: American Psychological Association.

Tomarken A, Holland J, Schachter S,Vanderwerker L, Zuckerman E, Nelson C et al. (2008) Factors of complicated grief predeath in caregivers of cancer patients. *Psychooncology,* Vol. 17, pp. 105-111

Walter (2000) On Bereavement: The culture of grief. *Palliative Medicine,* Vol. 14, No 1, pp 355

Worden JW. (1991/1997) *El tratamiento del duelo.* Barcelona: Paidós,.

Wortmann JH, & Park CL. (2008) Religion and spirituality in adjustment following bereavement: an integrative review. *Death Stud;* Vol. 32, No. 8, pp. 703-736.

Wortman CB; Silver RC; Kessler RC (1999) The meaning of loss and adjustment to bereavement. En: MS Stroebe, W Stroebe y RO Hansson (Ed.) *Handbook of bereavement: Theory, research, and intervention.* Cambridge: Cambridge University Press.

Yi, P., Barreto, P., Soler, C., Fombuena, M., Espinar, V., Pascual, L., Navarro, R., González, R., Bernabeu, J. & Suárez, J. (2006) Grief support provided to caregivers of palliative care patients in Spain. *Palliative Medicine,* Vol. 20, pp. 521-531.

Zhang B, Areej BS, & Prigerson H. (2006) Update on bereavement research: evidence-based guidelines for the diagnosis and treatment of complicated bereavement. *J Palliat Care;* Vol. 9, No. 5, pp. 1188-1203.

Zivin N. Christakis A. (2007) The emotional tool of spousal morbidity and mortality. *Am J Geriatr Psychiatry;* Vol. 15: 772-779.

6

The Place of Volunteering in Palliative Care

Jacqueline H. Watts
The Open University,
UK

1. Introduction

This chapter discusses the place and development of volunteering in palliative care in the context of hospice service provision in the UK. It draws on recent qualitative research undertaken in a large hospice in England. The research explored a range of issues connected to the process and experience of voluntary work in this setting including who volunteers, what roles volunteers take up, how they are trained and supported and the ways in which role boundaries are established and maintained. The research revealed that hospice volunteering is rewarding but often emotionally challenging and is now highly routinised and closely monitored in ways paralleling practices in the paid labour market. Although volunteers freely give their time to the work of hospice, their activities are subject to significant management prescription, with hospices increasingly adopting sophisticated business models to underpin their operation and, in many cases, their expansion (Watts, 2010).

As noted above, the discussion of volunteering in palliative care takes as its theoretical starting point the positioning of volunteering as work and the first section of the chapter briefly outlines the nexus of paid commodified work and the informal non-commodified work of volunteers. This discussion is pivotal in informing understanding about the motivation and commitment that underpins voluntary work in the hospice sector and wider palliative care. The discussion then moves on to outline the development of hospice and palliative care services in the UK highlighting the juxtaposition of hospice as a 'built' enterprise alongside the focus of palliative care in the community. The essential contribution made by volunteers to UK hospice services is drawn out suggesting that many hospices would not be able to offer the diversity and level of service without the huge amount of time and energy given by volunteer workers. Some brief commentary about other models operating in such countries as India and South Africa is the subject of the next section and is included to specifically highlight how volunteering in palliative care is culturally produced with operational models highly context dependant. Details of the research design and method comprise the next section foregrounding how empirical research in this area is sensitive work framed by a sense that all those engaged in hospice work are potentially vulnerable actors (Liamputtong, 2007). The accounts of research participants are explored in the next four sections focusing on the themes of motivation, training and support, role diversity, management and accountability and the trend towards professionalisation of volunteering in this context. Integral to these aspects are considerations connected to role boundaries and ethical conduct. The chapter closes with brief commentary about future directions for volunteering in palliative care.

2. Intersection of voluntary and paid work

Work, as paid employment, has long been understood to contribute to individual identity, particularly masculine identity, with the ideology of the male breadwinner still the focus of contemporary debates about the sociology of work (Mooney, 2004; Edwards & Wajcman, 2005; Warren, 2007). Work has also been found to have spiritual properties with Howard and Welbourn (2004) reporting that work is an important element in people's sense of meaning and purpose, contributing significantly to their spirituality and sense of 'self' in the world. The paid work sector has a number of connecting points with voluntary work and MacDonald (1997) notes that working in a voluntary capacity can be a source of experience, skills development, networking and the route to paid employment. It also can be the vehicle for enabling people to have structure in their lives and is a source of job satisfaction and individual fulfilment as is the case for paid work.

The concept of work is thus multi-dimensional. In recent times work, as paid labour, has undergone significant transformation, particularly in Western societies that have seen a decrease in manufacturing, the disappearance of a 'job for life', a huge increase in women's employment and, with the onset of the internet, a rise in home and flexible working (Bolton & Houlihan, 2009). A further change has been the growth of the voluntary sector that is characterised by a variety of organisations from large professional bureaucracies to small neighbourhood-based community groups (Newman & Mooney, 2004). Noon and Blyton (2007) argue that one of the long term factors stimulating the growth of both the voluntary sector and volunteering has been the rising cost of buying in services from the formal economy, leading to a form of local self-provisioning within communities. The range of activities that constitute voluntary work is vast incorporating informal tasks such as acts of kindness (for example, doing an elderly neighbour's shopping), social exchange activities (such as a baby sitting circle) as well as work in the more formally oriented health and social care field (Noon & Blyton, 2007).

Voluntary work, as uncommodified work, can be distinguished from paid commodified work in that it is freely undertaken for no financial payment and is often motivated by altruism shaped by a sense of wanting to 'give back' to the community. Noon and Blyton (2007) further characterise voluntary work as normally undertaken outside the family in the community, with its key feature as that of 'gift work'. A core value of volunteering is working for the good of others, expecting nothing in return apart from the emotional satisfaction that such efforts may bring. Stebbins (1996) draws distinctions between types of volunteering: career and casual, formal and informal, and occupational and non-occupational. Gender is also a factor with men and women tending to volunteer for different types of work. Noon and Blyton (2007) argue that women are more likely to undertake voluntary work in schools, with social welfare groups and to engage in fundraising activities. Men, on the other hand, are disproportionately active in voluntary work involving sports groups and committee work. Fink (2004) draws attention to the relational features of much voluntary work that she argues can be emotionally demanding giving rise to emotional distress with the need to develop appropriate coping strategies. Rojek (2010: 27) develops this theme arguing that 'the management of emotional labour does not stop when one leaves the workplace' such that issues of competence and the maintenance of credibility continue as an ongoing project across the life-course, with the undertaking of voluntary work as one strategy for maintaining personal congruence.

Voluntary work is thus very diverse and evokes many different forms of commitment, identification and allegiance with the debate about its role centring on the concept of active citizenship that, it is argued, cements social networks and relationships as well as enhancing the greater social good (Newman & Mooney, 2004). The promotion of the idea of an active civil society by successive UK governments has led to the professionalisation of some voluntary work as the product of a partnership between the voluntary sector, government and business. Within the UK during the 1980's and early 1990's, the voluntary sector began to have a key role in the delivery of a whole range of care services as part of the Thatcherite 'care in the community' policy. The significance placed on providing care in the community continues not least because of the general increase in life expectancy and a larger proportion of the population living into very old age.

Historically, caring for the elderly, the sick and the young has represented a major aspect of voluntary activity and currently volunteers can be found working in schools, day care centres, 'after school' clubs, hospices and hospitals and in charity shops that are now a familiar feature of many UK local high streets. Some ideas presented in the literature position lay care of the vulnerable as a privilege and Sinclair (2007: 76) notes that "philanthropic and voluntary involvement in palliative care confirms the archetypal notion of care as a privilege or gift". This notwithstanding, much voluntary work in the health field and in other sectors, too, has become characterised by more standardised working practices. Thus semi-formalised aspects of voluntary work have changed the experience of volunteering because as Morrison (2000: 109) argues 'there is a particular and very significant tension between a professionalised managerial approach and a more traditional volunteering ethos'. Operating within the 'professional' discourse of quality, accountability and regulated practice, some voluntary work has been made closer to the experience of paid work. Noon and Blyton (2007) suggest that in the broad care sector this may be particularly the case and point to issues arising from the relationship between voluntary and paid work. One they highlight is the extent to which voluntary care activity undermines or dilutes the role and status of those performing care tasks within their paid employment both in professional and non-professional roles. A further point is whether the expansion of unpaid voluntary work in the diverse field of health care has restricted the growth of occupations in this area.

These debates provide an underpinning empirical and theoretical thread to the discussion below and are useful in guiding understanding about hospice development and operation in the UK that is considered next.

3. Hospice and palliative care services in the UK

Much has been written about the development of the modern hospice movement, particularly the pioneering efforts of its founder, Cicely Saunders who formulated the vision of a haven where people could experience relief from pain and die with dignity within an atmosphere of calm and tranquillity. The services offered under the 'umbrella' of hospice now include day care, bereavement counselling, complementary therapies, day and night sitting services and terminal care both in the community and within the hospice for in-patients. This whole provision is seen as a 'high person, low technology and hardware system of health care' (De Spelder & Strickland, 2005) providing intimate care at scale. Its ultimate goal is the attainment of a 'good death' from the perspective of both the dying person and their family (Sandman, 2005), with the period before death characterised by the best possible quality of life (Randall & Downie, 2006). Whilst space does not permit an extended discussion of this concept, it is important to note that the 'good death' is contested; it is socially produced with, in the developed world, death often taking place over time as people live with life-threatening illness or slow degenerative conditions (Holloway, 2007). Furthermore, 'social death' may occur before 'biological death' when some people, such as those with AIDS (see below), are socially ostracised because of their illness (Auger, 2007).

The establishment in 1967 of St Christopher's in South London, as the first modern research and teaching hospice to cater specifically for the needs of the dying, was instrumental in raising the profile of terminal care. Previously end of life care had been peripheral to the agenda of the medical profession, mainly due to associated discourses of death as failure. In-patient hospices are the original model of palliative care delivery and by the year 2000, Britain had 400 hospices and palliative care units helping to provide a new model of death (Jupp & Walter, 1999). By the year 2008 this number had risen to 716 (Watts, 2010) and Clark (1993) comments that, although hospice is often described as a philosophy rather than a place (particularly by US commentators), the drive to build more hospices and establish professionally led dedicated palliative care units is very striking. Sinclair (2007) argues that this is hardly surprising given the primacy of the institutional model in establishing status, authority and credibility within the medical mainstream.

The expansion in the number of hospices, although ad hoc (Field & Addington-Hall, 2000) and therefore unevenly geographically distributed, has been significant and widespread. Hospices are now well established in the UK as the principal site for the practice of specialist palliative care and have traditionally operated outside direct mainstream National Health Service (NHS) control with many constituted as charities dependant mainly on fundraising initiatives for their income. Although mainly charity-based, hospices now operate on a business model raising funds from corporate sponsors as well as from sales in their high street shops and individual donations. Despite the continuing drive to maintain some autonomy, the independent feature of their operation is gradually being eroded within a culture of audit and evidence-based practice, as hospices increasingly are expected to demonstrate the effectiveness of services as part of the NHS referral system (Randall & Downie, 2006).

The original ideal of hospice, as the setting for a good death, is the creation of an extended family (Howarth, 2007), to act as a refuge or safe retreat for the dying and those close to them. Patients are encouraged to pursue their interests and pleasures as they would in their own home and, with extensive visiting hours, to spend as much time as they wish with friends and family members. Extending this familial idea, hospices see the patient's family as an integral part of the unit of care, involving them in all aspects of decision-making. The importance of the family is a recurring theme in the literature on the culture of hospice care, offering insight into the ways in which these institutions approach support of the dying, as one aspect of the holistic approach they advocate. This familial feature is especially reproduced in hospices dedicated to the care of children and young people and in recent years a number of these have been established across the UK to respond to what has been perceived as the special needs of families looking after a child with a life-limiting condition. The organisation, Children's Hospices UK, reports that there are now forty-one children's hospices in the UK (Watts, 2010).

The staffing profile of hospices is centred on a multidisciplinary approach to care with nurses, doctors, health care assistants, social workers, physiotherapists, chaplains and a range of complementary therapists working together to support the individual needs of patients. In addition, there is a growing emphasis on incorporating the skills of experienced managers to lead the hospice team as part of the ongoing drive for greater efficiency in all areas of service provision (Doyle, 2009). Alongside the paid and professional staff, hospices rely heavily on a significant volunteer workforce to help with the care of patients and their families both in the setting of the hospice and in the community with much care now taking place in patients' own homes (Armstrong-Coster, 2004; Howlett, 2009). Connor (2009), writing in the context of the USA, makes the further point that hospice and palliative care began there directly through the efforts of volunteers to create a new way of caring for dying people. Some of those efforts were inspired through religious belief and the development of the modern hospice movement has primarily been born out of a Christian tradition imbued with the principle of duty to others (Clark & Seymour, 1999). This sense of duty goes some way towards explaining the importance of the volunteer workforce to different aspects of hospice activities (Andersson & Ohlen, 2005) with Connor (2009: 117) pointing out that "the fact that people give of themselves to care for others has powerful significance to those who receive the care". He adds that people experience care given by professionals paid to deliver care differently than they experience the same care given by a volunteer arguing that the extra dimension of caring provided by volunteers has always been one of the unique features of hospice care.

The giving of self by the volunteer can result in the volunteer being the most significant person to the dying patient having devoted much one-to-one time to accompanying the patient as they face death. These interactions, supporting the work of paid staff, may be qualitatively different because of their 'gift nature' (see Noon & Blyton, 2007 above). The building of relationships between volunteers and users of hospice services is an important feature of high quality care and this is now seen as a characteristic of workforce excellence resulting in well-developed volunteer recruitment and training programmes. Given the ways in which specialist palliative care within hospices has evolved into a clinical set of disciplines whose emphasis is on pain control and symptom management in an approach similar to that found in mainstream clinical settings (Kellehear, 2005), the contribution of volunteers in 're-personalising' hospice care may be especially valuable. Sinclair (2007: 49), commenting on the pronounced voluntary staff component of most hospices, suggests that the population at large sees palliative care and the possibility of hospice support as a gift, and one to be both earned or repaid. This notwithstanding, volunteer work in this setting can be both stressful and emotionally demanding and can lead to 'burn-out' as may occur amongst members of the professional hospice workforce (Dein & Abbas, 2005). These and other aspects of the experience of being a hospice volunteer are explored more fully later in the chapter.

4. Other models of hospice and palliative care

Although the focus of the critique and research presented in this chapter is on hospice volunteering in the UK, there is merit in briefly considering some alternative models operating in other countries. The first of these is based in the state of Kerala in southern India and is characterised by Kumar (2009) as a neighbourhood network of palliative care. This network, that aims to develop a community-owned service, has grown out of pain clinics established as part of two cancer centres set up in 1990. The goal of the programme is the development of grass roots level sustainable and cost-effective care for patients with terminal disease. Its underlying premise is community participation with local people encouraged to train as community volunteers to offer emotional support to patients and families as part of a home care programme. In this model the work of volunteers operates alongside the clinical expertise of specialist doctors and nurses and has resulted in a combined workforce of 5000 trained community volunteers, 50 palliative care physicians and 100 palliative care nurses (Kumar, 2009).

There are criteria for the recruitment of volunteer workers onto the programme; they must be available to spend more than two hours per week to care for the terminally ill in their village and be prepared to undertake the 15 hour structured training before becoming a member of the volunteer network. Training covers the basic palliative care precepts including communication skills, emotional support, basic nursing skills and organisational aspects of care. Prospective volunteers also make home visits as part of their training with these led by either a doctor or nurse. The result is a well-developed and highly skilled local community palliative care network with trained volunteers able to perform a wide range of tasks including initiating and running palliative care units locally, raising funds for the network, advocating for patients and the network through mobilising support from governmental and non-governmental agencies and performing a range of essential administrative tasks. Organising awareness and training programmes in the community with the local governments and agencies are particularly important components of the work of volunteers focused on future sustainability and end of life care policy-making. Their central role, however, is to provide one-to-one help to patients in their home offering emotional and practical support. This initiative has been highly successful not least because there is no charge for the use of services provided by the network that does not aim to replace professionally led health care. Its emphasis on psychosocial and spiritual support provided by volunteers connects well with local cultural and religious frameworks and privileges a collective rather than an individual approach to palliative care drawing on a social rather than a medical model of health and disease.

A second model of palliative care services that relies heavily on volunteer support is that of the South Coast Hospice (SCH) located in the province of Kwazulu-Natal in South Africa. The hospice provides palliative care to a highly disadvantaged and impoverished population where there is 70 per cent unemployment and where the prevalence of tuberculosis is 116 per 100, 000 (Defellippi & Mnguni, 2009). However, it is the scale of HIV/AIDS in the area that has been the key challenge, with the social and psychological trauma associated with the disease for both sufferers and their carers an overwhelming problem. With anti-retroviral medication only very recently becoming available in South Africa, the hospice had to plan services with the prospect of huge numbers of AIDS patients requiring palliative care.

In the early 1980s during the first phase of SCH's development, services were planned broadly adopting the UK model of collaborating with primary health care clinics to provide holistic care mainly to cancer patients living in outlying rural areas. Care delivered by professionally qualified nurses was the foundation of an outreach programme that formed the basis for the integrated community home care model developed from the mid 1990s in response to the escalating HIV/AIDS epidemic. Within this model hospice care teams (salaried professional staff) visit patients in their home approximately once a week with interim support provided by trained lay volunteers who usually live within walking distance of the patients' homes. On average each volunteer is expected every week to visit about five patients and their families, and to make a report to the hospice's Voluntary Service Manager. This level of lay support has become necessary because the traditional care safety net of the extended family system in South Africa is being eroded by HIV/AIDS (Defellippi & Mnguni, 2009). Overburdened grandmothers, who are often frail and underfed, cannot cope with caring alone for their own sick adult children and young grandchildren, as well as inheriting the orphans many of whom are HIV positive.

The volunteer model of SCH is culturally located with some elements that differ from the community model of Kerala discussed above. In economically developed societies there is an assumption that volunteers work 'for free' and give their time with no expectation of financial remuneration. However, where people are living in impoverished circumstances, expectations may differ and motivations to volunteer can combine altruism and a sense of community service with hope that volunteering may lead to employment and be a vehicle to help alleviate their plight. These elements give rise to the concept of the 'paid volunteer' that is outside the traditional western model of voluntary work. Given the social context described above, SCH had to grapple with the issue of rewards for volunteers as part of a sustainable model of care delivery. Careful selection of volunteers is particularly important when payment of volunteers is involved especially in terms of identifying the motivation of any potential volunteer. SCH thus established a set of personal criteria for the recruitment of volunteers with most of these being in line with those adopted across all community palliative care programmes. Additional requirements were those seen as essential for the Southern African local context and include a track record of community involvement, an ability to communicate cross-culturally with sensitivity and respect and an ability to speak in an authoritative and compassionate manner about HIV/AIDS. The remuneration for this voluntary work ranges from financial stipends to food parcels, with the nature of the reward shaped by local conditions.

Nearly all the volunteers at SCH are women as it is women in African society who have the caring roles and responsibilities. Training, provided as induction to the volunteer role, incorporates a wide curriculum including behavioural conduct, psychosocial and spiritual support, pain and symptom control, paediatric AIDS and basic nursing skills that skill the volunteer to maintain basic hygiene and promote universal precautions in preventing the spread of infection as part of a health promotion approach. They also need to give sound nutritional advice to patients and families (Defellippi & Mnguni, 2009). This package of support can be understood as part of a wider programme of change that Kellehear (2005) sees as being intrinsically political, driving as it does, towards personal, local and, eventually, national change in particular behaviours.

A majority (60 per cent) of AIDS patients referred to the hospice are women who have contracted the virus from a male partner to whom they have been faithful, with the result that the skill level required by volunteers to initiate discussion about sexual health problems with both the infected person and their partner is very high. This is challenging work because, as Auger (2007) opines, HIV/AIDS is first and foremost a sociological issue with issues of stigma and social exclusion never far from view. Significant levels of supervision and mentorship are offered to volunteers in recognition of the stressful nature of this work. Evaluation and monitoring of the quality of support offered by volunteers is a feature of SCH's commitment to ensuring a high quality service drawing on the principle that feedback improves both practice and outcomes for service users. It also demonstrates to volunteers that they are valued and that their work is important and enables the hospice to extend its services to reach large numbers of people in need.

5. The study

The research, on which much of this chapter draws, was conducted in a large well-established hospice in England. Qualitative methods were used to explore a range of topics centred on developing understanding of the experience of becoming and being a hospice volunteer. Particular issues considered included volunteer motivation, previous and current occupational and professional roles, training and support programmes, rewards and benefits of hospice voluntary work and challenges associated with the role. This was a small-scale pilot study undertaken to inform the design of a much larger research project involving a number of hospices across the UK.

Access to the work of the hospice was facilitated by my role as a university educator in the field of death and dying and the associated practice visits made to a wide range of palliative care settings, positioning me as an insider researcher (Watts, 2006). My earlier research into labour market issues had made me aware of the growing importance of voluntary work within the economy and in the context of health care generally and death and dying, in particular, it was becoming clear that this was an area ripe for research. Locating the research in one hospice underpinned a case study approach that Simons (2009) characterises as being context-specific whether in terms of organisation or individuals or collections of individuals. The design of the small scale study required careful planning given that volunteers' time is limited and taking their time away from input to patients is one of a number of ethical issues in palliative care research (Addington-Hall, 2007).

The decision to run a focus group centred on their use as "ideal for exploring people's talk, experiences, opinions, beliefs, wishes and concerns" (Kitzinger, 2005: 57) and agreement for the involvement of a small number of volunteers to form the group was given by the Voluntary Service Manager at the hospice. Having circulated information to the large number of regular volunteers, she forwarded me details of potential participants who had expressed an interest in contributing to the study. From seventeen positive responses, eight participants were recruited to the study with them agreeing to take part in a focus group. Usual consent procedures were followed with me confirming full confidentiality and anonymity. A room in which to run the focus group was provided by the hospice and the session ran for almost two hours. Participants ranged in age from 41 to 77 years and all the participants were women.

I used a topic guide to conduct the session (Bryman, 2004) to facilitate a semi-structured approach as a way of grouping topics for discussion that quickly developed into a lively exchange. All the participants knew each other and some had become friends during their years of volunteering at the hospice resulting in an informal and comfortable atmosphere for the discussion. Kitzinger (2004: 270), writing about the dynamics of the focus group method, comments that "the fact that participants provide an audience for each other encourages a greater variety of communication" and the element of performance was very much evident in the session. Also evident was a high level of sensitivity and tenderness of emotion amongst the group, particularly during discussion of how individuals had been drawn into this voluntary role, with a majority talking about the death of a loved one whilst under the care of the hospice.

Focus groups are not a natural event (Kitzinger, 2004); they are social process and are necessarily contrived being strongly influenced by the presence and person of the facilitator who in this case was also the researcher. Considerable care was taken not to give too much direction beyond setting the ground rules at the outset and noting the topics. Rounding a topic off as away of moving the discussion on to the next subject was necessary to keep the flow focused and on track. The session was digitally recorded and subsequently transcribed and then thematically analysed using the topic guide as a framework. A rich body of data was produced highlighting the breadth of views of participants about their experience of hospice volunteering.

There is considerable debate in the literature about the mechanics, authenticity and rigour of this qualitative data gathering method and space here does not permit a developed critique of the key arguments except to say that focus groups are always context-situated and subject to the interaction dynamics of the group, with this aspect particularly challenging to address as part of the analysis (Wilkinson, 2011). Focus group data are not more or less authentic than data generated by other qualitative methods and they are often used as one component of a project. This, as it turned out, was the case in this study as two volunteers, who were unwilling to join the focus group, expressed an interest in being interviewed individually. These two interviews each lasted for approximately ninety minutes and were subject to the same ethical processes as for the focus group. The topic guide used for the focus group acted as the semi-structured interview schedule to try and bring a measure of content uniformity across the two methods. The interviews were digitally recorded, with transcripts produced and then sent to the two respondents. The texts were thematically analysed as for the main data set drawing on some of the principles set out by Braun and Clarke (2006).

A number of themes emerged from the data and the discussion below focuses on those most useful for the current purpose namely motivation to become a hospice volunteer, training and support, experience in particular roles and lastly, challenges of the work that was felt to be increasingly demanding. Threaded through the thematic discussion of the study's findings are the voices of participants; using their language enables a data-focused approach rather than one that is literature focused and this style of reporting accords with the ethical frame of the research that was grounded in a collaborative participatory model (Birch & Miller, 2002).

6. Becoming a hospice volunteer

Motivations to become a hospice volunteer are complex and varied and Howlett (2009) argues that there are almost as many motivations to volunteer, as there are volunteers. For participants in this research, however, volunteer motivations can be broadly characterised into the two categories of instrumental gain and altruism, with these not mutually exclusive. Howlett (2009) suggests that increasingly volunteers may expect to get something from their volunteering though, as demonstrated by this research, the rewards are very diverse and may well change over time.

In this context the concept of instrumental gain centres on fulfilling needs of the volunteer and for the older retired participants, the opportunity that volunteering affords to help organise time and give structure to weekly routines acted as a strong motivating force for their commitment to the work of the hospice. Joyce, a member of the focus group comments: "my Tuesdays here are sacrosanct so I organise everything else around that and I wouldn't be without it now". Lesley spoke similarly highlighting how, as she put it, "volunteering here helps to break up the week and sometimes when they are short handed I come in and do extra time". The temporal dimension was taken up by Joan who, recently retired, wanted to ensure that she had a balance in the way she used her newly acquired leisure explaining "I want to feel that my retirement is useful and enjoyable and I want to be able to expect to do different things on different days and then I won't feel that each day is just a blank".

The opportunity to mix and have social interaction with like-minded people was identified as another important instrumental motivation and Beryl, a focus group participant, spoke about how her life had seemed so empty after the death of her husband and of the way in which working at the hospice helped to fill the vacuum. "I feel part of something here and it helps with the loneliness". Lesley saw her work at the hospice as an enhancement to her social well being commenting: "I have made quite a lot of friends here and sometimes we meet up for coffee and have a good old natter". Commenting on the social contacts developed by volunteers working in the hospice bereavement service, Eileen, one of the two interviewees, explained thus: "we go out to lunch about once every two months and sometimes we go round to each other's houses and have lunch; we call it our self support group". The extent to which the social contact sustained motivation rather than initiated it was difficult to judge but as Howlett (2009) notes, volunteer motivations do change over time and this can make it difficult for Voluntary Service Managers to identify and respond to motives as part of their recruitment activities.

Others in the group spoke about having something useful and worthwhile to do beyond family interests and, of feeling valued. Eileen put it very succinctly thus: "you see it's all about feeling valued and valued on a professional level because you have a real contribution to make". She also added: "I was a social worker and volunteering here has been one way of keeping up some of those skills". This sense of being valued appeared to be of instrumental importance equally to those with a professional occupational background as for those who had not been in paid employment having been at home raising their families. They spoke about how their ideas and concerns were generally listened to, making them feel part of the hospice team, giving them status and self-worth.

Another instrumental motivation emerged from the comments of the youngest member of the focus group, Linda. She took up volunteer work at the hospice to gain experience of palliative care hoping to enrol as a mature student on a qualifying social work programme at her local university. Having been, as she put it a " stay at home mum" for many years, she was using her hospice voluntary work as an opportunity to acquire new skills and experience that would be of benefit in her future professional role. Barbara Monroe, CEO St Christopher's Hospice in London, is clear that hospice volunteering can act as a route into paid work and education, citing an increasingly diverse volunteer profile that now includes people with learning disabilities and men and women on licence from prison (Monroe, ADEC conference, 2011).

Altruism, as the second category of motivation, was an underpinning theme of why participants had chosen to volunteer at the hospice. Half the participants had initially come into contact with the hospice because of the terminal illness of a loved one and all expressed in different ways how impressed they had been by the quality of care on offer. Giving something back was thus very significant in stimulating a regular commitment of time, skills and experience to a number of the hospice's services. Molly, one of the focus group participants, spoke with emotion about her husband's care at the hospice and how she felt she wanted to make sure that others could have access to such high quality care and support. She said: "he was looked after so well and although it was awful, it somehow made it all bearable and now I feel ready to help out here so that all this fantastic work can go on and others can get help the way we did". Joyce also voiced a strong personal connection to the hospice saying: "my sister was in here, she died in here and they made it sort of peaceful and we all could come and go and be part of it.....I didn't think I could work here but then I thought I could maybe manage working in the coffee shop and even that can make a difference can't it?". Other comments from Joyce further point to the ways in which giving something back to the community, as part of a sense of duty, is an important motivation; she says: "giving up my time is the least I can do".

Although the two types of motivation discussed above are clearly significant in hospices continuing to recruit volunteers to their workforce, it is important to emphasise that sometimes those who apply to join hospices in a voluntary capacity, may not have a particular motive or aim but do so out of curiosity and good, if not clearly defined, intention. Others may want to undertake this work as part of their own recovery from bereavement or with the goal of converting others to a faith before they die (Connor, 2009). This raises the important issue of suitability for this role and the need for careful scrutiny of applicants with Voluntary Service Managers having an ongoing responsibility to ensure that volunteers are both appropriately supported in this work and that any changes to their personal circumstances do not negatively impact on their work in this setting.

7. Training and support

Although volunteers will have different perceptions of their role in the hospice ranging from those who see this work as a semi-professional 'job' to those who see this not as a job but more as providing informal help, all hospice volunteers are expected to undergo a period of training and induction (Spencer-Gray, 2009). Discussion about the training and support offered to participants centred mainly on the nature and extent of provision with an emphasis on the need for regular updates that could incorporate new research findings. Several participants had been volunteering for a number of years evidencing what Hamilton (2009) terms as 'the volunteer career' that is likely to have a number of stages of development. These long-serving participants found it difficult to recall the detail of the training they had received on joining the hospice. However, those more recently joined talked about the different components of their initial training that variously included death education, personal death awareness, principles of palliative care, social and psychological reactions to death, grief and loss and working effectively as a member of the multidisciplinary team. Training that addressed ethical issues such as patient confidentiality and maintaining 'working' boundaries was only briefly referred to in the focus group. One of the two interviewees, however, gave greater emphasis to this element of the training explaining: "I know it is important not to talk about patients to people and to keep their details private and confidential. I feel it's part of upholding their dignity and we know that keeping things confidential is one of the cardinal rules here. It was made very clear in my training and after a while it almost becomes second nature".

The topics covered in the training of these volunteers is broadly in line with what Connor (2009: 97) calls the 'basics', at least in relation to the western model of palliative care. The training model used with volunteers in the South Coast Hospice in South Africa (discussed above) also included basic nursing skills and knowledge about pain and symptom control such that they can, with supervision, administer prescribed medication. In the UK context, these skills are not expected of volunteers and there is a clear demarcation between the roles of professionally trained clinical staff and volunteers working alongside them. One of the reasons for this is the high level of regulation of health service provision to ensure clear lines of responsibility and accountability for those in professional practice.

In the focus group one of the prompts to develop discussion on the topic of training was the question "is there anything that you feel you would like more training on?". The areas of spirituality and diversity were identified as topics where there were knowledge gaps, particularly spirituality that seemed to present as a vague concept. Beryl, for example, commented: "I see spirituality as religion but these days a lot of people don't have a religion and so it is difficult to help people spiritually if you don't know how they see their spiritual needs. I suppose that is why we have the chaplain so he can look after the spirituality side of things". Directly following on, Joyce added: "yes, we could do with more training on spirituality so that we can be more confident about how to help people and understand what really matters to them". These points received general agreement amongst the group and both interviewees were also of the view that spiritual care was difficult to define and probably was best left to the chaplain.

The connection between spirituality, religion and cultural diversity was loosely made in the context of the gradually changing nature of the population in the locality of the hospice. Originally a white, prosperous middle class area, the population served by the hospice now included a growing south Asian population as well as a small but expanding eastern European community. The need for greater cultural awareness, particularly in relation to Hinduism and Islam was strongly articulated, with cultural competence seen as an important skill for volunteers working in the hospice. Diversity in palliative care, particularly in terms of access has long been debated (see, for example, Smaje and Field, 1997 and Firth, 2004) and participants' comments suggest that this still remains a deficit area.

Ongoing support for volunteers appeared to be organised according to their different roles but was mainly of two types: formal support from the hospice and informal peer support from fellow volunteers. Those working as part of the bereavement care team have a supervisor as well as a mentor with meetings with each on a monthly basis. In day care, support is provided by both the day care manager and the senior nurse who has responsibility for the organisation of activities and the overall care of patients. In day care there is a meeting between volunteers and the senior nurse before the start of each session to discuss any issues that may arise with particular patients and also to share updates that include information about patients who have died. Eileen comments: "we discuss who has died because that's upsetting because you make relationships in day care as you see them every week. Eventually the patients die and it is quite sad so you have to have somebody to discuss it with". These meetings are also the opportunity to discuss new patients coming into day care so that staff and volunteers can be fully prepared to welcome each new patient and meet their individual needs. It is this treating the patient as an individual that is the hallmark of specialist palliative care (Watts, 2010).

It was clear that volunteers who have the most contact with patients require the highest level of support because of the emotionally demanding nature of their work. Volunteers working in the coffee shop spoke about support that was mainly instrumental focusing on organisational matters such as work rosters and managing stock. Much of their contact is with hospice staff, visitors and family members of patients using the hospice. They do have contact with patients, but the opportunity to get to know patients in a personal way is limited as the coffee shop is generally busy with people waiting to be served, drinks to be made and tables to be cleared. Support in this role appeared to be mainly of the peer variety as the policy at the hospice is for the coffee shop to be staffed by two or three volunteers at a time. Joyce, who works in the coffee shop two days each week, explained how she gradually came to feel comfortable working the till and the coffee machine, because of the friendly help of a co-volunteer. She commented: "I found it all a bit confusing at first what with the till and the coffee machine that I had never used before but Sally (co-volunteer) was patient and kept showing me what to do and I really enjoy it. I think I would really miss it if I wasn't here those two days".

8. Experiences as a hospice volunteer

A variety of volunteer roles was represented amongst the ten participants in the study; two worked in the coffee shop, one on the main reception desk, three in day care, three in bereavement support and one as a volunteer complementary therapist offering reflexology to patients. All spoke with considerable enthusiasm about their work, particularly valuing the social aspects of their volunteering that Howlett (2009) argues can often be pivotal in hospices retaining their volunteers. Fiona, one of the interviewees, characterised the pleasure she gained from working in day care helping with arts and crafts activities as a privilege. In her early fifties, Fiona had left a high-powered post as a corporate chief executive and felt that her work at the hospice was rewarding because of what she described as its "high people content". Further comments from Fiona highlighted just what she meant by privilege in this context: "patients and their families come to the hospice often at a very desperate time when they are staring death in the face and what they generally find is that people here care and can give them their whole attention. Being part of that is so special and so very different from the business world where time is money and people matter less than the bottom line on the balance sheet".

An underpinning theme of much of the discussion, both in the focus group and with the two interviewees, was the practice and approach of *caring about* patients and families who come to the hospice. Beryl, recounting a recent conversation with one of the patients in day care, spoke about the patient's appreciation for the support volunteers provide and how the patient saw this as volunteers caring about patients as individuals. The ethos of care appeared to extend across different types of voluntary roles including those not represented in the study, such as those of driver and fundraiser and these were commented on within the context of care and relationships. Eileen referred specifically to the important caring role of drivers explaining: "of course we have volunteer drivers that go and collect people to bring them into day care and those volunteers get very close to the patients. I remember that one of our ladies from day care who died recently, I went to her funeral and her driver was there and he was in tears. I wondered then, if they (the drivers) get the support they need".

The activity of fundraising is central to the running of many hospices in the UK with most now part of the registered charity sector. Managing fundraising is a key role usually involving the initiation and co-ordination of a range of ventures. Participants referred to fund-raising activities in connection with contributions they found themselves making to particular events, with this seen as part of their wider relationship to the palliative care mission. Joyce commenting on a fundraising garden party, explained: "I don't know but I just seemed to get roped into helping. Joanna (fundraising manager at the hospice) was chatting to me one day and mentioned that they needed more help and asked me if I could help out. She is so nice and I didn't feel I could say no. It was fun, hard work, but fun and it took me a few days to get over it". This and other similar comments indicate that the work of volunteering at the hospice can be expanded beyond specifically assigned roles to take up a considerable chunk of time in volunteers' lives. The goodwill generated and reproduced through the highly valued care work of hospice is undoubtedly a resource for hospice managers. However, issues may arise about the extent to which the goodwill of volunteers can lead to their exploitation, with this as the unintended consequence of their deep and usually longstanding commitment to supporting this work.

9. Challenges

Hospice volunteering brings challenges both for volunteers and for Voluntary Service Managers. Data from the study reveal the concern of volunteers about maintaining appropriate functional and emotional boundaries, this despite the training and ongoing support they receive from professional staff. The emotional element of volunteer roles that involves close contact with patients was highlighted both in the focus group discussion and in the two interviews. The sensitive and potentially stressful nature of this work is illustrated by Fiona's comments: "we hear things that we don't quite understand or that we are not sure about and is this person telling you that they are going to commit suicide or are they not actually saying that and you think should I be telling someone or is it my job just to listen? Sometimes I wonder if I should have said more or something different but I am not a counsellor". Molly also talked about some of the boundary dilemmas she has had in her day care work: "sometimes I leave day care thinking what shall I do about this, did I ought to tell one of the managers and sometimes, though I don't take the patients' problems home with me, I do feel it and wonder if I did the right thing". Eileen was aware of the need to take responsibility for looking after herself emotionally and explained: "my theory about being a bereavement volunteer is that you have to have lots of empathy and lots of sympathy and love people but you have to have a hard centre. There has to be just that bit in the middle that they don't get through". These remarks demonstrate that careful management of emotions by volunteers is needed to prevent their negative impact and ensure this work does not spill over into other areas of life. In recognition of this, Dein and Abbas (2005) argue for more dedicated training on this topic for volunteers, with the aim of minimising the potential stress associated with the role.

Changes over time in the way in which volunteers are seen by the hospice management team was discussed within the focus group and attracted most comment from the longest serving volunteers. Eileen, for example, remarked: "when I was first here twenty years ago you couldn't stop hearing how much they needed us and what a difference we make. Now, though, you hardly ever hear that and I don't think it's because we are not valued, as I know we are, but it's just that everyone's so busy with paperwork and budgets and things like that. It all has got so formal somehow and maybe we matter less because of that". Connected to the issue of formalisation of procedures and bureaucracy is the sense of volunteering as a semi-professional role with an increased emphasis on continuity of care and the maintenance of high standards in all areas. Participants supported these values but some identified a gradual shift in the attitudes of department managers in relation to a less flexible approach to making changes to the days of work and in connection to taking extended holiday, particularly over the summer when three of the participants wanted to devote time to spending with grandchildren. Howlett (2009: 17), commenting on the growing formalisation of volunteering in hospice and palliative care, argues that 'we are seeing the expansion of the workplace model, in which volunteering looks like paid work, but without the pay'. He suggests that the trend towards a more formal style of organising and managing volunteers stems from two causes. The first is the drive by successive UK governments for the delivery of public services by the voluntary sector and the second is the growing risk and fear of litigation in which organisations fear being exposed to risk as a result of not having adequate management systems in place.

Volunteering in palliative care as discussed above is shaped by different motivations, with altruism and a wish to contribute to a high quality care service, dominant motives. Thorough volunteer recruitment processes operate in the sector that tries hard to match the skills of potential volunteers with the needs of the service (Spencer-Gray, 2009). One participant explained how important this is both for the volunteer and the hospice; she comments: "if people get the right job they stay; if they fit into a job that they like and can do they stay like people here in the bereavement service, most of them have been here a long time". Sometimes, however, this match is not successful and one challenge for Voluntary Service Managers is the task of ensuring that a probation period is just that, with the necessary support and advice in place as part of assessment of suitability in role. Here, features of the employment model come into play and this is another area where more formal processes have been widely introduced. Despite this, the task of informing an enthusiastic volunteer that they may not be right for a particular role is a sensitive one that requires careful handling. Where volunteers are introduced to the hospice through personal networks within the hospice, this can be especially challenging. Dismissing a volunteer who has successfully completed probation but later oversteps guidelines and boundaries such as, for example, becoming over-involved with patients, can be particularly difficult. O'Brien and Wallace (2009) correctly assert that the interests of patients are pre-eminent and they suggest that one approach might be to counsel a volunteer to leave.

A further issue raised by one of the participants is that of 'retirement' of volunteers and Eileen's words demonstrate that this can be another sensitive issue for Voluntary Service Managers. She says: "when I first came here people were told that they had to leave when they were seventy. Well, that's stopped now and the thing that concerns me is now there is no cut off point so what do you do when people should retire? We have a counsellor here who has forgotten what her job is and comes in for her own sake. At some stage people are going to get too old to do the job and they've got to be told somehow that they are too old".

The final challenge that I want to address here is that raised by Sinclair (2007) concerning demarcation between professional and volunteer roles. Taking the concept of multidisciplinarity that is a vital component of palliative care practice (Mitchell and Barclay, 2008), it is not difficult to see why on both a theoretical and practical level, volunteers should be treated as equal members of the multidisciplinary team. Sinclair (2007), however, drawing on Doyle (1995), asserts that the blurring of boundaries between professional and lay workers is not appropriate within palliative care that has continuity, high quality communication and professional cohesion as key precepts. He makes the further point that in the case of the UK, because volunteers in the hospice sector are predominantly white, more affluent and mainly middle class, vestiges of an earlier philanthropic model are retained with recipients of care not seen as worthy of the best and by implication, expert care. This thinking does lean towards positioning palliative care as something that only specialists can do, with the implication that the extensive use of volunteers in roles that involve close contact with patients, might lead to the deprofessionalisation of care for dying people that Sinclair (2007: 76) notes are already a 'devalued class'. Despite some resistance from the specialist palliative care lobby this emphasis on professional exclusivity is now being contested in the literature because of the growing diversity of palliative care models beyond the original UK form. As discussed above in relation to palliative care programmes operating in India and South Africa, the blurring of professional and volunteer boundaries is sometimes necessary in some models of palliative care and seen by some (Kellehear, 2005, for example) as a positive attribute in aiding both personal and community understanding of death and dying.

10. Conclusion

The discussion of the nature, extent and experience of volunteering in palliative care has revealed both the importance and complexity of this work. Patients and hospices benefit from the work of volunteers and there is now a wide understanding that professionals and volunteers, working in partnership, provide patients with a safe, relaxed and unthreatening package of care (Doyle, 2009). However, voluntary work in palliative care, as in other sectors, is changing and is now subject to health and safety regulation as well as a range of other management practices, many of which draw on approaches in the paid labour market. O'Brien and Wallace (2009) point to specific practices from the employment model that they see as potentially useful for developing the capacity and status of hospice volunteers. Annual appraisals, satisfaction reviews that consider the extent to which volunteers are getting what they want from their work and an opportunity for training and education to develop practice are all elements that may become a standard feature of volunteering in palliative care in the future. Much of this investment in volunteers is resource dependent and, with the drastic cuts to health and social care budgets currently ongoing in the UK, these measures may have to be deferred. Whilst UK hospices operate outside the statutory sector because of their charity status, they are recipients of significant amounts of income from statutory health care budgets and this does make continuity of current levels of funding subject to some uncertainty. Alongside and more generally, the broad mission of palliative care may be increasingly difficult for voluntarily funded organisations to continue to pursue, especially when it cannot be justified in terms of easily measurable outcomes that have an increased focus as part of the evidence-based system of health care now operating in the UK (Holloway, 2007: 95).

Despite this uncertainty, the place of volunteering in palliative care within the hospice context looks set to continue, particularly as the recruitment of paid professional staff may have to be limited due to budget constraints. The roles undertaken by volunteers of emotional comforter, spiritual supporter, palliative caregiver and therapeutic healer appear to play an important role in patients' psychosocial and emotional well being, with their work representing a division of 'healing' labour. Full recognition of these roles is proposed as a starting point for stronger collaboration between volunteer palliative care workers and professional clinical staff aimed at reducing patient and family distress. This notwithstanding, the extent of volunteers' contribution and the organisational value placed on their work will vary from hospice to hospice. Thus while the hospice setting for this research sees volunteers as essential to service provision, Sheldon (1997: 113) notes that in some palliative care settings volunteers are positioned 'as handmaidens to the professional team' and in some contexts are resented because of the substitution of volunteers for tasks previously done by professionals. In addition, broadening volunteering opportunities to draw in those from ethnic minority communities is a significant challenge for hospices to signal that hospice volunteering is not an elite activity practised by a privileged few. In an increasingly diverse society such as we have in the UK, it is important to have a volunteer workforce that caters for diverse local communities and client groups (Howlett, 2009). Dismantling the barriers that prevent those from diverse backgrounds seeking to become involved with hospice is a significant challenge within a culture that historically has managed to preserve a distinctly white middle-class image. Hospices are first and foremost care service providers but they are also employers, with responsibilities to promote anti-discriminatory policies and practices in all areas of their operation. Actively extending an inclusive approach to the recruitment of volunteers is an important initiative particularly for hospices located in inner city areas that have a culturally and ethnically rich and diverse population. Issues of diversity are now considered as part of the evaluation and audit of hospice services and the cultural profile of the volunteer workforce may in the future be incorporated within the overall picture of audited hospice activity in the way that patient diversity is currently.

All names have been changed to protect confidentiality

11. References

Addington-Hall, J. M. (2007) 'Introduction' in J. M. Addington-Hall, E. Bruera, I. J. Higginson and S. Payne (eds.) *Research Methods in Palliative Care,* Oxford: Oxford University Press, pp. 1-9.

Andersson, B. and Ohlen, J. (2005) 'Being a hospice volunteer', *Palliative Medicine,* 19(8), 602-609.

Armstrong-Coster, A. (2004) *Living and Dying with Cancer,* Cambridge: Cambridge University Press.

Auger, J. A. (2007) 2nd edition *Social Perspectives on Death and Dying,* Halifax, Canada: Fernwood Publishing.

Birch, M. and Miller, T. (2002) 'Encouraging participation: ethics and responsibilities' in M. Mauthner, M. Birch, J. Jessop and T. Miller (eds.) *Ethics in Qualitative Research,* London: Sage Publications, pp. 91-106.

Bolton, S C and Houlihan, M (2009) 'Work, workplaces and workers: the contemporary experience' in S. C. Bolton and M. Houlihan, M (eds.) *Work Matters: Critical Reflections on Contemporary Work,* Basingstoke: Palgrave Macmillan, pp. 1-20.

Braun, V. and Clarke, V. (2006) 'Using thematic analysis in psychology', *Qualitative Research in Psychology*, 3: 77-101.

Bryman, A. (2004) *Social Research Methods*, 2nd edition, Oxford: Oxford University Press.

Clark, D. (1993) 'Whither the hospices?' in D. Clark (ed.) *The Future for Palliative Care: Issues of Policy and Practice*, Buckingham: Open University Press, pp. 167-177.

Clark, D. and Seymour, J. (1999) *Reflections on Palliative Care*, Buckingham: Open University Press.

Connor, S. R. (2009) *Hospice and Palliative Care*, New York and London: Routledge.

Dein, S. and Abbas, S. Q. (2005) 'The stresses of volunteering in a hospice: a qualitative study', *Palliative Medicine*, (19)1: 58-64.

Defellippi, K. and Mnguni, M. (2009) 'Volunteers working in a community palliative care service' in R. Scott and S. Howlett (eds) 2nd edition *Volunteers in Hospice and Palliative Care*, Oxford: Oxford University Press, pp. 177-194.

DeSpelder, L. A. and Strickland, A. L. (2005) 7th edition *The Last Dance*, Boston: McGraw Hill.

Doyle, D. (1995) 'The future of palliative care' in I. Corless, B. Germino and M. Pittman (eds.) *A Challenge for Living: Dying, Death and Bereavement*, Boston, MA: Jones and Bartlett, pp. 377-391.

Doyle, D. (2009) 'Introduction' in R. Scott and S. Howlett (eds) 2nd edition *Volunteers in Hospice and Palliative Care*, Oxford: Oxford University Press, pp. 1-10

Edwards, P and Wajcman, J (2005) *The Politics of Working Life*, Oxford: Oxford University Press

Field, D. and Addington-Hall, J. (2000) 'Extending specialist palliative care to all?' in D. Dickenson, M. Johnson and J. S. Katz (eds.) *Death, Dying and Bereavement*, London: Sage Publications Ltd, pp. 91-106.

Fink, J. (2004) 'Questions of care' in J. Fink (ed.) *Care: Personal Lives and Social Policy*, Milton Keynes and Bristol: The Open University and The Policy Press, pp. 1-42.

Firth, S. (2004) Minority ethnic communities and religious groups in D. Oliviere and B. Monroe (eds.) *Death, Dying and Social Differences*. Oxford: Oxford University Press, pp. 25-41.

Hamilton, G. (2009) 'The support of volunteers' in R. Scott and S. Howlett (eds) 2nd edition *Volunteers in Hospice and Palliative Care*, Oxford: Oxford University Press, pp. 87-98.

Howard, S. and Welbourn, D. (2004) *The Spirit at Work Phenomenon*, London: Azure.

Holloway, M. (2007) *Negotiating Death in Contemporary Health and Social Care*, Bristol: The Policy Press.

Howarth, G. (2007) *Death & Dying: a Sociological Introduction*, Cambridge: Polity Press.

Howlett, S. (2009) 'Setting the scene: the landscape of volunteering' in R. Scott and S. Howlett (eds) 2nd edition *Volunteers in Hospice and Palliative Care*, Oxford: Oxford University Press, pp. 11-20.

Jupp, P.C. and Walter, T. (1999) 'The healthy society: 1918-1998' in P.C. Jupp and C. Gittings (eds.) *Death in England*, Manchester: Manchester University Press, pp. 256-282.

Kellehear, A. (2005) *Compassionate Cities: Public Health and End-of-Life Care*, London: Routledge.

Kitzinger, J. (2004) 'The methodology of focus groups: the importance of interaction between research participants' in C. Seale (ed.) *Social Research Methods*, London and New York: Routledge, pp. 269-272.

Kitzinger, J. (2005) 'Focus group research: using group dynamics to explore perceptions, experiences and understandings' in I. Holloway (ed.) *Qualitative Research in Health Care,* Maidenhead: Open University Press, pp. 56-70.

Kumar, S. (2009) 'Neighbourhood network in palliative care, Kerala, India' in R. Scott and S. Howlett (eds) 2nd edition *Volunteers in Hospice and Palliative Care,* Oxford: Oxford University Press, pp. 211-219.

Liamputtong, P. (2007) *Researching the Vulnerable,* London: Sage.

MacDonald, R. (1997) 'Informal working, survival strategies and the idea of an "underclass"' in R. K. Brown (ed.) *The Changing Shape of Work,* Basingstoke: Macmillan, pp. 103-124.

Mitchell, G. and Barclay, S. (2008) 'Enhancing the patient-clinician relationship' in G. Mitchell (ed.) *Palliative Care a Patient-Centered Approach,* Oxford: Radcliffe Publishing, pp. 127-138.

Monroe, B. (2011) Association of Death Education Conference, 22-25 June, Miami, USA.

Mooney, G (2004) 'Exploring the dynamics of work, personal lives and social policy' in G. Mooney (ed.) *Work, Personal Lives and Social Policy,* Milton Keynes and Bristol: The Open University and The Policy Press, pp. 1-38.

Morrison, J (2000) 'The government-voluntary sector compacts: governance, governmentality and civil society' Journal of Law and Society, Vol.27, No.1: 98-132.

Newman, J and Mooney, G (2004) 'Managing personal lives: doing 'welfare work'' in G. Mooney (ed.) *Work, personal Lives and Social Policy,* Milton Keynes and Bristol: The Open University and The Policy Press, pp. 39-72.

Noon, M. and Blyton, P. (2007) *The Realities of Work: Experiencing Work and Employment in Contemporary Society*, Basingstoke: Palgrave Macmillan.

O'Brien, S. and Wallace, E. (2009) 'Volunteers working in a tertiary referral teaching hospital' in R. Scott and S. Howlett (eds) 2nd edition *Volunteers in Hospice and Palliative Care,* Oxford: Oxford University Press, pp. 195-210.

Randall, F. and Downie, R. S. (2006) *The Philosophy of Palliative Care: Critique and Reconstruction*, Oxford: Oxford University Press.

Rojek, C. (2010) *The Labour of Leisure,* London: Sage Publications.

Sandman, L. (2005) *A Good Death: on the Value of Death and Dying.* Maidenhead: Open University Press.

Sheldon, F. (1997) *Psychosocial Palliative Care,* Cheltenham: Stanley Thornes (Publishers) Ltd.

Simons, H. (2009) *Case Study Research in Practice,* London: Sage.

Sinclair, P. (2007) *Rethinking Palliative Care,* Bristol: The Policy Press.

Smaje, C. and Field, D. (1997) 'Absent minorities? Ethnicity and the use of Palliative Care Services' in D. Field, J. Hockey and N. Small (eds) *Death, Gender and Ethnicity.* London: Routledge.

Spencer-Gray, S-A. (2009) 'The training and education of volunteers' in R. Scott and S. Howlett (eds) 2nd edition *Volunteers in Hospice and Palliative Care,* Oxford: Oxford University Press, pp. 63-86.

Stebbins, R. A. (1996) 'Volunteering: a serious leisure perspective', *Nonprofit and Voluntary Sector Quarterly,* 25(2): 211-224.

Warren, T (2007) 'Conceptualising breadwinning work', *Work Employment and Society,* 21(2): 317-336.

Watts, J. (2006) 'The outsider within: dilemmas of qualitative feminist research within a culture of resistance'. *Qualitative Research*, 6(3), 385-402.

Watts, J. H. (2010) *Death Dying and Bereavement: Issues for Practice*, Edinburgh: Dunedin Academic Press.

Wilkinson, S. (2011) 'Analysing focus group data' in D. Silverman (ed) 3rd edition *Qualitative Research*, London: Sage, pp. 168-184.

Part 2

Challenges in Practice

7

Dilemmas in Palliation

Deepak Gupta
Wayne State University/Detroit Medical Center, USA

1. Introduction

The term 'palliation' by Latin origin meaning 'cloaking' (Stolberg, 2007) of symptoms of disease would seem to be most relevant at the end-of-life. However, palliation by essence does not preclude the use of 'cloaking' at other time-points of disease management, wherein a pallaitive approach may provide deep insight into realistic goals of medicine and consequently result in long-lasting changes in individual patient care. Additionally the dilemmas in applying the essence of the palliative care model to the art of medicine as a whole may lead to substandard medical care out of ignorance. The present chapter will attempt to cover some of the different aspects/dilemmas in palliation from this author's perspective.

2. Dilemmas

2.1 Palliative care diagnoses

Since the advent of the concept of modern palliative care in the United Kingdom (Saunders, 2002), palliation services have primarily covered cancer and cancer-related diagnoses because cancer was supposedly considered to be a terminal illness with the only difference being the speed of progression of various cancers. Slowly with time, other medical diagnoses with similar clinical profiles of variable progression but eventual terminal end-point found their desirable places in palliative medical care (Addington-Hall & Higginson, 2001, as cited in Weatherall, 2001). Paradoxically, the improved survivorship of the cancer patients perpetrated the need of delayed palliation for these cancer patients. So the big question is which all medical diagnoses need palliation as part of their ongoing medical care when death is ultimate truth of all life and irrespective of any medical diagnosis, all patient populations may require palliative services at different time points in their medical lives.

Let us try to understand this with a clinical scenario. When this author proposed for inclusion of moribund obesity as a palliative care diagnosis in the medical literature (Gupta, 2009), this author had variable responses from the medical community. This author's perspective for this inclusion was based on the chronicity of this disease as well as its terminal outcome with variable rate of progression. However, the medical community needs to understand that the inclusion of a medical diagnosis under the spectrum of palliation does not mean the end of the road for the patients suffering from that particular disease. Rather the inclusion is meant to target those patient populations who will be in dire need of palliative services in due course of time; and the underlying intent for these inclusions will be patient advocacy for better quality of life instead of quantity of life. The early recognition of palliative care needs in a patient population does not mean the preclusion of curative medical care because palliation is not synonymous with the end-of-life care but is a model based on the realization and following of realistic goals and outcomes by both patient and medical team at any given time-point of patient care.

In summary, all medical diagnoses except acute and spontaneously resolving diseases or acute and completely curable diseases without any long-lasting sequelae can be included in the palliative care diagnoses' spectrum.

2.2 Disease stage and introduction to palliation

The next big question is related to the appropriate timing for the introduction of palliation in any disease state. The palliation as a concept can be instilled in the medical care as soon as it is recognized that the disease state will be running a chronic course that will require psychological, social and spiritual care besides the attempts at curative physical care. The dilemma is that based on the present understanding of the society about the palliative care, the early introduction of palliation model will confuse the patients, their families and the medical caregivers about the appropriateness of palliation. However, the answer does not lie in deterring the palliation till the very-end-of-life. Instead pioneering an education and awareness initiative for both patient population as well as medical community to realize the role of palliation in almost all disease stages will establish achievable prudent holistic care.

Let us try to understand this with a clinical scenario. It is always amazing that the focus of present medical care is on the innumerable attempts at curing the not-so-curable diseases and in turn providing false hope of longevity without paying attention to the adequacy of quality of these long lives. Peripheral vascular diseases are widespread medical phenomenon with the progressively worsening epidemics of morbid obesity and unrelenting cigarette smoking. As the primary involvement of the lower limbs with deteriorating symptoms usually bring the patients with the hope of curative surgeries to save the dying lower limbs, the limbs that are dying at variable rates of progression or are already dead undergo staged revascularizations that fail requiring staged resections. Though these lines of management may appear to be curative to both patients and medical caregivers, however, this has palliation written all over it as the underlying disease with non-resolving modifiable risk factors cannot be undone and in time, the formal transfers to palliative services are ascertained by the medical teams when there is no more dead limb to be saved. It may be easy for palliative care advocates to propose that the patient needed an early review of the patient's medical goals and needs in regards to helplessly trying to maintain a painless lower limb without actually losing it; however when the end of the limb is inevitable and the goal of revascularizing a dying limb becomes almost analogous to attempting the revascularization of dead bowel, it is already delayed dawning on the medical caregiver team that although the limbs do not have as much length as bowel that can be harmlessly resected, the end of all types of tissues require identically appropriate communication of palliative considerations for adjusted goals and achievable outcomes so that no one loses the perspective for effective patient care.

In summary, the stage of the disease does not matter for efficient enrollment of the patient for palliative care services; however, this will require the mass awareness programs to impress upon the patient and caregiver (family and medical) populations alike that although the palliation has its origin as a specialty to tender services to the abandoned patient populations at their end-of-lives, the palliation has enough potential to mature into a consulting, educating and caregiver specialty rendering the black-and-white medical care along with a good coverage of the gray zones in the patient care needs.

2.3 Interaction of curative and palliative care teams

The modern medicine has become so sophisticated that the complexities of patient care provisions cannot be accomplished without adequate compartmentalization of the medical care into specialty and sub-specialty care. However, this specialist based care model is bound to fail without sound and constant interdisciplinary discussions and interactions for a common goal of good quality holistic care. This becomes more cumbersome when palliative services are branded as subspecialty catering a very small proportion of the patients who are in dying stages even though palliation as a medical concept is continually practiced across the spectrum of all medical specialties without clear-cut perception of the irony in their 'curative' medical care.

Let us try to understand this with a clinical scenario. When on professional palliative care providers' initiative the liberal use of the opioids for pain management became one of the pillars stones of the modern patient care, the medical society was skeptical that high doses of the opioids may hasten patient's death by their sedative and respiratory depressant effects. However, the semi-centennial experience of the modern palliative medicine affirms that early institution of palliative care can actually prolong life, minimally but by definite amounts (Bourseau 2011; Temel et al. 2010). If this is the unexpected transformation of the palliative ideology, this author does not see any harm in this ideology's analogous application for all inexplicably incurable diseases where medication based symptomatic management ensures patients to live longer with delayed complications of lesser severities. The examples include and are not limited to diabetes mellitus and hypertension. Herein, the primary care physicians including primary specialists caring for the patients' special medical needs can come on level grounds with the palliative care teams who can guide and educate them and their patients based on the long experience of palliation in understanding the societal fears and concerns about the agonies related to the dying and the uncertainty related to the dreams of a peaceful death whenever it happens.

Let us try to understand this with another perspective. This author proposed that whenever the true potential of a medical diagnosis since its inception entails the long term prognosis of a patient ending up in the laps of palliative care teams, it is the humane duty of the medical care providers to realize the potential of preemptive palliation (Gupta 2010a) as a resourceful involvement and input of the palliative care teams for making patients understand that early involvement of the palliation in their medical care is analogously nothing more than the provision of advance care directives or living will that are a common place in present day medical care. The early inclusion (and not exclusion) of palliative care team in the patient care will enhance the patient care with palliative care teams' experiences in regards to enormous evidence based understanding of patients' goals when they are dealing with a lifelong suffering secondary to their unrelenting chronic diseases. This inclusion at early stages of diseases will relieve a major burden from other medical teams because they may not be well experienced in dealing with the complex questions of "why me" and "what next" and hence may have been actually avoiding them rather than dealing with them by including the experts for these apparently trivial but still complex clinical scenarios. This author propose that if the word 'palliation' itself interferes with the deserved inclusion of palliative services at so-early stages in the medical care, then for the sake of surrendering to the complacent society, the palliation can be offered at all patients under the disguised name of 'supportive care' that will still maintain the essence and experience of the palliation for a complete holistic patient care.

In summary, it is not at all about the timely transition of medical care from curative to palliative ideology but it is about sharing the patient care between the medical teams who are working to cure the diseases and the palliative care teams who help patients understand how to live with their diseases.

2.4 Curative needs at the end-of-life

This discussion now leads us to the reciprocity of the clinical scenario at the end of life where the patients have now become the complete responsibility of palliative care teams and are almost abandoned by their primary care providers with minimal if any involvement of their primary specialists. This understandable abandonment secondary to 'nothing more to offer' reasoning may leave the palliative care teams unwary to the curative needs of their patients at their end of lives. The palliative care teams may not be hesitant in asking for second opinions for the acute and curable diseases of their patients even if it involve the short term but best possible specialist care at that point of time. The lists of such scenarios may be short but definitely include the broad spectrum and bug-specific antibiotics for difficult infections, interventional angioembolizations of the acute bleeders that may be very acutely hastening the death, curative amputations of dead and septic limbs, short term ventilator support for acute but resolvable pneumonias and the possible percutaneous coronary revascularization in the event of the acute transmural myocardial infarction.

Let us try to understand this ambiguity with a clinical scenario. The patient is suffering at the end of life waiting for inevitable death. Though the body has advanced stages incurable and terminal disease, the tissues are susceptible to common bacterial attacks. These infectious diseases may become difficult secondary to the underlying advanced stage illness and hence requiring advanced generation antibiotics for resistant organisms. The dilemma is whether to hold those expensive antibiotics and avoid their likely adverse effects in a frail body or to provide the known cure for these infections that may have definite improvement in quality of life with possible prolongation of life. In due course, if it is the septic limb that is the source of this difficult infection, the curative amputation may be the best possible medical decision for prolonged life. The pain and symptoms associated with curable pneumonias and unanticipated acute myocardial infarction in an otherwise healthy heart must have the possibility considered by their palliative teams for consultations and management by the intensivists and cardiologists.

In summary, the patient management at the end-of-life by palliative care teams not only involves the symptomatic care but also the aggressive counter-action to the acute but potentially distressing ailments with all potential resources of curing them if there is a feasible and efficient cure available for the ailment at that point of time. In other words, the combined and shared team approach of curative and palliative care teams all through the course of disease is essential to maintain a dignified medical care for the patients since the inception of the disease process till the peaceful end of life.

2.5 Patient's choices or family's wishes

Patient autonomy is integral part of modern medicine and especially palliative care medicine because in the present form of palliation, a lot of decisions are related to negotiating a cost-effective medical care without prolonging a life that is poor in quality. The definite and transparent patient autonomy can only be exercised when the patients make some future decision in regards to their medical care like in advance care directives at a point of life when they are hail and healthy. Even though during these advance decisions documentation all possible clinical scenarios are brought up for clear cut discussions about the patient's destiny, still these scenarios are figments of patient's future and the patients may decide differently when these clinical scenarios become a reality of their lives. At such point of times of reality, the patients' autonomous decisions are certain to be colored with their fears, their love-hate relationship with their family and the uncertainties of the medicine. This level of uncertainty in autonomous medical decision-making becomes more complex when the family has to act as a surrogate decision maker for the patients who become incompetent secondary to their terminal illnesses.

Let us try to understand this ambiguity in patient autonomy with a clinical scenario. In the zeal of their healthy times and as a proponent of the total control on their body, life and death, the advance care directives are documented. However, as the life evolves, the medical science advances and the personal life experiences and observations of surrounding death accumulates, the documenter's perspectives may change and become completely opposite to the documented wishes. Moreover, when the time comes for making the end-of-life decisions, the emotional status of the sufferer is clouded by 'why me' that may not allow the sufferer an appropriate amount of time to understand the inevitability of the ensuing dying and death or to peacefully accept the turn of events in his life that brought the patient to this terminal event. Additionally, the families may not agree with the decisions made by the patients whether they are vocal or subtle about their own preferences in regards to the turn of events. Eventually, the mental status changes in all the patients rendering them incompetent at the very end-of-life; and all final decisions are to made by the families or surrogates who if emotionally attached to their patients cannot escape the coloring of their decisions based on their love-hate emotions for the patients and if emotionally detached to their patients cannot be acting more than a legal writer for the consent that allows the patients in question to die within a pre-decided time-frame after the withdrawal/withholding of life-sustaining treatments.

In summary, the care for the families and emotionally attached surrogates is integrated in the art of modern palliative medicine because the palliative medicine is not only meant to care for the dying but the survivors of deaths in the family; however, it will be a misnomer when we accrue medical decision-making of the patients as autonomous because the families and surrogates covertly or overtly influence in the medical decision making of and for the patients.

2.6 Patient's choice to embrace death NOW

The intent to restore total control over their lives and extending that control to end the life at the time pre-determined by the patient is one big controversial and debatable topic in modern medical science. The reasons may differ why the terminally ill patients may decide that why wait for death to embrace them when they can embrace the death at their own preferential times. The legal and ethical system does not endorse this ideology because their understanding is that the modern palliative medicine can overcome the patients' fears of loss of control over their terminal symptoms by effective and aggressive palliation. Still a very few states respect persons' decisions to end their lives at their own free will and practice euthanasia and/or physician assisted suicide including Netherlands, Belgium, Luxembourg, and Oregon (United States) and Washington (United States); as well as Switzerland as a state allowing assisted suicide only if the executor does not have selfish motivations to assist suicide. This very small percentage of global community practicing the debatable palliative concept may represent the analogous very small percent of terminal patients who if given the opportunity, will decisively complete their wishes for death despite aggressive palliative support.

Let us try to understand this debate with a clinical scenario. At the time of diagnosis of their terminal disease, the patients decide to end their lives because of their poor understanding of the disease and its terminal symptoms and the failure of medical care teams to pursue timely efficacious discussions about their diseases. As the disease evolves, the patient understands their diseases and the supportive care offered and rendered by the palliative care teams; and at this point of time, they may decide that this may be the right time to take the final flight at their own leisure because they feel that it may be the right thing to do. However, eventually, the patient despite attempting to sell their thought for dying at their chosen time ends up losing their full competence or control on their mental status; and are left at the mercy of their family or surrogate decision maker to decide for what they have beem asking all the time: timely death. Additionally, even though the surrogate decision making endorses the withdrawing and withholding the life-sustaining treatments as terminal palliative management protocols, however, instead of the pre-determined times by the patients' choices, now the death is happening when the surrogates and medical teams based on their understanding and perception of the progressive terminal disease decides to let go the patient.

In summary, if the time of flight and the time to embracing the death can be determined by the medical futility and difficult but allowed surrogate decision making, constantly debating the euthanasia or physician assisted suicide may be unnecessarily delaying the appropriate incorporation of these concepts in the armamentarium of modern day palliative care practitioners; this may be ironic when the modern medicine holds patient autonomy in such high regards and pledges to uphold it under all circumstances.

2.7 Choices and cost to the society

The evolution of the medicine has been an uphill task and the new heights to scale keep becoming more tedious with stringent hardships involved. In historical times, the rewards for the practice of medicine by the practitioners was the job satisfaction involved with the patient care with secondary gains involving better hierarchical position in the society with or without financial gains. However, with the increased sophistication and the complexities of the diseases and their management involving the soaring costs of the research for new medicines to continually ensure sound medical care under the fear of the litigating patient population has increased the financial burden of maintaining health. These costs are directly or indirectly bore by the productive sections of the population even though it may appear that the government or the insurance companies are paying for it. Therefore when a poor person decides to surrender to death believing that there is no accesible hope against the terminal disease in the circumstances of personal poverty, this personal choice is no different than a case of an insured person whose timely death happens under the circumstances of the surrogate decision making that withholds or withdraws the costly but medically futile life sustaining treatments. The medical costs are contained either by the patients' personal choices or the family's/society's surrogate choices because the quality of life matters more than the quantity of life, and the decision makers realize that the survivors with very poor quality of life accrue financial as well as non-financial costs for the patients, families and the societies.

In summary, the direct and indirect cost-bearing and cost-sharing of palliation guide many decisions in the palliative care scenarios and the guilt and/or the grudge for the inability to appropriately provide for medical care with or without palliation to a patient should not prevent the patient, the family or the society to decide for the most cost-effective medical solutions for the patient's terminal illness.

3. Innovative perspectives

3.1 Pre-emptive palliation

This goes without saying that palliation is not terminal care. Similarly, the encompassing of some preventive case scenarios or pre-emptive care scenarios under the cloak of palliation is not ambitious overreaching efforts on the part of the palliative care provider community. The only proposition by the proponents of palliative care model is that the medical care team realizes the abovementioned facts and incorporates the ideologies of the palliative teams when they care for their patients since the inception of the diagnosed diseases. Recognizing the palliative virtues of the diseases, risk factors, treatment plans and prognosis of the diseases treated by non-palliative care teams will go a long way in ensuring the thorough understanding of the disease and the realistic expectations about the management with specific answers for patients' fears related to the disease prognoses. Pre-emptive palliation is the concept of initiating these early interventions in all non-palliative care practitioners' settings so that patients can gain from the abundance of knowledge and experience of the palliative care teams which they purport to share and educate for the direct and indirect care of the potential patients who may need traditional end of life care in future. One good example can be the regular and non-hesitant deliverance of Life is a Gift talk as proposed by this author (Gupta, 2010a) for all the potential patients who are identified during their hospital stays or recurring emergency room visits as at-risk population unresponsive to non-pro-active life style discussions that are affecting the prognoses of their diseases and interfering their appropriate, timely and efficacious medical care.

3.2 'Considering' do-not-resuscitate

The life span of a human life keeps growing with advanced medical practices and development of new and sophisticated life-sustaining treatments. The ratio of the productive life span to the total life span keeps decreasing even though the total numbers of both productive and total life span years keep increasing. The life span as a species has been growing with contributing evolutionary factors like grandmother hypothesis (not grandfather hypothesis) effect (Lahdenperä et al. 2004, 2007, 2011) as well as technological factors like improved medical care; however, the quality of this increased life span may be scarred by the cultural factors like alienating family constituents and psychological factors like loneliness and abandonment. The lonely long-living controlling human being has the responsibility by choice and by reason to choose for the end of life decisions and document in the ways best known to human society including family if any, friends if any, attorneys if any, family physicians if any or imprinted on their body parts as tattoo flash as suggested by this author (Gupta 2010b) so that even though the people may die alone but the consent, the choice and the control at the final moments will be theirs that has already been communicated to the caregiver team in multiple and variable ways. At the end, it is the people's choice and people's say in their times of death that are endorsed, followed and executed by the people surrounding them including medical and non-medical caregiver teams based on the system devised as per the cultural, social, ethical and legal standards.

3.3 Paradox of slippery slope

Debate for and against euthanasia and assisted suicide at the end of life is analogous to the hot debate between the pro-lifers and pro-choicers at the beginning of life; the only differences being that though the fetus in question has no say in these decisions, the society is almost equally divided in their propositions for two different types of fate for them; however, the terminally ill population, who can have insight and understanding to make the choices regarding end of life conditions, are deemed unfit to choose death over life in almost 98% countries of the world and many of these societies who do not allow euthanasia or assisted suicide accept withdrawal and withholding life sustaining treatments at such point of times when the terminal patients can no longer decide on their own and the family and society decide based on their perceptions of what the patient would have decided under the conditions of the medical futility of their conditions. There is always a big concern for endorsing the death-by-choice in regards to association of slippery slope to it; however, there is no single ideology (dominant or oppositional) where the society does not reach a slippery slope when it is critically overdone leading to counter-productivity because of a lack of the dialogue between the antagonizing ideologies. The only variation in the incidence of slippery slope with any ideology is the lag time in achieving the critical break-point and subsequent tripping to slippery slope. Additionally, when ideologies obsessively highlight the slippery slope of their oppositions, they suffer the paradox of the slippery slope secondary to over-zealously even so ignorantly or arrogantly overlooking their own approaching critical break-points to slip. The only possible answer is continuity in a dialogue between the supposedly antagonizing ideologies when they may be actually two sides of the same coin to decide for each clinical case scenario on case-by-case basis. The important thing for the conflicting ideologies is to share the pedestal and work in the best interests of the patients', families' and societies' choices, dignities and duties. It took long time for palliation to be accepted as a patient care specialty when the dominant ideology of curing the diseases was at its peak and ended up overdoing the search for 'cures' by enrolling the terminal patients to non-salvageable treatments and non-curative life-sustaining methods. Similarly, the time may have come for the palliation to remember its hardships as a clinical ideology in infancy and henceforth, share some of its newly-found recognition in the society with the advocates of euthanasia and assisted suicide because there is always enough space for all types of ideologies to survive and flourish as long as they do not go overboard their critical points for slippery slope. The understanding of paradox of slippery slope for conscientiously accepting modality of death may not be as difficult to understand as it appears because in the analogous social scenarios, brain dead patients undergo organ harvesting for living through the fellow human beings even when few question if brain dead are actually 'dead' (Banja, 2009), and convicted felons on death row are executed by lethal injections when the civilized society recognizes that their lives pose more risk to fellow human beings than their deaths to human civilization.

4. Conclusion

In summary, per this author (Gupta, 2008), we die in the system we create; and it is not about right to live or right to die but the best negotiable ideology for each individual case scenario to render the most appropriate medical care for the patient in question by maintaining an open-ended continuous dialogue among the conflicting medical ideologies that prevents and/or resolves the dilemmas for the medical care providers and avoids the confusion in the patients, families and societies. Whether it is inclusion of new palliative care diagnoses, pre-emptive palliation, considering do-not-resuscitate directives or societal acceptance for euthanasia/assisted suicide, palliation provides a perfect floatation for a patient to achieve a state of seamless flying in their living, in their dying and into their death above the rocky mountains of pain and despair associated with chronic diseases, advanced stages, unrelenting end-of-life symptoms and terminal state of life.

5. Acknowledgment

This author is deeply indebted to the inspirational mentors, Sushma Bhatnagar, MD, and Seema Mishra, MD, Institute Rotary Cancer Hospital, All India Institute of Medical Sciences, India as well as Michael Stellini, MD, and Harold Michael Marsh, MBBS, Wayne State University/Detroit Medical Center, United States.

6. References

Banja, J.D. (2009). Are brain dead patients really dead? *The Journal of Head Trauma Rehabilitation,* Vol.24, No.2, (March-April 2009), pp. 141-4, ISSN 0885-9701

Bourseau, M. (2011). Early access to palliative treatment prolongs life. *Revue de l'infirmière,* No.168, (February 2011), pp.33-4, ISSN 1293-8505

Gupta, D. (2008). We will die in the system we create. *Journal of Palliative Medicine,* Vol.11, No.8, (October 2008), pp. 1155, ISSN 1096-6218

Gupta, D. (2009). Moribund obesity as a palliative care diagnosis. *Journal of Palliative Medicine,* Vol.12, No.6, (June 2009), pp. 515-516, ISSN 1096-6218

Gupta, D. (2010)."Life is a gift": a vision for preemptive palliation. *Journal of Palliative Medicine,* Vol.13, No.2, (February 2010), pp. 109, ISSN 1096-6218

Gupta, D. (2010). Tattoo flash: consider "do not resuscitate". *Journal of Palliative Medicine,* Vol.13, No.9, (September 2010), pp. 1155-1156, ISSN 1096-6218

Lahdenperä, M.; Lummaa, V.; Helle, S.; Tremblay, M. & Russell, A.F. (2004).Fitness benefits of prolonged post-reproductive lifespan in women. *Nature,* Vol.428, No.6979, (March 2004), pp.178-181, ISSN 0028-0836

Lahdenperä, M.; Russell, A.F. & Lummaa, V. (2007). Selection for long lifespan in men: benefits of grandfathering? *Proceedings. Biological Sciences / The Royal Society,* Vol.274, No.1624, (October 2007), pp.2437-44, ISSN 0962-8452

Lahdenperä, M.; Lummaa, V. & Russell, A.F. (2011). Selection on male longevity in a monogamous human population: late-life survival brings no additional grandchildren. *Journal of Evolutionary Biology,* Vol.24, No.5, (May 2011), pp.1053-63, ISSN 1010-061X

Saunders, C. (2002). Hospice: a global network. *Journal of the Royal Society of Medicine,* Vo.95, No.9, (September 2002), pp.468, ISSN 0141-0768

Stolberg, M. (2007). "Cura palliativa". The concept of palliative care in pre-modern medicine (c. 1500-1850). *Medizinhistorisches Journal,* Vol.42, No.1, (2007), pp.7-29, ISSN 0025-8431

Temel, J.S.; Greer, J.A.; Muzikansky, A.; Gallagher, E.R.; Admane, S.; Jackson, V.A.; Dahlin, C.M.; Blinderman, C.D.; Jacobsen, J.; Pirl, W.F.; Billings, J.A. & Lynch, T.J. (2010). Early palliative care for patients with metastatic non-small-cell lung cancer. *The New England Journal of Medicine,* Vol.363, No.8, (August 2010), pp.733-742, ISSN 0028-4793

Weatherall, D.J. (2001). Palliative care for non-cancer patients. *Journal of the Royal Society of Medicine,* Vo.94, No.11, (November 2001), pp.600-601, ISSN 0141-0768

8

Breaking Bad News to Families of Dying Children: A Paediatrician's Perspective

M. P. Dighe, M. Marathe, M. A. Muckaden and M. Manglani
Tata Memorial Centre,
India

1. Introduction

"The death of a loved one is a highly emotional and stressful experience for families and the death of a child, in particular, is one of the most painful bereavements for families and also for professional care givers." (Stevens, 2004) According to Fallowfield, "The physicians' behavior and communication of caring and competence at the end of life are known to have a major influence on the ability of patients and families to assimilate the news, consider options, and adapt and adjust to what lies ahead." (Fallowfield, 2004) It follows therefore that communication at the end of a paeditaric patient's life is an important area of general paediatric practice.

1.1 Deaths in childhood

The mortality rates in childhood show a wide difference globally. In India, the under-5 mortality rate in 2009 was 66 as compared to 6, in the UK. Infections and malnutrition are the leading causes of deaths in India while accidents, congenital anomalies are the main causes in the UK. (UNICEF) This chapter has been written based on a recent study by the authors in the Paediatrics department of a tertiary general hospital in Mumbai, India.

1.2 Relevance of the study

The study is relevant not only to palliative care but also to the field of Pediatrics because the overall aim is to obtain an in-depth understanding of the perspectives of resident paediatric doctors about factors that affect the communication of the child's actual or impending death to the family care givers. In Palliative medicine as a specialty, much emphasis is laid on the provision of high-quality physician-family communication at the end of life. Palliative care professionals can be instrumental in offering constructive criticism about communication issues in other specialty settings like Paediatrics. A study by Pan et al. clearly showed the presence of a palliative care service improved the confidence of fellows in end of life care. (Pan et al., 2005) As one of the primary aim of paediatric palliative care is "the provision of care through death and bereavement" (Association for Children's Palliative Care/Royal College of Paediatrics and Child Health, 2003), a study of the perspectives of resident paediatric doctors about breaking bad news to families of dying children is clearly relevant to palliative care.

1.3 Background

Previous studies have identified some of the factors that affect the process of communicating the death news to the paediatric patient's family. These factors may be broadly divided into those related to the doctors, factors related to the patient and the family and to factors in the work environment.

A qualitative study by Contro et al. from a Children's University hospital, in an urban setting (Contro et al., 2004) described the perspectives of families of deceased children and of staff members of the hospital and community physicians, on the quality of Palliative Care. The study employed two diverse approaches- family caregivers of children who had died at the hospital were interviewed on a face to face basis while staff members and community physicians filled up a written survey. Communication between staff and families of dying children was one of the problem areas marked by the staff members who reported feeling "inexperienced" in communicating with families about end of life issues. Lack of experience was associated with feeling distressed in communicating with families and patients. Staff members perceived that "emotional, psychological and social support was lacking or nonexistent" within their work environment. "Personal pain and the lack of support" were related to staff members' most difficult experiences of caring for dying children. Majority of the staff members including 85% of the residents said that they would "welcome consultation with a palliative care team."

A part of the same study which relates to the experiences of bereaved families has been published in another paper. (Contro et al., 2004) Sixty-eight family members of 44 deceased children were interviewed by clinical social workers and a psychologist. The views of the families corroborate those of the staff members- feeling distressed due to uncaring delivery of bad news and careless remarks made by staff members and lack of support from the staff. Besides non-English speaking families reported that the language barrier greatly affected their ability to comprehend the information given by the doctors. The above study explains the relevance of preparation, language, staff training and support to how resident doctors communicate with families of dying children. In a study from another specialist paediatric centre in the USA, Kolarik et al. also demonstrated the lack of effective palliative care training in paediatric residency programmes; the authors attribute this to the absence of specific mentorship and role modeling during their residency and to the absence of a formal palliative care service in the hospital. (Kolarik et al., 2006)

Clark, in a lucid commentary outlining specific concerns about residents' and interns' training in a neonatal intensive care unit, points out to factors in the work environment that affect communication between residents and families. (Clark, 2001) He identified long work hours, lack of clear institutional policies and doctors' fear of litigation which negatively affect interactions between them and parents of dying children. The doctors' personal attitude that death is an enemy leads to inappropriate therapies and "distancing" behaviour with the parents.

Previous interactions of the residents with the family and the patients are also known to affect their manner of breaking bad news. Sahler et al. interviewed 31 interns after the death of a child in their care so as to understand the factors that determined their interaction with the patient and his family. (Sahler et. al., 1981) The authors identified that the major patient related factor that determined their interaction was the ability of the children to have a meaningful interaction which was dependent on the child's age and neurological status. The interns failed to develop an active relationship with parents of children who were unable to interact with them. The interns' relationship with the parents of the dying child was affected by the duration of the child's illness- having cared for a long time for an ill child helped the intern to understand the child's place in the context of the family and also increased their empathy towards the parents when it became clear that the child was dying. Interns "actively avoided" parents of children who died suddenly sensing the hostility that parents felt towards the interns.

Previous studies have identified some significant factors that are likely to affect communication with families of dying children. We believe that a qualitative research methodology based on the grounded theory will enabled us to obtain an in depth understanding of the subject.

None of the above studies specifically explored the issue of breaking the news of the actual or impending death of the child to the family. The practice of death declaration is one of the most sensitive areas in general paediatric practice and one in which research is greatly lacking.

It became clear from the review of existing literature that the factors which are likely to affect the practice of breaking bad news to families of dying children. These factors were explored in our study.

1.4 Objectives of the study

The overall aim of this qualitative study was explore the perspectives of Paediatric resident doctors about breaking bad news of the actual or impending death of a dying child to the family, in an urban Government run general hospital in Mumbai, India, with respect to the following.

- Physician related factors e.g. training, experience and knowledge and attitudes
- Patient related factors such as age, gender, cognitive ability or type of illness, duration of care provided
- Family members' characteristics such as gender, educational status
- Environmental factors within and outside the residents' work such as patient load, availability of space and privacy, support

2. Study methodology

This was a qualitative study based on the grounded theory approach. Strauss and Corbin, define qualitative research as "any type of research that produces findings not arrived at by statistical procedures or other means of quantification. It allows the investigator to research about persons' lives, lived experiences, behaviors and emotions."(Strauss and Corbin, 1998) In Health care, qualitative research methods have been applied to study subjects such as the organization of health services, interactions between doctors and patients, and the changing roles of the health professions. (Pope and Mays, 1995)

The qualitative research method was suitable for the present study as it allowed the investigators to obtain an in depth understanding of the topic and to interpret data in terms of the meanings attached by the residents.

The investigators used a naturalistic inquiry process in which they attempted to discover the perspectives of the residents without affecting any change in the environment. Data obtained through "naturalistic inquiry" manner is more likely to reflect the "real world" situation. (Patton, 2002) The interviews were conducted by MD who was unknown to the residents and did not work at the site of data collection. This decreased the bias that the interviewer brought to the interview process. The tool for data collection was the semi-structured interview which was based on the interview guide. This type of interview allowed the interviewer to explore in depth and ask questions to illuminate a particular subject *within* each topic area specified in the interview guide.

The sample for the study was drawn from the pool of Resident doctors in the department of Paediatrics at Lokmanya Tilak Municipal General hospital, Mumbai. These resident doctors included those who were in a residency program either a post graduate degree (MD) in Paediatrics or a Fellowship in Pediatrics. The points of divergence were- gender, current posting (ward, paediatric intensive care, neonatal intensive care), marital status and being a parent. These specific points of divergence were included as each of these characteristics was thought to have an effect on the communication with families of dying children. Residents who had declared death a family at least once during their training were included in the study. Even though the expected sample size was approximately 10, seven interviews were conducted as thematic saturation was achieved within this number having met all the points of divergence.

Prior to starting the study, the proposal was ratified by the Institutional review board of the first author's host institution and the Human Ethics committee of the Institution where the data were collected. Each participant received the "participant information leaflet which contained the details of the study. They were given a 'sleep over time' of at least twenty four hours prior to obtaining a valid consent. All the interviews were conducted on site by MD. Five interviews were recorded on a digital audio recording device. For two respondents who refused audio recordings, notes were taken during the interview. Demographic data were collected at the time of the interview. These included age, gender, marital status, number of own children and any personal bereavement in the past two years, average number of occasions when bad news has been broken by the doctor.

The interviews were transcribed verbatim and narratives were written for each respondent on the basis of the interview, demographic data and any additional notes made by the interviewer during the interview. Confidentiality was ensured by keeping the consent forms separate from the data sets. The narratives were analyzed for emerging subthemes by MD and MM.

3. Results

Three major themes emerged from the data- Practice, Attitudes and Interpersonal relationships.The major themes were divided into subthemes as follows-
Practice- Preparation, Language, Setting and Training and Support

Attitudes- Emotional responses, Coping, Influence of personal life, Roles
Interpersonal Relationships- Resident- patient relationship, Resident- family member relationship.

We discuss each theme in detail in the section below.

3.1 Main theme: Practice

The theme Practice addresses the actual practice of breaking bad news in the study setting.

3.1.1 Preparation

Preparation refers to the communication between the doctors and the families prior to the declaration of the patient's death. The content of this communication revolves around giving information about the clinical condition, ongoing treatment and mentally preparing the family for the child's death.

The following is an example of how doctors "prepare" the families to receive the bad news.

RD6: "The usual practice of breaking bad news is….. when a child is serious; the poor prognosis is explained to the family. We explain what the problem that the child ….then what we are doing to improve the child's condition. We explain in such a way that they realize that everything possible is being done to salvage the child. If the child continues to deteriorate and finally dies, the family is explained that despite the maximum medical support, the child could not be salvaged."

Giving detailed information is considered important for gaining the trust of the family, which in turn facilitates breaking bad news. Families must have sufficient time to prepare themselves mentally to hear the bad news; families who have not had enough time to come to terms with the impending death, experience much psychological distress. The other reason that emerged was that the doctors felt that the family would "blame" them or become "aggressive" if they were not adequately aware of the efforts being made by the doctors to save their patient's life as is evident from the above response.

The setting of the Neonatal Intensive Care Unit (NICU) is different as compared to the general ward setting. RD5, a registrar in the Neonatal Intensive Care unit points out to the distress of families suffer while having to face an unexpected turn of events when a newborn is admitted to the intensive care unit. She says-

RD5: "And a... it's like especially in NICU it's like a small baby and it's a generally like a time of joy when they know that the baby has been delivered now and so but instead of that if they get this news that the baby is really sick and…….."

Thus preparing the families is emphasized by all residents so as to gain trust, allow time for the family to be mentally prepared and to avoid blame.

3.1.2 Language

Patients from diverse socioeconomic, linguistic and educational backgrounds are treated in the present study setting. The sub theme language looks at the way the doctors use language to effectively communicate with families of dying children from such dissimilar backgrounds.

According to the doctors, families with poor educational backgrounds are unable to grasp certain medical terms that may be used in the context of the patient. Hence given the importance of communicating appropriate information, resident doctors emphasized the use simple terms while conveying information about the patients' crucial condition to the families who are often poorly educated.

Also relevant to the subtheme "language" is the exact use of words that the doctors use to describe the dying patient. Some of the descriptors used are "serious", "things going out of hand" and "not going to make it" rather than using the word "dying".

RD1: "We never saying "dying"- even after the first cardiac arrest we say that we are doing everything ventilator, injections..........."

RD7: "I tell them whether the patient is serious I usually tell them before hand that you know that like the patient is getting serious, you know, things are getting out of hand. We don't know there are very less chances of his survival and we are trying our best. "

Most of the doctors preferred not use the term "dying" to describe the patient's condition but rather to use various euphemisms to convey the information. The one respondent who would actually use the word "death" while preparing the family probably had enough rapport to explain the situation and the prognosis to the family beforehand. He would use the actual words "possibility of death" while talking about a future outcome.

Sharing a common language with the family is viewed as an effective tool for rapport building with the family. The doctors and the patients come from diverse linguistic backgrounds as the hospital in which the study has been done is located in a large metropolis in India.

To summarize, the subtheme "language" focuses on the use of simple, non medical words while informing poorly educated families about the patients' condition and ongoing treatment. The use of terms such as "dying" or "death" is considered inappropriate by all but one of the doctors. Sharing a common regional language with the family helps doctors to build rapport in the setting where there is significant linguistic diversity.

3.1.3 Setting

The subtheme "setting" includes the perspectives of the resident doctors about the various factors within the local environ, that affect the way they break bad news to the families.

All the respondents pointed out to the limitations of resources they faced in their setting. These included lack of availability of beds in the intensive care unit and limited financial resources of the families. Limited human resources in relation to the number of patients are also viewed as a problem which affects the work. Some of the following examples illustrate these problems.

RD1: "The problem here is that other municipal or government hospitals often do not have vacancies and the private setups too expensive for our patients. In such a situation patients end up in the ward where they die. Also since Sion is a tertiary hospital, patients come here in a bad shape".

RD2: "Unfortunately in other places like the ICU it becomes difficult (To break bad news) "- due to the design of the place, constraint of space."

All the doctors acknowledge that the lack of availability of beds on the Intensive Care Unit does affect the care delivery to the patients. Limitation of space also compromises the privacy that is needed while breaking bad news to the family.

Limitation of human resources means that the doctors often do not have fixed duty hours. The setting of the study is a busy Paediatric tertiary unit catering to thousands of patients annually. The resident doctors have a very busy work schedule. The following examples provide an insight into the work that they put in during their training as resident paediatricians-

RD1: "In my first post I worked without off call for 3 months ---"

RD7: "we used to have work like anything in Sion Hospital.."

Overall the resident doctors' work during their training is quite grueling. Despite this, the respondents felt that it may affect other areas of their work but not the way they broke bad news.

Within the subtheme "Setting", the impact of the institution's policies on the doctors' practice is discussed in the subsequent paragraphs. The doctors are bound to follow certain institutional procedures which affect their interaction with the family of the deceased child. One such procedure is related to having to ask for a mandatory post mortem examination when a patient dies soon after getting admitted. This is viewed as a particularly distressing process for the grief stricken family.

Currently, there are no clear policies about withholding futile treatments.

RD5: "a…what Dr. M. (senior neonatologist) feels that we should give them (all babies who are critically ill) 100 percent chances and put him on the ventilator and try our level best. But from whatever I've seen I've like baby 700 gms I don't think that we should really be aggressive… depending on how preterm the baby is…..being really aggressive to save the child at the cost of all the other babies especially in our setting."

RD5's response reflects her feeling that scarce resources must be used optimally and the policy of resuscitating every neonate, irrespective of the outcome may compromise care for other patients.RD3 who is a Fellow in Haematology and Oncology also felt that the likely prognosis should determine the priority the patients receive for their treatment.

RD3: "But what happens ki (that) when we have a..'N' number of children, and we have to prioritize a few….So definitely we would like to prioritize the ones who are salvageable."

To summarize, the doctors' practice is guided by the policies and procedures of their institution. They perceive some of these procedures, such as seeking the bereaved family's consent for a post mortem examination, as unduly distressing for the family and to an extent, even for the doctors. The issue of appropriate policies about resuscitation of neonates at the edge of viability and just allocation of scarce medical resources based on the prognosis was also discussed here.

The question "What kind of changes would you like to see in your setting about the practice of breaking bad news?" elicited somewhat similar responses from all the doctors. One area of change was related to having a "designated person" to support the families after bad news was broken to them. However there were some differences in the perception of the exact role of this person.

RD3: "There is no emotional support in our part of the setup and it is definitely very important.........That emotional support maybe some counselors should be there."

RD6: "Ummm……The overall practice of breaking bad news is good as it is…….but it is better to have a dedicated social worker or counselor for the PICU. This individual can support the bereaved family immediately after the patient's death."

Residents would value a dedicated person who would provide emotional support to the family while the doctors should be the ones to break the bad news. Three of the respondents also pointed out to the need for private space where families may receive bad news.

3.1.4 Training and support

In this subtheme, the level of training that the resident doctors have in communication skills, specifically in end of life issues, is discussed. The support that is available for doctors from staff members in their institution and colleagues, while communicating with families about crucial issues, including breaking bad news is also described under this subtheme.

General communication skills workshops are conducted for the resident doctors in the study setting for the past three years. These workshops include didactic teaching and discussions. Not all doctors have completed this training- in fact only five out of the seven doctors interviewed have completed the training. The training has been in the form of "stand alone" teaching sessions without any refresher or follow up sessions. The impact of the communication skills training was perceived quite variably among the residents. While one of the doctors who had not received training himself but had seen his juniors being trained felt that they were fortunate to have been trained formally in communication skills. He said-

RD1: "The new batch of residents is lucky- they have orientation communication training etc. We had to learn on our own."

RD4 had received some communication skills training at the centre where she worked previously. She felt that the formal training that she had received was good but she could not incorporate the skills into her routine practice. She said-

RD4: "Ya it was helpful, but that I forgot after that. I didn't practice…didn't practice much."

It is evident that the even though the doctors had received some formal training in communication skills the impact of such training on actual practice was not significant. One of the reasons could be that most of the doctors had been trained in "stand alone" sessions without any follow up or reinforcement and this may be a possible reason why the impact of the session on practice was insignificant.

Besides formal communication skills training, other sources for learning also emerged-such as studying for foreign medical examinations, books and television. Observing senior colleagues and faculty members as role models and experiential learning were the other important ways of inculcating communication skills. Nurses were also considered as a source of support in difficult situations of breaking bad news. This is an example where the supportive role of nurses becomes evident-

RD6: "Nurses do not directly declare death but they help by supporting the female family members like the mother or the grandmother. They talk to the family, call other family members who may not be in the hospital at the time of death and give first aid to the bereaved person if required."

The presence of a "mob" of relatives is perceived as a threat and the presence of security personnel at the time of death declaration was considered to be appropriate. This opinion is the result of the episodes of abuse that resident doctors have faced in the recent past in the centre where this study has been carried out.

In summary, training has minimal effect on the practice of breaking bad news to families of dying children. Senior staff members as role models and one's own experiences are important sources for learning communication skills. Staff members like nurses and security personnel are supportive in difficult communication situations.

3.2 Theme - Attitudes to death of children

The main theme "Attitudes to the death of children" was divided into the following sub themes-Emotional responses, Coping, Influence of personal life and Role.

3.2.1 Emotional responses

All the Resident doctors perceived the death of their patient as "saddening". In fact RD2 describes the death of the patient as "devastating" while RD3 admitted that he "felt depressed" following the death of a paediatric patient. The respondents also pointed out that their reactions to the deaths were more intense during the initial part of their training but over the course of time, the intensity of their emotional responses has diminished and that they have come to accept deaths of patients as an inevitable part of their work. The following is an illustration of this point:

RD3: "At a personal level ..umm..actually during the initial part of my training I used to feel a bit depressed but a..Gradually over the years I am training I have gone to several institutes. I have seen multiple deaths." "deaths are bound to happen and we have to accept it that is what I have realized over several years of my working".

Thoughts about the death of a patient affect the resident doctors' work for some period of time but having to get on with the tasks of caring for other patients is a distraction. An example of this is given below:

RD2: "Over a period of time you can get into the care of other patients that is the best thing to do..get into your work, dedicate yourself to your work..and may be in an hour or two you can be totally out of it."

Respondents whose interaction with the patient was more personal were emotionally more affected by the death of that patient. Also a longer period of caring and a better rapport with the patient or the family led to the death being viewed as saddening. Specifically, playing with the children was viewed as a "bonding activity". Excerpts from interviews highlight this point.

RD2:" As a paediatrician, there is a tendency to get bonded with the patient. May be that is there in medicine also but it is more so in paediatric age group. We play with those kids and it does affect you mentally somewhere."

RD4: "we are…we are also emotionally attached. The small babies… we means…. play sometimes with them and chat with them; they suddenly go bad so………really we feel bad."

RD6: "When the patients are suffering from a chronic disease, they have a long follow up. So we become more attached to such patients. When such a patient dies we feel worse. There was a leukemic girl who was not responding to treatment. We knew that she was dying but felt that she should not die. We had made a lot of efforts to let this child to pull on."

One of the respondents, RD6 perceived that doctors may make greater efforts to save the life of a particular patient to whom they have become "attached".

Six out of the seven respondents mentioned that they "blamed themselves" for the death of the patient when they were unable to save the life either due to lack of medical resources or due to their clinical inexperience.

RD1 who is a registrar in the Paediatric Intensive care unit said that, "I feel bad when a patient who is salvageable, dies because there were no resources. I feel bad at a personal level…. like I have the knowledge but am helpless……….. Sometimes it is depressing……….. I try not to blame myself for the death."

All the respondents mentioned that they reflected about each death clinically and tried to understand what could have been done differently.RD5, a junior registrar in the Neonatal Intensive Care Unit, mentioned that the Mortality meetings in the Neonatology department every month were helpful in this respect.

To summarize, Paediatric resident doctors view the death of their patients as saddening. The emotion was stronger when the residents had become "attached" to the patient. They also experience some guilt about the death of patients but consider each one as a clinical learning opportunity in their practice.

3.2.2 Coping

The busy ward and large number of patients under their care helps the doctors to take their minds off a patient's death.

RD5 points out to lack of time –"We don't really keep thinking about it there is so much happening that you can't really sit and think about one patient that you've lost. We don't get that sort of time here."

Four out of seven respondents said that they spoke to friends or family members when they were upset about a patient death. It was particularly helpful if the person were a doctor as they felt that such a person would understand them better. Watching movies or going out with friends also helped.

There is no formal structured support for resident doctors who may face emotional distress as a result of their work.To illustrate the point, excerpts from the interview with RD3 are given below.

RD3: "For Doctors, (laughs), it will take a hundred years to happen, in India."

Another respondent felt that staff members actually offered support and advice to the resident doctors about patient deaths. In this regard, he said that-

RD7:" I am down after a patient's death, madam sees ___ why you are worried. This is you know just part and parcel of life. So----yeah, obviously I do get support from all of them. "

One of the respondents volunteered that being spiritually inclined helped him keep his peace of mind and get on with the numerous roles he had to play on the professional and the family front.

To summarize, the resident doctors coped with patient deaths in different ways. The most common mechanism was to become involved in caring for other patients. The lack of formal mechanisms for psychological support in the work place was recognized but senior staff members were viewed as being helpful. Watching movies, talking to family or friends and spirituality were also considered helpful in coping with the deaths of paediatric patients.

3.2.3 Impact of family life

In this study specific factors related to the family lives of the residents were explored to ascertain whether they had an influence on the practice of breaking bad news. A general question to this effect was "Sometimes, factors in our life, outside our work environment may affect our work. Do you think that there are any such factors that affect your communication with families of dying children?" Specific prompts were used to elicit issues regarding the influence of their family lives on their professional practice.

RD1 had experienced a recent bereavement and also had a close family member who was suffering from advanced cancer. RD1 appeared uncomfortable while answering this question but he acknowledged that on certain occasions his personal experiences may have affected how he broke bad news to the family. However he tried consciously to prevent this from happening.

RD7 is the only doctor in the setting who has a child. He thinks that he may become more "emotional" while breaking the news of death of a child to the family because he is able to identify himself with the parents of the patients.

All the other respondents were asked a hypothetical question related to the issue- "How do you think having one's own children would affect the way in which they broke bad news to the family?" The male respondents were not sure whether having their own children would make a difference to the practice of breaking bad news. The remaining two female respondents were divided in their opinion- one of them felt that there would be a difference in the way they broke bad news while the other (RD5) felt otherwise.

RD5: "Umm…in the medical a…field I don't think it would make a difference because we've been trained and groomed over the so many years. It doesn't make so much of an impact."

From the ongoing discussion, it is evident that doctors' communication with families is affected by certain situations in their personal life, however they make a deliberate attempt to keep their personal and professional lives separate.

3.2.4 Roles

Here we discuss the doctors' perceptions about the role that they play in the in the care of the paediatric patient. The doctors view that their main responsibility is to be involved in the physical aspect while the psychological care is largely considered to be outside the scope of their job.

The following examples illustrate the doctors' views about their role in care giving.

RD3: "I strongly feel that this (psychological support) is one domain where this one thing is that clinicians don't have so much of time as I told you."

Even though residents realize that psychological support is important for bereaved families, they would not be in a position to do so themselves because the doctors are too busy. Besides, the task is viewed as both time consuming and emotionally taxing. Residents would rather hand over the care of dying patients to another professional care giver.

RD3: "So I would like ki (that) maybe I can invest more time in the ones who..(Pause 2seconds) In whom I may get the fruit out of my efforts rather than those in whom I know a… that my limitations will not allow me to take the child for long."

While the above response reflects RD3' s personal opinion about caring for children who have poor chances of survival or improvement, his comment also highlights the ethical issue of distribution of scarce resources in his local setting. This issue of resource availability is further elucidated in the theme "setting".

Like the above two respondents, RD4 a female registrar in the NICU, puts her feelings about breaking bad news as follows-

RD4: "Ya it's the worst part. I hate that means I hate I *literally hate* it I can do every work. I can do as much hard work as I can but I hate means declaring to the patient and writing a Death Certificate."

The reason for RD4' s aversion to breaking death news of neonatal patients is probably related to the fact she has been in this setting for several months, at a stretch, without respite from frequent patient deaths which happen.

Overall, the doctors regard breaking bad news of the patient's death as an emotionally draining task. They also acknowledge that due to constraint of time, they would rather entrust the task of providing emotional support to the families to another professional, a specialist in caring for dying patients and their families, while they would invest their energies in caring for patients who are more likely to get better.

Only one of the doctors mentioned the term "Palliative care" to describe the care that dying patients should receive. This respondent, unlike others, is probably aware of palliative care because he has worked in a large cancer institution which has a specialist palliative care team. This fact clearly points to a lack of awareness about palliative care among the doctors. However the descriptors used by the others to describe the desirable care for dying children, are actually related to the essential principles of palliative care practice indicating the need for palliative care provision in this setting.

3.3 Main theme-Interpersonal relationships

3.3.1 The patient

In this sub theme, the perspectives of the doctors about the paediatric patient, within their role as professional care givers and outside that role, are described. The impact of these perspectives on the practice of breaking bad news to the families is also described.

Children, even as patients, are viewed as endearing and innocent by the respondents. Here are some of the responses to the question "How are paediatric patients different from adults?"

RD2: "Their innocence..ya ..unlike adult patients may vocalize to you all findings ..there may be some abstract things affecting you but in the pediatric age group....even pain for that matter..if a child is in pain he will immediately vocalize it out...while an adult might keep it subdued."

Doctors share the view that the loss of a child who is able to talk and to communicate is viewed as greater than that of one who is not able to do so, both by the doctors and by the families. The following are some examples that illustrate this view point-

RD1: "Children who are about 4-5 have cognitive abilities.... They are able to communicate..so the bond of these children is more than with very small babies."

RD6: "Families react more intensely when an older child dies."

The child's ability to communicate appears to be central to the bonding that families and even the doctors share with the child. The other aspect that doctors consider important while developing a "bond" with their patient is when they play with the patient. This is discussed in detail under the subtheme "Role".

Within their practice, the doctors often have to care for children whose limited cognitive ability precludes any meaningful communication. The doctors agreed that patients with abnormal cognition are unable to communicate well and hence it is difficult to "bond" with them; however these children are still considered to be "special".

RD2 says, "No even those -you may not be having interactive sessions but you will feel sorry - humanity comes in the picture. You feel that as it is he is in pain, as it is he is dying, unfortunately he cannot vocalize. So then you get puzzled-what is the best thing you can do."

Most doctors felt that the gender of the patient makes difference while breaking bad news because the reactions of families were likely to be stronger when it was a male child rather than a female.

RD2: "Ya at least in our community it does to be honest......we have seen that at times if it is a female child people are accepting while if it is a male child, people might create a lot of.............we have seen that at times ya so at least in the Indian setup it does."

RD5: ": a…first of all a…when you tell them the sex of the baby that might be a problem if it's a female child. A…specially there are no male children already there in the family so that's kind of like really sad to know that they still feel like that of girl child and all that."

The doctors witness gender discrimination against the female child, by the family, within their practice setting. They also point to specific situations or groups where such discrimination is more likely to occur.

RD1: "Rarely, in cases of neglected children or orphans with HIV, neglected children with cerebral palsy- female children were at a disadvantage."

RD2: "On the other hand there may be someone from the lower socioeconomic strata who are desperately wanting a male child and that particular male child is sick then they will be affected more………"

A child who is socially "at risk" is more likely to face the brunt of gender discrimination. Only one of the respondents RD5 remarked that she was saddened by the discrimination; the other doctors seemed to look upon the issue as inevitable fallout of the general societal norms in their setting.

Neonates are a specific subgroup within the paediatric patient population. Two of the doctors interviewed were working in that unit at the time of their interview. Their perceptions about their very young patients are presented here-

RD5: "And a... it's like especially in NICU it's like a small baby and it's a generally like a time of joy when they know ki the baby has been delivered now and so but instead of that if they get this news that the baby is really sick.."

In the NICU the patients are often brought in almost immediately after their birth. In this scenario, the anticipated joy turns into a stressful situation for the family, as is evident in RD5's response.

RD4: "Clearly means it feels like as if a part of our family member is going it's like that only…(pause 1 second)…Because it really feels bad. It feels like all our hard work is wasted and we are…we are also emotionally attached. This small babies we means play sometimes with them and chat with them they suddenly goes bad so really we feel bad."

RD4's response gives an indication of the sense of loss that she herself feels when a newborn baby dies. Playing with the patient emerges as a source of "bonding" once again from RD4's response.

To summarize, the paediatric patient is perceived quite differently from the adult. The doctors find themselves becoming emotionally attached to their paediatric patients; the child's ability to communicate is an important factor in developing this attachment. Even children who are not able to communicate are considered to be special and the doctors are more sympathetic towards them. The doctors recognize a difference in the manner in which families react to deaths of children, depending on their gender. This is probably considered as an expected outcome of the existing societal attitudes. In case of the newborn patient, the family often witnesses a joyous situation turn into a stressful one and for the residents; the "involvement" with these young patients seems to be more marked.

3.3.2 The family

The practice of breaking bad news to the families seemed to depend to a large extent on the expected reactions of the family members and on the previous interaction between the families and the doctors. The expected reactions described by the doctors ranged from acceptance of the child's death to anger and aggression. The following are examples of the different reactions described by the doctors.

RD7: "They talk about everything you know… how much care they have taken about this child. What that child meant to him or to her or to them. And yeah I mean they really break down I mean…. They were through a lot and when they see this I mean obviously you know the sky breaks for them."

RD3: "The most important thing which I have felt the parents feel is that, they feel that they have not done enough for the child because they are, usually the patients at Sion Hospital are very poor non – affording kind, So they feel that they a.. a lot of time there are financial constraints. When they are not able to arrange then they feel guilty that because of not getting this medicine my child expired. So that guilt feeling... if I'm able to take it out from their mind that is also a big achievement so that life long they should not feel guilty "That our child expired because we could not get the medicine." So I generally make them understand that if you even tried to get the medicine the disease was such and a.. the child was so sick that a.. we have limitations, we are not God."

Grief and guilt are common reactions of the families to hearing the death news. However families may sometimes respond with anger directed at the doctors. The following are some examples-

RD2: "They were always under the impression that whatever happens however bad our child is he is going to come back again ..but here accepting the fact that the child had died……..the dad became very volatile."

RD2: "They are so used to hospitalization, child deteriorating, going to intensive care and coming back.So might be somewhere they have this idea that this is a routine thing. And this particular thing happening-child not shifted to the ICU but dying in the ward….so they might feel because of those elements not happening ……so they start comparing- this time the child was not sent to the ICU. So was it a mistake on part of the doctors?"

The doctors have experiences- their own or those of their colleagues where family members have become aggressive or abusive. All the respondents who mentioned such experiences attributed them to the family's lack of mental preparation for the death or of their denial of the possibility of death.

Conversely, doctors find that trust and having a good rapport with the family facilitate breaking bad news. The following examples illustrate this point.

RD6: "Most of the times, the families accept the situation because they generally trust the doctors."

RD7: "I have a lot of rapport with all of my patients since beginning since I was the houseman. The patients, their relatives tend to relate with me. I tend to listen a lot that is one way. I have seen many resident doctors have altercations with the family but I never had to face that problem. So if you have that rapport things become easier."

To summarize, lack of acceptance of the bad news and aggression by the family are the difficulties that the doctors face while breaking bad news. It was "easier" to break bad news to families which trusted the doctors or with whom the doctors had a good rapport.

3.3.3 Gender

All the respondents felt that the gender of the family member to whom they broke the bad news affected their practice. All but one of the doctors remarked that they would rather avoid breaking the bad news to female relatives in general and to the mother specifically. RD1: "I do not break news of death to female relatives like the mother or the grandmother. We usually tell male relatives like the father or the grandfather."

RD3:" And therefore he (the patient) is there like that, so it was easier for the parents to accept or the whosover is receiving this death news. It would be easier for him to accept. And then I would tell them that a..a they should first take care of the mother and console her properly and then slowly break the news to her."

RD4: 'Umm... so initially whatever happens to the newborns na we keep on informing to the relatives. A…not to the mother usually to the male relatives."

RD6: "I try to avoid giving bad news to the mother unless there is no one else. I would try to break bad news to male relatives like the father or the grandfather."

All the above responses reflect reluctance to break bad news in general to the female relatives and in particular to the mother of the deceased child. Some the reasons are evident from these responses-

RD3: "In India definitely it makes a difference because a… females maybe they are not able to accept the news so early this is particularly about death news I am telling. Whereas males…… they, means they try to understand a situation, they're not so emotionally labile particularly at that moment so I prefer first telling to the male member so that they can dilute it and then convey it to the other members of the family including females."

RD5 : " Ya…a…that's just because the bond unknowingly whatever …….even if the mother has not been with the baby……since the baby was born. But a…we don't really want the mother to collapse or something just hearing the news that the child is no more."

The strong emotional response expected from the mother is a deterrent to breaking bad news directly to her. On the other hand, men are perceived as being more composed and in control of the situation. The doctors therefore prefer to break bad news to the male family members.

While the gender of the family member was an important factor in breaking bad news, the gender of the doctor who broke bad news did not seem to affect breaking bad news to the family, in the opinion of all but one of the respondents.

In the present study setting, there are many patients who come from poor socioeconomic and educational background. Each doctor was asked whether the educational level of the family made a difference to breaking bad news. All of them felt that the level of education of the families variably affected their emotional responses to the bad news but made a difference in how they perceived the patient's condition.

RD3: "Ya...ya it affects a lot because a... a...because what happens...depending on the literacy level they have other beliefs also, like a few families are there who feel that some other therapies and some other faith healers or ayurvedic (traditional Indian medicine) and like that."

RD6: "When the families are poor and there are several children in the family their reaction to the death may not be very intense, in fact they may not be too bothered by it. A poor family who has a past experience of losing a child may not be too bothered by another child death."

RD7: ". Sometimes uneducated people will you know accept it, some educated people will not accept it."

To summarize, the educational or socioeconomic levels of the family may affect their understanding of the patient's condition prior to death. Poor families with a previous loss of an offspring may react less intensely to the bad news. Lack of education may also lead families to refuse medical treatment and to opt for traditional therapies or faith healers thereby endangering the patient's life.

The significance of the gender of the family member became clear as all but one of the doctors expressed reluctance to break the bad news to the patient's mother. This may reflect the doctors' unwillingness to handle strong emotional reactions or their perception that providing support to the female family members who were viewed as more "emotional" was not a part of their job. The educational level of the families has a variable impact on the way that the resident doctors break bad news. The less educated families are viewed as more "accepting" in their attitude.

4. Discussion

4.1 Main theme: Practice

The descriptions of the resident doctors about the actual process of breaking the news of the death of the child to the family were quite similar. All the respondents emphasized that the families must be "prepared" to receive the news of the child's death in a gradual stepwise manner. The doctors usually begin by explaining to the family the nature of the child's illness and his present clinical condition and then go on explain in detail the measures and treatments that are being done to save the child's life. "Preparation" emerged as an important subtheme within the main theme "practice". Preparation referred to - giving the family time to come to terms mentally with the reality of the child's impending death, making the family aware of the ongoing treatments and helping the family members to understand the limitations of doctors and medical interventions in prolonging the child's life.

Preparing the family was seen as an important step towards gaining the trust of the family members and doctors found it easier to break bad news to families who trusted them. The doctors believe that families who receive the news of the child's death without any warning suffer greater psychological distress. When families understand that everything possible is being done to save the child's life, the chances that they will blame doctors for the patient's death are reduced.

The residents stressed the need to not merely convey information to families but also to use language that the family members could comprehend. Most families who receive treatment at the centre of the study often come from poor socioeconomic backgrounds. They are unable to understand medical terms. Hence the residents make sure that the words that they use while explaining the situation to the family are common terms used typically by the people. The residents consciously avoid using medical jargon while speaking with patients' families.

The centre of the study is in a cosmopolitan area where people often come from other parts of the country to find a livelihood. Hence the patients coming here are from diverse linguistic backgrounds and sharing a common language with the family is thought to enhance rapport building. In contrast, a language barrier is a major obstacle to conveying information effectively.

There is reluctance to use the term "death" or "dying" and this probably reflects a general reluctance to openly discussing issues related to death, among the common people as well as the residents in our study setting.

Some factors in the local environment that affect the process of breaking bad news to the families. Despite grueling work hours and lack of time for self care, none of the residents feel that these factors affect the way they break bad news to the family. Certain institutional procedures that have to be followed after the death of a patient are perceived to be distressing for family members. Among the changes that the residents would like to see in their workplace as regards to the practice of breaking bad news are- adequate privacy for the family and a designated person to provide psychological support to the bereaved family.

Five out of the seven respondents had received some formal training in communication skills but none of them found that it affected their practice. Stand alone training sessions without follow up were ineffective in producing any change in practice. Informal methods such as learning from one's own experience and by observing senior staff members as role models were considered to be important in learning communication skills.

Nurses are viewed as playing a supportive role in caring for families of dying children. Some of the residents find it desirable to break the news of death to the family in the presence of security personnel-reflecting that the residents sometimes feel threatened by the families.

4.2 Attitudes

The emerging subthemes here are- Emotional responses, Coping, Influence of personal life and Role.

The residents describe feeling saddened by the death of the paediatric patient, one of the residents reported feeling "devastated" by the patient's death. These emotional responses are more acute during the initial part of the residency training.

Residents felt sadder when they had a better rapport with the patient and the family or had been involved in caring for a longer duration. Playing with the children was seen especially as a bonding activity. One respondent observed that residents may make heroic efforts to save the life of a child to whom they had become attached.

All the residents reflected on a patient's death as a professional learning experience.

The doctors coped with patient deaths by becoming involved in caring for other patients and by talking to their friends and family members. Even though there was no formal mechanism to support the doctors emotionally, senior staff members were sympathetic and this seemed to help the residents.

Residents acknowledged that experiencing a recent personal bereavement or having one's own child probably affected the way they broke bad news to the family; however they consciously tried not to let their personal feelings affect communication with families.

Residents perceive that their main role in caring for the patient is restricted to the physical domain and providing emotional support is seen to be secondary due to lack of time and the emotionally taxing nature of the task.

The need for an additional service that supports families facing the death of child is expressed by all the residents. This may well reflect the felt need for palliative care in the study setting.

4.3 Interpersonal relations

The relationships that the residents form with the patient and the family affect the way that they break bad news of death to the family. Children are considered to be "endearing" unlike adult patients. A child's ability to talk and communicate typically around the age of 4-5 years, increases the bonding with the child. The loss of such a child is considered greater than that of a preverbal child. Even though children with cognitive deficiencies are unable to communicate much with the doctors and the families, such children are considered to be special and evoke more sympathy than other patients. The loss of a neonate is felt more acutely by the residents possibly because they feel that a time of anticipated joy for the family turns into grief.

Residents remark that the loss of a male child is considered by some families to be greater than the loss of a girl child. The attitude is more prevalent among poorer uneducated families where the male child is valued for his potential to add to the family's earning. For the doctors themselves children of either gender are equal. Children who are socially "at risk" are more likely to face gender discrimination. The discrimination against the girl child witnessed by the residents in our study is part of a general societal trend in the country which has seen a falling sex ratio over the past few years.

Factors related to the family which affect death declaration are the expected emotional reactions of the family members, the gender of the family member to whom the bad news is broken and the socioeconomic factors. Doctors are better able to deal with families who trust them and accept the situation as against those who seem to deny the reality of the loss and become aggressive or abusive. All the respondents have either themselves been involved in or have seen colleagues been involved in situations where family members have become abusive.

There is almost a uniform reluctance to break bad news to the female relatives specifically the mother of the child as the mother is expected to become very emotional on hearing the bad news. On the other hand, men are perceived to be in better control of the situation and it is easier to declare death to male relatives.

Some families from a poor socioeconomic background may not be able to fully understand what is going on with the patient. These families may sometimes refuse proper medical treatments and instead go to faith healers. This can be frustrating for the residents who may be unable to save the child's life. However there are often poor families who can comprehend most of the information given to them by doctors as long as medical jargon is avoided.

Based on the above discussion we were able to identify relationships among the various themes and subthemes. As the data were analyzed simultaneously with further data collection, certain emerging themes from the preliminary interviews were explored further in the subsequent interviews. For instance, the strong reluctance to declaring death to the patient's mother emerged in the very first interview. Even though we had included "gender of the family member" as one the prompts in the interview guide, we probed further about the residents' perspectives of breaking bad news to the mother in subsequent interviews. Thus "iterative approach" allowed the investigator to refine data collection based on emerging themes fits the paradigm of grounded theory. (Lingard, et al., 2008).

As data collection and analysis were done in tandem, comparisons within data sets were made constantly. For example, the subtheme "preparation" emerged prominently within the data sets and there was uniform emphasis on preparing the family prior to death declaration. One of the "background assumptions" when we started the data collection was that formal training in communication skills would help residents in breaking bad news to families of dying children. The responses showed that there was divided opinion about the value of training. A closer look at the data showed that the doctors who thought that training was useful were in fact those who had not received the training themselves but presumed that it would be helpful in dealing with families. Hence we conclude that training in communication skills was not helping residents to break bad news to families of dying children.

Interrelationships among the various themes and subthemes emerged and are described in the subsequent paragraphs.

The subthemes "preparation" and "language" are interrelated and are in turn related to the subtheme "Family" as follows. Both the subthemes preparation and language refer to communicating information about the patient's critical condition in a manner that the family can understand. Gaining the families' trust or failing to do so is determined by the efficacy of the doctor-family communication. Families that do not trust doctors may become aggressive or abusive. Thus effective communication is indirectly related to the family's expected reactions to the bad news.

In the subtheme "Roles", it emerges that even though residents believe their role in care giving is mainly limited to the physical aspects rather than the psychological, the need for having an additional person(s) for providing support for families was recognized and a recommendation for such was noted in the subtheme "setting". The subtheme "Roles" is also connected to the subtheme "Patient". When residents see themselves outside the role of professional caregivers, they tended to develop a more personal involvement with the patient e.g. by playing with the child.

Support from senior staff members, categorized under the subtheme "Training and Support" was linked to the subtheme "Coping" as it was considered helpful in dealing with patient deaths. Feelings of sadness or guilt after a death was included in the subtheme "Emotional responses". The various measures that the residents took to overcome these feelings such as sharing with family members or friends were described in the subtheme "Coping".

Predictably enough, personal experiences of bereavement or parenthood seemed to make residents more emotionally sensitive while breaking bad news. Hence the subthemes "Influence of personal life" and "Emotional responses" are interconnected.

5. Limitations of the study

The results of this study are context-specific and hence may not be generalizable to other settings, where patterns of patient load and medical resources may be different. The results of the study are influenced by factors such as the socioeconomic background, gender issues which are characteristic of the patient population served by the centre.

We did not attempt to validate the research findings as it was considered beyond the scope of the present study.

A paediatric palliative care service is in the initial stages of establishment at this centre and this is likely to significantly change the residents' perspectives of breaking bad news to family caregivers of dying children.

6. Future research

This study has helped in identifying several factors which affect communication between resident doctors and families of dying children. Findings from this study may be used to develop a quantitative measure which may be used across similar settings to gain an understanding of the important end of life communication in the general paediatric setting.

It would also be interesting to repeat a similar study in the same setting so as to assess the impact of the new paediatric palliative care service.

7. Conclusions

The process of breaking bad news of the death of the paediatric patient is an important area of practice. A number of factors which affect this process have been identified in this study. The findings of this study can form the basis of further research on the topic and can be used to develop recommendations for improving communication between resident paediatricians and families of critically ill children.

8. References

[1] ACT/RCPCH. 2003. A guide to the development of children's palliative care services: report of the joint working party. 2nd ed. London: ACT/ RCPCH.

[2] Clark, P. 2001. What residents are not learning: observations in an NICU. Academic Medicine 76(5), pp. 419–424.

[3] Contro, N. et al. 2002. Family perspectives on the quality of pediatric palliative care. Archives of Pediatrics and Adolescent Medicine 156(1), pp. 14-19.

[4] Contro, N. et al. 2004. Hospital staff and family perspectives regarding quality of pediatric palliative care. Pediatrics 114(5), pp.1248-1252.

[5] Fallowfield, L. 2004. Communication with the patient and family in palliative medicine. In: Derek, D. et al. eds. Oxford textbook of palliative medicine. 3rd ed. New York: Oxford University Press, pp. 102-108.

[6] Kolarik,R., et al. 2006. Pediatric resident education in palliative care: a needs assessment. Pediatrics 117(6), pp. 1949-1954.

[7] Lingard, L., et al. 2008. Grounded theory, mixed methods, and action research. British Medical Journal 337(7665), pp.459-461.

[8] Maguire , P. and Pitceathly , C. 2002. Key communication skills and how to acquire them. British Medical Journal 325(7366), pp. 697-700.

[9] Pan C. et al. 2005. There is hope for the future: national survey results reveal that geriatric medicine fellows are well-educated in end-of-life care. The Journal of the American Geriatrics Society 53 (4), pp.705–710.

[10] Patton, M. 2002. Qualitative research and evaluation methods. Thousand Oaks: Sage publications.

[11] Pope, C. and Mays, N. 1995. Reaching the parts other methods cannot reach: an introduction to qualitative methods in health and health services research. British Medical Journal 311(6996), pp. 42-45.

[12] Sahler, O. et al. 1981. Factors influencing pediatric interns' relationships with dying children and their parents. Pediatrics 67(2), pp.207-216.

[13] Stevens, M. 2004. Care of the dying child and adolescent: family adjustment and support. In: Derek, D. et al. eds. Oxford textbook of palliative medicine. 3rd ed. New York: Oxford University Press, pp.807-822.

[14] UNICEF. 2009. UNICEF Statistics and monitoring. [Online]. Available at: http://www.unicef.org/infobycountry/india_statistics.html [Accessed: 15 August 2011].

Palliative Care in the Muslim-Majority Countries: The Need for More and Better Care

Deena M. Aljawi[1] and Joe B. Harford[2]
[1]King Faisal Specialist Hospital and Research Center,
[2]National Cancer Institute,
[1]Saudi Arabia
[2]USA

1. Introduction

The need for palliative care around the world is immense. In round numbers, approximately 60 million deaths from all causes will occur worldwide this year. Of all global deaths, approximately 80% will be in low- and middle-income countries (LMIC's). The majority of those dying in LMIC's would be expected to benefit from palliative care, but palliative care services are lacking in most places. Although palliative care is much more than pain relief, palliative care cannot be adequate if pain is going unrelieved. The World Health Organization (WHO) has gone so far as to assert: "A palliative care program cannot exist unless it is based on a rational drug policy including…ready access of suffering patients to opioids." (WHO, 2002). WHO has estimated that 5.5 million people with terminal cancer are not receiving the pain relief they need. In addition, 1 million late-stage HIV-AIDS patients, 800,000 people with injuries lack adequate pain relief (WHO, 2009).

The barriers to the rational use of opioid analgesics are varied depending on location but certain barriers are common. Barriers to accessing oral morphine identified in a survey of healthcare workers, and hospice/palliative care staff in Asia, Africa and Latin America include excessively strict national drug laws and regulations, fear of addiction, poorly developed health care systems, and lack of knowledge at all levels including healthcare providers (Help the Hospices, 2007). Barriers to accessing palliative care in Pakistan, for example, appear similar to those identified elsewhere (Shad et al., 2011). To address and reduce these barriers, changes will need to be affected not only in laws and policies but also in knowledge, attitudes, and behaviors of medical practitioners as well as among patients and their families.

Palliative care involves much more than the alleviation of physical pain but rather encompasses "total pain" as conceptualized by Dame Cicely Saunders, founder of modern hospice care, with total pain including emotional, psychological, social, and spiritual pain (Saunders, 1976; Mehta & Chan, 2008). Issues regarding to spirituality including existential beliefs regarding the meaning of life and extending to include religious beliefs and practices can come to the forefront in patients advanced illnesses (Williams, 2006). Spirituality and religion are coping mechanisms, and where the question has been examined, reports suggest that many patients may wish to discuss their beliefs with their healthcare providers (Ehman et al, 1999). It would appear obvious that for these discussions to be optimally useful, healthcare providers should possess cultural and religious knowledge and sensitivity relevant to the patients being treated.

A report was recently published on the size and distribution of the world's Muslim populations (Pew, 2009). There are currently approximately 1.6 billion Muslims in the world representing 23.4% of the world's population. This number is projected to increase to over 2.2 billion representing 26.4% of the world's population by 2030. Nearly 75% of Muslims live in the 49 Muslim-majority countries (MMC's). Only about 3% of the world's Muslims live in non-Muslim-majority countries of the more-developed world such as Europe, North America, Australia, New Zealand, and Japan. However, many of the health care workers in MMC's are trained in or sent from these countries having relatively small Muslim populations. As such, their exposure to Muslim perspectives on illness and death may be inadequate.

In this chapter, the current situation regarding palliative care services in MMC's will be reviewed. Special attention will be paid to those features of palliative and end-of-life care that have some distinctive in the Muslim culture that ought to be included in any training of healthcare providers. While these issues are perhaps of most relevance to those healthcare workers in MMC's, these considerations are certainly relevant to those working elsewhere. Seventy-two of the world's countries have Muslim populations of more than one million, and this number is projected to rise to 79 countries by 2030. For example, the Muslim share of the US population is expected to more than double by 2030 and will exceed 6 million, making Muslims roughly as numerous as Jews or Episcopalians in the US today. In Europe, there are ten countries including Russia, France, and Belgium where Muslims represent more than 10% of their total population. In the UK, more than one-quarter of new immigrants this year are expected to be Muslim (Pew, 2011). Muslims live and die in every region of the world (see Figure 1), and so healthcare workers in every region of the world should be prepared to provide them with palliative care and end-of-life care in a culturally sensitive way.

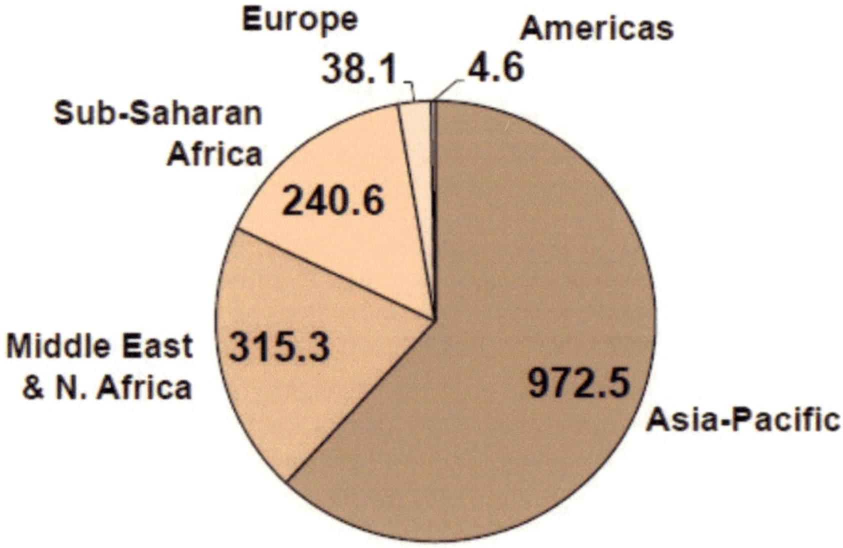

Fig. 1. Distribution of Muslims in the major regions of the world. Numbers shown represent millions of Muslims in each region. (Based on data from Pew Research Center on Religion & public Life: *The Future of the Global Muslim Population*, January 2011).

It is certainly recognized by the authors of this chapter that every human being is unique and that adherents to any religion vary in their beliefs and practices. Islam is no exception. It is a monotheistic religion, but it is not monolithic in terms of knowledge, attitudes, and behaviors as these relate to healthcare more broadly or palliative and end-of-life care in particular. There are two major schools of thought in Islam (Shia and Sunni). Nearly 90% of the world's Muslims are Sunni with most Shia Muslims living in four contries (Iran, Pakistan, India, and Iraq). In certain parts of the world (e.g., Africa), Sufism, which focuses on the mystical elements of Islam exists, and Sufis can be Shia or Sunni. Within any given branch of Islam there is diversity of thought, traditions, and voices. One of the authors (DA) is Muslim and serves as Clinical Nurse Coordinator within the Palliative Care Unit of the King Faisal Specialist Hospital and Research Center in Riyadh, Saudi Arabia, a predominantly Sunni country. This hospital has been at the forefront in developing palliative care services in Saudi Arabia (Gray et al., 1995). Most patients receiving palliative care at this hospital have cancer.

2. The current state of palliative care in Muslim-majority countries

The ability to assess the state of palliative care in a given location is a complicated process and the comparison of one location to another even more complicated since comparable data are not always readily available. Guidance for implementing quality palliative care exits, but the application of these guidelines appears to be predominantly at the level of individual organizations seeking to define themselves in terms of quality rather than as an internationally recognized "model of standard care" (Ferris et. al., 2007). Outcome measures that have been developed for evaluating palliative care have been reviewed (Jocham et. al., 2009). Many of the studies cited by these authors suggest that there is a lack of good quality evidence upon which to base conclusions regarding the appropriate measures for palliative care assessment. Most of the studies covered are from North America and western Europe.

Group as Defined by IOELC	Muslim-majority Countries
No known activity	Afghanistan, Burkina Faso, Chad, Comoros, Djibouti, Guinea, Libya, Maldives, Mali, Mauritania, Niger, Senegal, Somalia, Syria, Turkmenistan, Western Sahara, Yemen
Capacity building	Algeria, Bahrain, Brunei, Kuwait, Lebanon, Oman, Palestinian Authority, Qatar, Sudan, Tajikistan, Tunisia, Turkey, Uzbekistan
Localized provision	Albania, Azerbaijan, Bangladesh, Egypt, Indonesia, Iraq, Jordan, Kazakhstan, Kyrgyzstan, Morocco, Pakistan, Saudi Arabia, Sierra Leone, The Gambia, United Arab Emirates
Approaching integration	Malaysia

Table 1. Distribution of Muslim-majority countries according to the typology of the International Observatory on End-of-Life Care (data from Wright et al., 2008).

Several years ago, the U.S. National Cancer Institute commissioned a survey by the International Observatory on End-of-Life Care (IOELC) of palliative care services within the jurisdictions of the Middle East Cancer Consortium (MECC) and published a monograph containing the results of this analysis (Bingley & Clark, 2008). Four of the members of MECC have Muslim-majority populations (Egypt, Jordan, Palestinian Authority, and Turkey). A summary of the situation analyses conducted by IOELC has also been published (Bingley & Clark, 2009). More recently, the MECC Palliative Care Steering Committee has published country-specific situation analysis for the MECC membership as well as two additional MMC's (Lebanon and Saudi Arabia) (Moore et al., 2011). These situation analyses, while useful, were based on input from a relatively small number of healthcare workers from each jurisdiction.

The IOELC has also published a survey of palliative care services around the world (Wright et al., 2008). The countries of the world that were analyzed were placed by the IOELC into four categories of palliative care activity. The four-category typology depicts levels of hospice-palliative care development with "approaching integration" being the most advanced category. Countries in this category are characterized by a critical mass of activists; multiple providers and service types; an awareness of palliative care on the part of health professionals and local communities; the availability of strong, pain-relieving drugs; an impact of palliative care upon policy; the development of recognized education centers; academic links forged with universities; and the existence of a national association (Wright et al., 2008). Of the 234 countries analyzed by the IOELC, 35 countries (15%) were placed in the "Approaching integration" category. Of Muslim-majority countries that were analyzed, only Malaysia was characterized as being in this most advanced category (see Table 1). Seventeen MMC's were placed in the "No known activity" category, 13 in the "Capacity building" category, and 15 in the "localized provision" category. In general, the countries in Group 4 ("Approaching integration") tend to have higher GDP per capita than in those in the other three groups suggesting that palliative care services might be a prerogative of high-income countries. However, the more wealthy MMC's with GDP per capita in excess of $20,000 (Bahrain, Brunei, Kuwait, Oman, Qatar, Saudi Arabia, and United Arab Emirates) are absent from Category 4. Five of these countries are in Category 2 ("Capacity building") and 2 are in Category 3 ('Localized provision").

This situation analysis enabled its authors to calculate the ratio of services to the population of the country providing a measure of how many thousands of persons would theoretically be served by each service. These ratios for selected MMC's are provided in Table 2 along with comparators of the United States and the United Kingdom. The MMC with the most favorable ratio was again Malaysia wherein 37 services were identified, and there was an average of 685,000 persons per service. This ration compares to 43,000 for the UK and 90,000 for the US. The least favorable ratio was seen in Pakistan where only 1 service was identified for a population of 157,935,000. With the exception of Malaysia with 37 services, no other MMC had more than 3 services identified. As an example of the disparity in hospice/palliative care services, Egypt with a slightly larger in population than the UK was found to have 3 services whereas the UK had nearly 1400 services.

Palliative care services can take the form of palliative consulting services within a hospital, dedicated palliative beds within a hospital, a stand-alone hospice facility, and homecare palliative/hospice services. One of the principles of a "good death" from the Muslim

Region	Country	Services	Ratio 1:1000's
Europe	Azerbaijan	1	8,411
Western Asia	UAE	2	1,344
	Jordan	2	2,852
	Saudi Arabia	3	8,191
	Iraq	1	28,807
Asia Pacific	Malaysia	37	685
	Bangladesh	3	42,274
	Pakistan	1	157,935
Africa	The Gambia	1	1,517
	Sierra Leone	1	5,525
	Egypt	3	24,678
	Morocco	1	34,487
Comparators	UK	1,397	43
	US	3,300	90

Table 2. Hospice-palliative care services and indicative ratios of hospice-palliative care services to populations in selected Muslim-majority countries with comparison to the United Kingdom and the United States (data from Wright et al., 2008).

perspective would be to have access to hospice services in any location, not only in the hospital (Tayeb et al., 2011). Reflective of the extended family structure that is typical in Muslim families, it has been reported that most Muslim families would prefer to care for relatives at home and that patients would prefer to die at home (Gartrad, 1994; Gardener, 1998; Sarhill et al., 2001), although there has been little or no research on this topic in most MMCs. Muslim families may feel that sending a relative to a hospital without curative intent may be a form of shirking of the responsibility to care for family members at the end of life. In one study, some participants in a survey stated that they preferred to die in a holy place like a mosque or in Makkah or Medina (Tayeb et al., 2011), but this may reflect religious idealism rather than practicality. Historically, care for the dying has been seen as a family responsibility and death has been generally managed at home (Gatrad & Sheikh, 2002). However, the lack of home care services in most MMC's can lead to return trips to the hospital and/or extended stays and death in a hospital. This dilemma may also be exacerbated by the long distances that more rural patients may need to travel to get to hospitals that are usually located in urban settings. Expansion of palliative care and hospice services including access to opioid analgesics in the home setting has the potential of relieving the patient load on in-hospital services.

Another measure of palliative care activity is provided in analysis of the use of opioid analgesics. Palliative care involves, of course, much more than pain relief. Indeed, advanced cancer patients experience a range of symptoms that require medical management. Cancer patients tend to experience multiple symptoms including what has been termed "symptom clusters" i.e., two or more symptoms that present together (Fan et al., 2007; Jimenez et al., 2011). Symptom clustering has also been documented in Muslim patients in Kuwait (Alshemmari et al., 2011). Granting that pain control is not synonymous with palliative care, use of opiod analgesics nonetheless provides a "barometer" for palliative care, and data on opioid consumption are available. The amounts of opioid analgesics consumed in a year are monitored by the International Narcotics Control Board (INCB), an agency of the United Nations located in Vienna, Austria. There are a number of ways in which opioid analgesic consumption might be compared among countries. The website of the Pain Policy Study Group (PPSG) of the University of Wisconsin (see http://www.painpolicy.wisc.edu/) presents data collected by the INCB. Given that there are many forms of opioid analgesics (e.g., fentanyl, hydromorphoe, methadone, oxycodone, pethidine, in addition to morphine itself), the PPSG website has converted the quantities of each form into "morphine equivalents". This enables one to compare consumption between countries that may utilize different forms of opioid analgesics for whatever reason. The use of fentanyl transdermal patches has become increasingly popular. For example, over 50% of the morphine equivalents in Egypt and Saudi Arabia and more than 90% of the morphine equivalents in Turkey are fentanyl according to the INCB database for 2008 (see http://www.painpolicy.wisc.edu/). Fentanyl transdermal patches are a rather expensive form of opioid analgesics, and it would be of interest to explore the reasons for increasing use of fentanyl in MMC's.

Using the INCB data, countries can be compared for total morphine equivalents consumed per capita. Not surprisingly, the range is very large with most of the world's morphine consumed by countries representing a relatively small fraction of the world's population. In general, there is a correlation between a country's income and it use of opioid analgesics. Indeed, approximately 80% of morphine is consumed by 7 high income countries representing <10% of the world's population. Developing countries, which represent >80% of the world's population, account for <10% of global morphine consumption. In about 150 countries, the use of morphine is severely restricted. Palliative care services in most MMC's countries in the world are indeed quite limited. It is noteworthy, that among the exceptions to the correlation between income and opioid analgesic usage are the relatively wealthy countries of the Arab Gulf where opioid use is low despite a high average income.

Perhaps more meaningful than opioid consumption would be evaluation of consumption of opioids in comparison to the need for pain relief. Recently, a study was published by Seya et al. (2011) that proposed a rough but simple way for estimating the total population need for opioids for treating moderate to severe pain. The authors calculated the needs for terminal cancer patients, terminal HIV patients and lethal injury patients and corrected for the needs associated with pain from other causes (e.g., nonlethal cancers, nonlethal injuries, non-end-stage HIV, surgery, sickle cell episodes, childbirth, chronic nonmalignant pain). The calculation resulted in an "adequacy of consumption measure" (ACM). Based on these methods an ACM of 1.00 or more was deemed to represent "adequate" access to opioid analgesics relative to need. An ACM between 0.30 and 1.00 was considered to as "moderate" consumption relative to need; an ACM between 0.1 and 0.3 as "low" relative to need; an ACM of between 0.03 and 0.1 was deemed to be "very low" relative to need, and an ACM of under 0.03 was deemed to be "virtually nonexistent" consumption of opioid analgesics. The study was based on morphine equivalents and so represented use of all forms of opioids. Globally, this analysis of 188 countries painted a very bleak picture with only 7% of the world's population judged to have adequate access to opioid analgesics. The situation in MMCs was even more grim. No MMC was found to fall into the adequate, moderate, or even low categories i.e., all were in either the very low or virtually nonexistent categories. Figure 2 is based on these data for the fifteen MMCs with the largest populations and ordered in the figure according to decreasing ACMs.

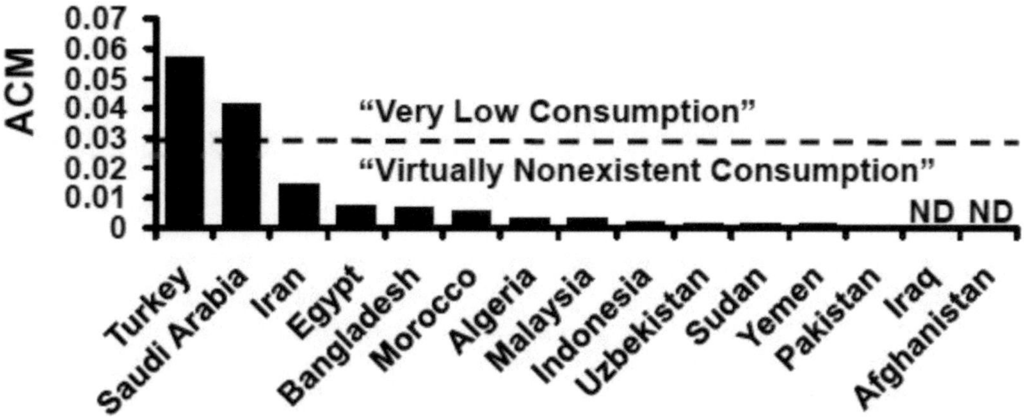

Fig. 2. Consumption of opioid analgesics in the fifteen largest Muslim-majority countries ordered by decreasing ACM. The dashed line represents the boundary between "very low consumption" and "virtually nonexistent consumption" based on the data and definitions of Seya et al. (2011). ACM = adequacy of consumption measure. ND = no data. By comparison, the ACM for the US was calculated to be 2.48.

The extremely low consumption of opoiods in MMC's is very troubling because it means that most dying patients in these countries are suffering unnecessarily. Considering cancer patients alone, the MMCs represent approximately 835,000 deaths from cancer (all cancer sites excluding non-melanoma skin) each year according to the GLOBOCAN 2008 database of the International Agency for Research on Cancer (www.iarc.fr). Physical suffering of cancer patients has been addressed and the prevalence of various symptoms including pain documented (Teunissen et al., 2007). In a small survey of adult patients in Kuwait, pain was the most common and most distressing symptom with 82% of the patients having physical pain (Alshemmari et al., 2010). It is estimated that adequate pain relief can be achieved in up to 90% of patients using existing WHO treatment guidelines available in multiple languages including Arabic (Sepulveda et al., 2002).

There is a paucity of research in MMC's on the barriers to opioid use that might exist in MMC's. As in other settings, the barriers are likely to be a multifaceted and complex mixture of legal/policy aspects combined with lack of knowledge and misguided attitudes on the part of policy makers and healthcare providers in addition to patients and their families. Fear of diversion of narcotics from patients is one concern, but it has been found to be rare or non-existent in one MMC (Malaysia) (Devi et al., 2008). It has been suggested that Muslims may perceive suffering as a means of atoning for ones sins (Al-Shahri & Al-Khenaizan, 2005). To the extent that this interpretation exists among Muslim patients, it may contribute to low opioid usage in MMC's. It should be noted that clearly not all Muslims adhere to this idea, and the linkage of suffering and atonement is not unique to Islam but is also a belief held by some Christians for example. More research is needed to understand the barriers to opioid usage in MMC's. It is likely that there will be distinctions found from country to country even within the MMC's, so local research would be most appropriate. Once the barriers are better understood, educational efforts aimed at overcoming the barriers can be designed, evaluated, and implemented. Since 2006, the INCB has requested annually that all governments promote rational medical use of opioid analgesics, and there is recognition that pain relief is a component of the human right to the highest attainable standard of mental and physical health or a human right on its own (Help the Hospices, 2007; Seya et al., 2011).

The Global Access to Pain Relief Initiative (GAPRI) is a joint programme of the Union for International Cancer Control and the American Cancer Society to make effective pain control measures universally available to cancer patients in pain by 2020, in line with Target 8 of the World Cancer Declaration. GAPRI's projects are designed to address these key objectives: creating stronger collaboration between cancer and HIV communities around pain treatment; improving the market for essential pain medicines; empowering governments to take the lead in expanding access to pain relief; addressing health systems challenges at multiple levels; and mainstreaming the issue of pain treatment in global health efforts (see http://www.uicc.org/programmes/about-gapri).

3. The need for additional healthcare workers trained in palliative care

The need for additional healthcare workers trained in palliative care was recognized for the U.S. in 1994 when the NCI noted, "There are few formally structured programs for training in palliative patient care available in the United States" and issued a request for applications "To stimulate medical schools…to design methodologies for the education and training of health care professionals in hospice and palliative care." Nonetheless, even in the U.S., a minority of medical schools appear to require training in palliative care and to evaluate students in their care of patients with advanced, incurable conditions. Nursing training in palliative care in the U.S. is also inadequate. Although comparable assessments of professional school training in palliative care within LMICs are sparse, it would not appear that the topic is covered even remotely in proportion to the need for palliative care in these venues.

Several years ago, the U.S. National Cancer Institute (NCI) commissioned the U.S. Institute of Medicine to produce a publication entitled "Cancer Control Opportunities in Low- and Middle-Income Countries." (Sloan & Gelband, 2007). Among the statements made in this publication was "Ideally, medical, nursing, and social work students (and other relevant health care workers) will receive training in palliative care and practitioners will incorporate palliative care into routine practice." Unfortunately this is not yet the reality. Contributing to the lack of palliative care services in MMC's is a paucity of healthcare workers with knowledge of the basic principles and specific skills of palliative care delivery.

Recognizing the importance of palliative care education and the advantages of distance learning, the Institute for Palliative Medicine in San Diego, CA, with support from the U.S. National Cancer Institute's Office of International Affairs, has launched a website through which healthcare professionals worldwide can access training resources in palliative care. It is hoped that this web portal [referred to as the *International Palliative Care Resource Center* (IPCRC)] will contribute to the desperate need for additional capacity for palliative care service delivery and palliative care research not only in MMC's but in LMICs more generally (see www.ipcrc.net).

An optimal situation would be for all healthcare workers to have basic knowledge and skills in palliative care, those treating cancer, AIDS, and geriatric patients to have more advanced skills, and those members of specialist palliative care teams to possess expert skills. While there are a number of educational materials available for healthcare workers in different disciplines (e.g., under "Education" at www.ipcrc.net), most of these resources address more advanced or specialist skills and virtually all are in English. While these materials are quite useful in many venues, there are other locations where English language skills of nurses, in particular, are limited so as to render these educational materials of limited utility. It is also the case that educational materials that are currently available have not generally been tailored so as to include considerations of religious and cultural distinctive of Muslims.

As part of an effort to address this issue and to build capacity for palliative care services in the Arab world, a course for Arabic-speaking nurses was created to be pilot tested in Tanta, Egypt. This course targets all nurses not only those working or aiming to work in a palliative care unit, consulting service, or hospice. The course is designed to convey the basic knowledge and skills in palliative care that would be beneficial to all nurses. It is anticipated that subsequent to this basic training, a subset of nurses will be selected for more advanced and ultimately specialist training. The basic skills course for nurses may be of use throughout the Arab-speaking world. In addition, such a course could be adapted to meet the needs of nurses who speak languages other than Arabic.

There have been publications regarding palliative care in Muslim patients that have attempted to address distinctives of Islam and Muslim culture that should be understood by healthcare workers who are treating Muslim patients (Al-Shahri & Al-Khenazian, 2005; Gatrad, 1994; Gatrad & Sheikh 2002a, 2002b; Sarhill et al., 2001; Sheikh, 1998; Tayeb et al, 2010). In one instance, over 250 Muslims in Saudi Arabia were surveyed and some interviewed as to what constitutes a "good death" starting with the elements identified in Western communities (Tayeb et al, 2010). These authors found that participants identified elements in three main domains: 1.Faith and belief; 2. Self-esteem and image to friends and family; and 3. Satisfaction about family security after the death of the patient. Given the centrality of the family in the Saudi culture, it is not surprising that two of the three domains were family-oriented. An attempt has been made to incorporate these and other Muslim-centered elements into the Arabic nursing training in palliative and end-of-life care described above. In most instances, the Arabic-speaking nurses being trained are themselves Muslims as are the vast majority of the patients they are serving. The Muslim-centered elements that have been included will only be summarized briefly here.

Modesty is a highly regarded value in most Muslim cultures. For example, in Saudi Arabia, an *abaya* (full body cloak) and *tarha* (head covering) is nearly universal, and many women also cover their faces. Unnecessary touching between unrelated adults of the opposite sex is considered highly inappropriate. In some cases, a Saudi woman, for example, might be uncomfortable even communicating with an unrelated man and may be more comfortable if discussions with a male healthcare provider were carried out through a close male relative. Once again, we would note that discomfort with a healthcare provider of the opposite sex is not unique to the Muslim culture. It may be more common in Muslim cultures however, and it should not be disregarded in the delivery of care. Asking permission to touch for hands-on medical care may not be the norm for Western-trained physicians and nurses but it would be considered appropriate in the case of a Muslim patient of the opposite sex.

One very fundamental tenets of Islam based on the Noble Qur'an is that the death of every individual is predetermined by Allah, and only Allah knows when that death will occur.

Conversations with patients and families regarding prognosis and life expectancy need to recognize this belief, and be in general terms describing the natural history of the given terminal illness. Nonetheless, the family would likely appreciate knowing when death appears imminent, so they can be around the patient in his/her final hours and be prepared for the Muslim funeral rites that aim for speedy burial.

When Muslims are sick, their friends and relatives tend to visit and sometimes in rather large numbers for rather extended visits. Western trained healthcare workers may find this somewhat unusual, but consideration should be given to the point where the visitors are in someway impeding the delivery of care. Near the end of the patients life the family may wish to read passages from the Qur'an or recite *Shahadah* that bears witness to Allah being the only God and Muhammad (pbuh) being the messanger of Allah. The *Shahadah* is one of the five pillars of Islam, and it is generally desired that these be the last words heard by and on the lips of the patient in this life. One concern regarding the use of opioid analgesics may be that morphine-induced sedation might interfere with the ability of the patient to recite the *Shahadah* or hear the Qur'an being read.

Some families may not wish their dying relative to be fully informed regarding his/her illness. While this is certainly not unique to Islam, it is perhaps somewhat more common in Muslim families than in Western families today. In some instances, the patients and relatives may be engaging in what has been termed "mutual pretense" (Bluebond-Langer, 1978) i.e., both the patient and his/her family know that the patient is dying but the topic is avoided with each pretending that the other doesn't know the real situation.

Another of the five pillars of Islam is the *Salah,* five daily prayers, and these are to be performed in sickness and in health if the patient is cognitively able. Accommodation of the patient's ability to perform the *Salah* should be made if at all possible. If bed-ridden, the prayers can be performed in bed. Muslims usually prefer that the prayer times be in a quiet environment, and the patient should be facing Makkah. In a hospital located in an MMC, the direction of Makkah would be known, but Muslim patients in a non-Muslim setting may need assistance in identifying the direction to pray and orienting their bed so as to allow them to face Makkah. It is desirable to time medical interventions so as to avoid the time of prayers. Another aspect of the daily prayers that has implications in a hospital setting relates to cleanliness. The clothes and body of the patient should be free of urine, stool, vomit, and blood at the time of the prayers. Washing before prayers may also require that special accommodations be made and assistance rendered. Another concern regarding the use of opioid analgesics may be that morphine-induced sedation might interfere with the ability of the patient to pray.

Muslim dietary considerations also may come into play in caring for the terminally ill Muslim patient. Here again, the basic dietary restrictions of Islam would be less of a concern in a care facility located in an MMC but could be an issue in a non-MMC setting such as in the US or Europe. Ramadan is celebrated by Muslims in the ninth lunar month of each year, and during Ramadan, the *Sawm,* another pillar of Islam is observed. This requires abstinence from food and drink during the daytime. Although the sick can be exempted from the mandate to fast, many Muslim patients will desire to keep Ramadan. Adjustment of meal times is one accommodation that can be made. Perhaps more challenging is that the restrictions of Ramadan may be interpreted to include certain medical interventions relevant to palliative care e.g., oral medications, blood transfusions and intravenous fluids, although injections, transdermal patches (e.g., fentanyl), enemas, and suppositories are permissible (Al-Shahri, 2002).

Another pillar of the Muslim faith is the *Hajj*, a pilgrimage to Makkah once in life. As Muslim patients come to appreciate that their life is approaching its end, they may well wish to go to Makkah prior to dying. The *Hajj* rites may take days to complete and may be quite strenuous for an ailing patient. Planning for a *Hajj* (or an abbreviated pilgrimage called *Omrah*) is likely to require cooperation between the family of the patient and the palliative care team.

When death of the patient occurs, it is important to assist the family in preparation for burial which is to be performed as quickly as possible. Autopsy is not generally done except for legal or possible public health reasons. Immediately following death, the eyes and mouth of the deceased should be closed, the body freed of all needles, tubes, etc., and the limbs straightened. Generally, members of the family of the deceased perform a ritual washing and shrouding of the body in preparation for burial. The major assistance to be rendered to the family by the healthcare team is the timely completion of necessary paperwork (e.g., the death certificate) so as to release the body to the family as quickly as possible for burial.

4. Conclusions and recommendations

Muslims make up nearly one-quarter of the people on earth and are in the majority in 49 countries. Based either on assessment of available palliative care services or on the consumption of opioid analgesics, it is very clear that palliative care is severely lacking in MMC's. This is true not only in the low- and middle-income MMC's (e.g., Pakistan, Bengladesh, and the MMC's of Africa) but also in the higher income countries of Arab gulf. More research is needed to understand the barriers to the use of opioid analgesics in MMC's. At least one of these barriers may have ties to Muslim concepts of suffering and death, and these can be addressed. In Saudi Arabia, for example, a fatwa (a legal pronouncement in Islam, issued by a religious law specialist on a specific issue) has been issued that supports the use of opioid analgesics for relief of pain.

The paucity of palliative care services in MMC's clearly needs to be addressed, although this an issue that goes far beyond MMC's (Wright et al., 2008). Ideally, these services would encompass consultative services within each hospital, dedicated beds for a palliative care unit, stand-alone hospices, and home-care palliative care and hospice services. The ideal set forth by the IOELC is "integration" into the healthcare system. Were this to be achieved in MMC's, the deaths of the over 800,000 individuals who die each year from cancer in MMC's as well as those from other causes would approach a "good death." This integration would mean that palliative care would be a part of multidisciplinary case management from diagnosis and not merely appended at the end of life.

A clear barrier to the desired integration of palliative care into healthcare is simply the shortage of physicians and nurses with specialized or advanced training in palliative care delivery. Clearly, training and capacity building in palliative care should be a high priority of the governments of the MMC's as well as the international community as a whole. While there are existing educational material and curricula in palliative care (see www.IPCRC.net under "Education"), almost all of this training material is in English. It should also be a priority to produce educational materials in other languages (probably via translation and adaptation of existing content). This issue is of particular importance when it comes to training nurses, since it is often the case that their English skills as a group are on average less advanced than those of physicians in the same country.

It is, of course, also important that material in all languages, including English, reflect cultural sensitivity and recognize that certain aspects of the Muslim religion and/or culture have an impact on delivery of healthcare more broadly and on palliative and end-of-life care in particular. In some MMC's, many or even most of healthcare workers are either trained in or come from Western countries. Despite the fact that the vast majority of the patients they treat are Muslims, their training and experience in a Muslim-minority setting may have left them poorly equipped to deliver high quality palliative and end-of-life to their Muslim patients. It is clear that modules related to cultural and religious distinctives should be added to palliative care training courses and programs. Such modules would benefit not only those healthcare workers who practice in MMC's but also those working in settings where the Muslims are a minority (e.g., the US and Europe). In many of these settings, the fraction of the population represented by Muslims is projected to rise in the future.

5. References

Al-Shahri (2002). Culturally sensitive caring for Saudi patients. *J. Transcult. Nursing* 13, 133-138.

Al-Shahri, M.Z. & Al-Khenaizan, A. (2005) Palliative care for Muslim patients. *J. Support. Oncol.* 3, 432-438.

Alshemmari, S., Ezzat, H., Samir, Z., Sajnani, K. & Alsirafy, S., Symptom burden in hospitalized patients with cancer in Kuwait and the need for palliative care. *Am. J. Hospice & Palliat. Med.* 27:446-449.

Bingley, A. & Clark, D. (2008). *Palliative care in the region represented by the Middle East Cancer Consortium: A review and comparative analysis.* National Cancer Institute. NIH Pub. No. 07-2630, Bethesda, MD.

Bingley, A. & Clark, D. (2009). A comparative review of palliative care development in six countries represented by the Middle East Cancer Consortium (MECC). *J. Pain & Symptom Manage.* 37, 287-296.

Bluebond-Langner, M. (1978) Mutual pretence: cause and consequence. In: *The Private Worlds of Dying Children*. Princeton University Press, Princeton, NJ: 210-230.

Devi, B.C.R., Tang, T.S. & Corbex, M. (2008). Setting up home-based palliative care in countries of limited resources: A model from Sarawak, Malaysia. *Ann. Oncol.* 19, 2061-2066.

Ehman, J.W., Ott, B.B., Short, T.H., Ciampa, R.C. & Hansen-Flaschen, J. (1999). Do patients want their physicians to inquire about their spiritual or religious beliefs if they become gravely ill? *Arch. Intern. Med.* 159, 1803-1806.

Fan, G., Filipczak, L., Chow, E. (2007). Symptom clusters in cancer patients: A review of the literature. *Curr. Oncol.* 14:207-282.

Ferris, F.D., Gomez-Batiste, X., Furst, C.J. & Connor, S. (2007). Implementing quality palliative care. *J. Pain & Symp. Manege.* 33, 533-541.

Gardener, K. (1998). Death, burial and bereavement amongst Bengali Muslims. *J. Ethn. Migr. Stud.* 24:507-521.

Gatrad, A.R. (1994). Muslim customs surrounding death, bereavement, postmortem examinations, and organ transplants. *BMJ* 309, 521-523.

Gatrad, A.R. & Sheikh, A. (2002). Palliative care for Muslims and issues before death. *Int. J. Palliative Nursing* 8, 526-531.

Gatrad, A.R. & Sheikh, A. (2002). Palliative care for Muslims and issues after death. *Int. J. Palliative Nursing* 8, 594-597..

Gray, A.J., Ezzat, A. & Volker, S. (1995). Developing palliative care services for terminally ill patients in Saudi Arabia. *Ann. Saudi Med.* 15, 370-377.

Help the Hospices (2007), Access to Pain Relief—An Essential Human Right. URL: http://www.helpthehospices.org.uk/our-services/international/resources/developing-services/drugs-and-pain-control/

Jimenez, A., Madero, R., Alonso, A., Martinez-Marin, V., Vilches, Y., Martinez, B., Feliu, M., Diaz, L., Espinosa, E. & Feliu, J. (2011). Symptom clusters in advanced cancers. *J. Pain & Sympt. Manage.* 42, 2431.

Jocham, H.R., Dassen, T., Widdershoven, G. & Halfens, R. (2009). Evaluating palliative care—a review of the literature. *Palliat. Care Res. & Treat.* 3, 5-12.

Mehta, A. & Chan, L.S. (2008). Understanding the concept of total pain: A prerequisite for pain control. *J. Hospice & Palliat. Nursing* 10, 26-32.

Moore, S.Y., Pirrello, R.D., Christianson, S.K. & Ferris, F.D. (2011). Strategic planning by the palliative care steering committee of the Middle East Cancer Consortium. *J. Pediatr. Hematol. Oncol.* 33, Supplement 1, S39-S46.

Pew Research Center on Religion & Public Life (2009). *Mapping the Global Muslim Population.* October, 2009. URL: http://www.pewforum.org/Muslim/Mapping-the-Global-Muslim-Population.aspx

Pew Research Center on Religion & Public Life (2011). *The Future of the Global Muslim Population.* January 2011. URL: http://www.pewforum.org/The-Future-of-the-Global-Muslim-Population.aspx

Sarhill, N., LeGrand, S., Islambouli, R., Davis, M.P. & Walsh, D. (2001) The terminally ill Muslim: Death and dying from a Muslim Perspective. *Am. J. Hospice & Palliat. Care* 18, 251-255.

Saunders CM. (1976). The challenge of terminal care. In: Symington T, Carter RL, eds. *Scientific Foundations of Oncology.* London, England: Heinemann. p. 673 -679.

Sepulveda, C., Marlin, A. Yoshida, T. & Ullrich, A. (2002) Palliative care: The World Health Organization's global perspective. *J. Pain Symptom Manage.* 24, 91-96.

Seya, M.-J., Gelders, S.F.A.M., Achara, O.U., Milani, B. & Scholten, W.K. (2011). A first comparison between the consumption of and the need for opioid analgesics at country, regional, and global levels. *J. Pain & Palliative Care Pharmacotherapy* 25, 6-18.

Shad, A., Ashraf, M.S. & Hafeez, H. (2011) Development of palliative-care services in a developing country: Pakistan. *J. Pediatr. Hematol. Oncol.* 33, Supplement 1, S62-S63..

Sheikh, A. (1998) Death and dying—a Muslim perspective. J. Royal Soc. Med. 91, 138-140.

Sloan F.A. & Gelband H. (2007) *Cancer Control Opportunities in Low- and Middle-Income Countries.* National Academies Press (US), Washington, DC.

Tayeb, M.A., Al-Zamel, E., Fareed, M.M. & Abouellail, H.A. (2010). A "good death": Perspectives of Muslim patients and health care providers. *Ann. Saudi Med.* 30, 215-221.

Teunissen, S.C., Wesker, W., Kruitwagen, C., de Haas, H.C., Voest, E.E. & de Graeff (2007). Symptom prevalence in patients and incurable cancer: A systematic review. *J. Pain Symptom Manage* 34, 94-104.

World Health Organization (2002). National cancer control programmes: Policies and managerialguidelines (2nd ed.), World Health Organization,Geneva, p. 87. URL: http://www.who.int/cancer/nccp/nccp/en

World Health Organization (2009). Access to Controlled Medications Programme. Improving access to medications controlled under international drug conventions. World Health Organization briefing note 2009. URL: www.who.int/medicines/areas/quality_safety/ACMP_BrNoteGenrl_EN_Feb09.pdf

Williams, A.L. (2006). Perspectives on spirituality at the end of life: A meta-summary. *Palliat. Support. Care* 4, 407-417.

Wright, M., Wood, J., Lynch, T. & Clark, D. (2008). Mapping levels of palliative care development: A global view, *J. Pain Symptom Manage.* 35, 469-485.

10

Challenges in Advanced Dementia

Esther Chang and Amanda Johnson
University of Western Sydney,
Australia

1. Introduction

This chapter presents the significant challenges in practice health professionals' face in providing care to people with advanced dementia. These challenges constitute all facets of care giving inclusive of physical, psychological and spiritual care. Worldwide advanced dementia is an increasingly burdensome health issue. People with advanced dementia have substantial care needs at the end of their life (Birch & Stokoe, 2010). The Alzheimer's Disease International report (2010) stated there were 35.6 million people living with dementia. The report estimates the number of people living with dementia worldwide will increase to 65.7 million by 2030 and 115.4 million by 2050 (Alzheimer's Disease International, 2010). Further the majority of people will live in low and middle income countries (Alzheimer's Disease International, 2010). In 2010, the financial burden of dementia was costed at US$ 604 billion (Alzheimer's Disease International, 2010). The Alzheimer's Disease International, 2010 report predicts that "these costs account for around 1% of the world's gross domestic product, varying from 0.24% in low income countries, to 0.35% in low, middle income countries, 0.50% in high, middle income countries, and 1.24% in high income countries" (Alzheimer's Disease International, 2010, p.5).

A high proportion of people with dementia need some level of care to supplement their cognitive decline. This care can range from minimal support of individual activities for example, shopping to a full range of personal care. As the person declines and the disease progresses total supervision necessitating 24hr care across 7 days per week, of all activities of daily living, is required. The Alzheimer's Disease International, 2010 report states that the cost of informal care (unpaid) provided by families and the direct costs of care by health professionals in residential aged care facilities, equates to being the world's 18th largest economy (Alzheimer's Disease International, 2010). Evidence also suggests that a lack of training, education and support for both health professionals and informal caregivers is still present (Chang, et al., 2005; Chang, et al., 2009). Thus the challenges before the community are significant and need to be responded to in a planned, informed and educated manner so that people dying from dementia can be the recipients of quality care at the end of their life.

2. Dementia

Dementia is a progressive, incurable disorder severely limiting an individual's functional ability and quality of life (Access Economics, 2009). It is a collective term used to describe a series of symptoms resulting from impaired cognitive function that affect the person's memory, thinking, behaviour, psychological capacity and the ability to perform activities of daily living (Emre, 2009; Sampson, 2009). After age 65, the likelihood of developing dementia roughly doubles every five years (Alzheimer's Disease International, 2010). For people aged 65 years or older, more than 10% are affected by dementia (McKeel, Burns, Meuser & Morris, 2007). Alzheimer's disease is the most frequently experienced type of dementia [31%] followed by: vascular dementia [22%], dementia with Lewy bodies [11%] and the fronto-temporal lobar degeneration dementias [7.8%] (Sampson, 2009). The disease trajectory for dementia is protracted and is considered to unfold over a series of stages. These stages consist of mild, moderate and severe. The proportion of Americans aged 65 years and older with mild dementia represented 28% in 2010 (with a projected decrease to 23% in 2050); moderate dementia represented 31% in 2010 (with a projected decrease to 29% in 2050) and severe dementia represented 41% in 2010 (with a projected increase to 48% in 2050) (Alzheimer's Association, 2010). These percentages provide insight into not only the prevalence of the disease but also the escalating need for palliative care to play a role.

2.1 Advanced dementia

Advanced dementia is the term used to denote a combination of both the severe and end stages of this disease. This term refers to progressive immobility and reduced capacity for self care; poor nutrition resulting from reduced fluid and liquid intake; infections related to immobility; skin breakdown and general debilitation (Shuster, 2000). Recognition of dementia as a terminal disease has been slow and it is only now that a body of evidence is emerging upon which to base practice (Chang et al., 2008; Hancock et al., 2006). In the USA, Alzheimer's disease ranks as the sixth leading cause of death (Alzheimer's Association, 2011). Of greater significance and impact on the worldwide community is the reported 66% increase in death rates from dementia as compared to all other leading causes of death which have declined (Alzheimer's Association, 2011). Further people dying from dementia are reported to have the presence of a co-morbid condition in 19% or higher of cases (Moss, Braunschweig, & Rubinstein, 2002). Thus the provision of care in this context is multifactorial and complex (Sampson, 2010). This context demonstrates the requirement for an educated and skilled staff in the provision of palliative care principles to provide care to the person dying from dementia to ensure their needs and those of the family are adequately met (Chang, et al., 2005; Chang, et al., 2009; Chang & Walter, 2010; Johnson, et al., 2009).

Recent acknowledgement of dementia as a terminal illness has been made by recognising that it is a disease in which a steady deterioration occurs that leads to death (Albinsson, & Strang, 2002; Mitchell, et al., 2009). This recognition has come about because advanced dementia is now perceived to have a similar symptom burden and prognosis to advanced cancer (Sampson, 2010). Further acknowledgement of dementia as a terminal illness is made with researchers providing evidence of the need for the principles of palliative care to be applied to those suffering from dementia along with those who have a diagnosis of incurable cancer (Fulton et al., 2011). It is argued that the application of palliative care principles makes an important contribution to the comfort of the person with dementia and the family's wellbeing and that this introduction should occur much earlier on in the dementia illness trajectory (Fulton et al., 2011). However Chang and Walter (2010) assert that few people in nursing homes or long term care facilities with advanced dementia are recognised as being 'at risk' for death. They claim that until advanced dementia is formally diagnosed as a terminal illness, the lack of prognostication will serve as a barrier to the principles of palliative care being applied in this context (Chang & Walter, 2010). Banerjee &

Owen (2009) report that only 1/3 of people are ever formally provided a diagnosis of dementia which therefore exacerbates an already difficult care situation for health professionals to know when to intervene with palliative care principles, as it lies substantially unacknowledged.

2.2 Palliative care

In the following section we will examine the dying trajectory for a person with advanced dementia. The trajectory presents a multitude of symptoms and behaviours affecting the person's mind, body and spirit which poses many challenges for family members and health professionals. Failure to identify and address these needs may mean the person dying and their family will have unmet needs leading to physical, emotional, mental and spiritual distress and the diminished capacity for healthy bereavement in family members following the death of the person with dementia. Incorporating a holistic approach to care ensures that these unmet needs are addressed and appropriate interventions implemented to promote quality care at the end of life for all involved.

2.2.1 Holistic approach to caring for a person with advanced dementia

In striving for a holistic approach to care and a healthy state we need balance and harmony in all aspects of the person's life - physical, social, emotional, cognitive and spiritual to be present irrespective of the presence or absence of physical disease and mental illness. A person's wholeness is the dynamic interaction of the mind, body and spirit components within the person, between and among others and with the universe (Erickson, 2007, p.140). When a holistic approach to care is adopted in advanced dementia the journey taken by both the, informal carer, health professional and the person is of a healing nature. Healing is a core element to a palliative care philosophy which promotes harmony and balance in the terminal phase of a person's illness.

Adopting a holistic approach in caring for the person with advanced dementia necessitates health professionals responding also to the needs of family members. Providing palliative care is centred on the family unit and involves those individuals who are defined by the dying person as being significant to them (Johnson, 2012). The dementia trajectory frequently means family members have been involved over a long period of time and provided much of the care until relocation to a residential aged care facility. The constant exposure by family members to the person's declining cognitive state may be expressed as anticipatory grief or pre death before the actual physical death of the person occurs (Sampson, 2010). Recognising how families are feeling and coping with their loss and grief has a direct impact on the person with dementia which often contributes to their anxiety, depression, wandering and other displays of behaviour. Addressing the physical, intellectual, emotional and spiritual needs, within the cultural context of the family unit, is as equally important as those of the person dying (Johnson, 2012). The relationships fostered between the health professionals, the person with advanced dementia and their family may facilitate healing restoring a degree of harmony and balance. If a holistic care is not adopted significant levels of distress and suffering may be experienced by the person and their families (Maher & Hemmings, 2005) which may manifest as behavioural issues in the person with advanced dementia and unhealthy bereavement in family members. Practising in this way demonstrates a shift of care from being disease orientated to prioritising the needs of the person and their family above all else (O'Brien King & Gates et al., 2007).

Principles underpinning holistic care involve the understanding of the person as a unique human being who interacts with their environment and recognises a need for healing in cases where there is no cure but where the emphasis is on promoting comfort and alleviating suffering (Mitchell et al., 2009). Most importantly for the health professional is giving care that values compassion, respect, trust, and authenticity to promote healing. Johnson et al (2011) suggest that the role of the health professional should initially focus on managing the physical symptoms because if these needs are not addressed it would be problematic to address their psycho-social and spiritual needs. Health professionals who take account of the complexity of need manifested in the person with advanced dementia demonstrate their commitment to the concept of holism.

The pathology of advanced dementia means that there will be many challenges and disruptions along the illness trajectory resulting in the manifestation of several symptoms and behaviours that can affect the body, mind and spirit of the person (Johnson et al., 2011). These symptoms and behaviours are further exacerbated by the presence of co-morbid conditions that culminate in death (Evans & Goodman, 2009). Dementia often follows functional decline with the person suffering disability throughout the last year of life with substantial impact on activities of daily living. Maximising the person's quality of life is the primary goal for health professionals. This can be better supported by more accurate prognostication of the need for palliative care intervention and recognising the value of palliation at different points of the trajectory (Fulton et al., 2011; Hallberg, 2006).

2.2.2 The application of palliative care principles

The provision of palliative care to people dying only with a cancer diagnosis has shifted. In Australia, the provision of quality care at the end of life must be available for all people regardless of location, age, income, diagnosis and prognosis, social and cultural background (Palliative Care Australia[PCA], 2008). The Australian view expressed resonates also with the UK, USA and many other countries (Birch & Stokoe, 2010). Research provides evidence that the symptoms experienced by a person dying are similar regardless of the underlying pathology (Sampson, 2009). This evidence suggests the broadening of palliative care to include all life limiting illnesses in practice is warranted. Dementia is one of those chronic life limiting illnesses now seen as benefiting from the application of palliative care principles (Birch & Stokoe, 2010; Chang et al., 2009). Escalation of numbers of people dying worldwide from dementia also means a heightened interest in palliative care in this context (Birch & Stokoe, 2010; Sampson. 2009). Further with a greater emphasis on symptom management and supportive care, the role of palliative care is recognised as being instituted as early as the time of diagnosis and at any other point along the illness trajectory, in accordance with the needs of the person dying and their family. No longer is it confined to the 'terminal phase of an illness' or 'at the end of life' as palliative care has much to offer in alleviating the suffering and promoting comfort of a person in a multitude of disease trajectories. Specifically Panke & Volicer (2002), confirm that the most critical symptoms decreasing quality of life and comfort in people with advanced dementia are behavioural symptoms and pain. Implementing care underpinned by this broader view means the principles of palliative care can be provided within a variety of care settings: acute care, aged care, community and hospices (Haley & Daley, 2008) supplemented by assistance from specialist palliative care services and colleagues (Johnson et al., 2011). This is particularly so for people with advanced dementia. Chang & Walter (2010) highlight that the symptoms exhibited by a person in the terminal phase of dementia required nursing home intervention on 90% of occasions, and 70% of all dementia related deaths, in the USA occur in nursing homes (Fulton et al., 2011). In Australia over 50, 000 older people die in residential aged care facilities annually (Australian Institute of Health and Welfare [AIHW], 2010a) and the government response has been to target better end of life care through the up skilling of the aged care workforce through education to meet this need (PCA, 2011). These figures provide evidence of the escalating need for sound knowledge and skills in palliative care to have a presence in settings where people with a non-cancer related diagnosis are cared.

Thus palliative care, as described by the World Health Organisation [WHO] (2005), is an approach to care that improves the quality of life of patients and their families facing the problem associated with a life-limiting illness, through the prevention and relief of suffering by means of early identification and impeccable assessment and treatment of pain and other problems, physical, psychosocial and spiritual and:

- provides relief from pain and other distressing symptoms;
- affirms life and regards dying as a normal process;
- intends neither to hasten or postpone death;
- integrates the psychological and spiritual aspects of patient care;
- offers a support system to help patients live as actively as possible until death;
- offers a support system to help the family cope during the patients illness and in their own bereavement;
- uses a team approach to address the needs of patients and their families, including bereavement counselling, if indicated;
- will enhance quality of life, and may also positively influence the course of illness;
- is applicable early in the course of illness, in conjunction with other therapies that are intended to prolong life, such as chemotherapy or radiation therapy, and includes those investigations needed to better understand and manage distressing clinical complications.

Chang et al (2009) have long advocated the need for staff to have superior skills in assessment, pain and symptom management and negotiation of care with family. Further improved knowledge about the dementia trajectory, the principles of palliative care and advance care directives and their role in caring for the person dying with dementia are needed (Chang, et al., 2009). Fulton et al (2011) argue that people dying with dementia are a highly vulnerable group because of a high rate of co-morbidity, inability to participate and understand their care situation and a reliance on caregivers to act as their advocates. The need therefore to keep people dying from dementia in an aged care setting (nursing home, residential aged care facility or long term care) with appropriate palliative interventions is paramount to eliminating the need to transition to other care settings. Transitioning to other care settings in this group is identified as a major complication (Fulton et al., 2011) that might precipitate adverse events culminating in death. In summary the importance of recognising dementia as a life limiting illness and the benefits afforded by the application of palliative care principles to this group of people cannot be underestimated (Sampson, 2010; van der Steen, 2010).

3. Symptom management

Dying in the 21st century has become more complex and protracted as a result of modern medicine typically taking 30 months from the time a terminal diagnosis is confirmed to die (Old & Swagerty, 2007) . However, a person dying from dementia has spent many years in a progressive and steady functional decline leading to an increased dependency on caregivers to support them in their activities of daily living. This functional decline may also manifest in the person as suffering with a severe disability. Further, given the age of the person with dementia, it is highly probable that at least one co-morbid condition is present concurrent to their primary dementia diagnosis (AIHW, 2010b). The breadth of symptoms displayed combined with their presentation, reveals caring for the person dying from dementia to be a challenging and complex environment requiring a knowledgeable and skilled workforce to deliver care (Hennings, Froggatt & Keady, 2010). The symptom breadth and presentation are magnified as a consequence of the person being older person with the high probability of co-morbidity and a reduced reserve capacity combined with a disease which manifests with severe functional decline. Therefore instituting a philosophy of palliative care into practice has the potential to promote quality of life by mitigating the impact of factors that may reduce quality of life (Hallberg, 2006). The focus of care becomes reorientated to managing symptoms as opposed to the actual disease itself (Hallberg, 2006).

People dying from a chronic, life limiting illness, such as dementia, where curative and restorative outcomes are no longer viable frequently share a common cluster of symptoms at the end of their life regardless of the underlying pathology (Johnson et al., 2006). This cluster of symptoms include: fatigue, pain, nausea with or without vomiting, constipation and dyspnoea (Johnson et al., 2006). If left unmet these symptoms have the greatest potential to adversely affect the quality of living the person dying experiences and limits the capacity of their family to engage in normal grief (Johnson, et al., 2006). Evidence is now emerging which shows that the symptom burden between those dying with dementia to be comparable to those dying with a cancer diagnosis. A retrospective study identified pain, dyspnoea, agitation, fatigue, eating problems such as difficulty in swallowing (McCarthy et al., 1997) to be present in those dying from dementia. More recently Mitchell, et al's (2009) 18 month prospective study of 323 nursing home residents confirmed that advanced dementia is a terminal illness which leads to aspiration pneumonia or eating difficulties in the final stages and last few months of life. Specifically while much commonality exists, Pautex et al's (2007) study showed that fatigue is frequently not reported in dementia patients and suggests this is because it is less prevalent or infrequently noticed. It may however be that the person dying with dementia is unable to express this need and therefore it goes unreported. Many studies report that pain and shortness of breath (dyspnoea) to be the most frequently occurring symptoms commonly experienced by people dying from dementia (Fulton et al., 2011; McCarthy et al., 1997; Pautex et al., 2007). The complexity in which care is delivered is magnified further by the person with dementia's cognitive impairment acting as a significant impediment to discerning what the symptoms are, how best to manage them and if they remain unmet. This impediment to symptom management lies primarily in those who are dying from dementia (though other neurodegenerative diseases and cerebral cancers may also fit into this category) making them a highly vulnerable group not able to access and be recipients of quality symptom management. This vulnerability further heightens the need for a superior skilled aged care workforce to deliver palliative care (Chang et al., 2009; PCA, 2011).

The following section provides a brief overview of the symptoms commonly experienced in a person with advanced dementia.

3.1 Pain

The presence of pain or discomfort in the person dying from dementia is further complicated by the individual's inability to articulate their pain. Pain has been reported to occur in 21% to 83% of all dementia patients, at some point along the disease trajectory

(Zwakhalen et al., 2009). Further the presence of pain is identified as increasing as death approaches (Williams, et al, 2005). Pain may be displayed by the person with advanced dementia in the form of: agitation; restlessness; facial grimacing; moaning or an alteration in their respiratory rate and pattern and resistive behaviours (Panke & Volicer, 2002; Sampson, 2010). However, while pain is common in people with advanced dementia it frequently goes under-detected and under-treated (Fulton et al., 2011; Sampson, 2010). Two main reasons co-exist for this under-detection and under-treating. The first is poor assessment knowledge and skill in the health professional and the second is the communication difficulties a person with advanced dementia experiences which become further magnified as the disease progresses (Sampson, 2010). While a complex entity, this should not mitigate this symptom being adequately managed (van der Steen, 2010).

3.2 Eating and swallowing

Difficulties with eating and swallowing usually signify the person with dementia has transitioned into the final stage of the disease trajectory with months to a year of life remaining (Fulton et al., 2011). Mitchell et al's (2009) revealed an eating problem was present in 85.8% of 323 nursing home residents that they studied. The study further identified that in the last 3 months of their life the prevalence of an eating problem rose to a level of 90.4%.

3.3 Dyspnoea

Shortness of breath or dyspnoea increasingly appears in people with advanced dementia as they approach death in half to three quarters of all individuals (van der Steen, 2010). This rate of prevalence is comparable to those people with a terminal cancer (van der Steen, 2010). Shortness of breath in the person with advanced dementia is attributed to pneumonia as consequence to aspiration (Mitchell et al., 2009; van der Steen, 2010). Mitchell et al's (2009) study reported high and increasing level of aspiration were present as the person with dementia neared death. For families, as well as the person shortness of breath causes much discomfort and distress (Johnson, et al., 2006; Johnson, 2012).

3.4 Behavioural

The presence of behavioural and psychological symptoms is as high as 90% of people with dementia at some point in their illness trajectory (Sampson, 2010). It remains a challenging problem in caring for people with dementia in general (Bidewell & Chang, 2011). In advanced dementia specifically Mitchell et al., (2009) identified over half of their study participants remained agitated and distressed. Behavioural symptoms may be displayed as passivity and withdrawal, resisting care in a verbal and or physical manner and may constitute an expression of discomfort within the person's environment and or actual physical discomfort (Panke & Volicer, 2002) that they are unable to express due to an impaired communication ability resulting from dementia. Examples could include but are not limited to: feeling cold; hungry; in pain, constipated or having a full bladder. A person with advanced dementia is unable to verbalise their feelings and therefore the presence of these stimuli indicate a level of discomfort escalating to pain which necessitates an alternative means of expression usually displayed in the form of aggressive and resistive behaviours (Sampson, 2010). Of interest is that agitation is less frequently assessed for in the final stage of a person's life with advanced dementia as pain and shortness of breath became the overriding symptom family members in particular are concerned about (van der Steen, 2010).

3.5 Infections

In people with advanced dementia the presence of infections becomes more prevalent (Sampson, 2010). Mitchell et al's (2009) study revealed over an 18 month period pneumonia (41%) and a febrile episode (53%) were most common. Sampson reports that the febrile episode is mostly likely to be a urinary tract infection. Burns et al (1990) had previously reported that up to 71% of deaths in people with advanced dementia were most likely attributed to these two infections (Burns et al., 1990). The presence of infections in people with advanced dementia, are attributed to the person being immobile, bed bound, at increased risk for aspiration and an impaired immunological system (Sampson, 2010).

To illustrate the comparable nature of symptoms experienced by a person with advanced dementia and someone dying from cancer the following case study is presented:

> Caroline Hegarty is my patient today. She is a 70 year old woman. On reading her notes I know she is dying. A cascade of symptoms is present which provide me with the trigger indicating she is dying. The staff are increasingly needed to perform and or support her Activities of Daily Living and now she is completely dependent on them. Her appetite has been intermittent for weeks and has now declined to the point where she is unable or unwilling to eat. An assessment on other causes for a depressed appetite has been conducted and there is little evidence of swallowing difficulties present. Two weeks ago she commenced on thickened fluids but since Monday Caroline has displayed little interest in these. Further she has become increasingly lethargic and has been difficult to arouse in the last 48hours. Previously Caroline had been very restless and would frequently walk the corridors but now she seems to have lost her restlessness and seems at peace. When I last saw Caroline two weeks ago she could raise her head to take the thickened fluids now she doesn't have the energy to hold her head up and to swallow.

In summary this case study attempts to illustrate that regardless of the underlying pathology, in essence when a person is actively dying a common cluster of symptoms are present for all people to a lesser or greater degree.

3.6 Management of symptoms

Under treatment of symptoms at the end of a person's life with dementia is a major concern (van der Steen 2010). This is largely due to the lack of recognition of dementia as a terminal illness and the person's cognitive decline and impaired communication. While Mitchell et al's (2009) study confirmed that advanced dementia was indeed a terminal illness it also highlighted the lack of referral to hospice as compared to those with another terminal disease despite the obvious presence of pain and dyspnoea in the last 3 months of life. In her study only 29% of the cohort received hospice intervention (Mitchell, et al., 2009). This poses significant challenges for family and health professionals in managing the symptoms, as a result of the dying process. Chang & Walter cite as evidence of the lack of application of palliative care interventions as: the underuse of advanced care planning; the overuse of tube feeding; the inadequate management of dyspnoea, pain, agitation and aspiration symptoms (2010, p. 1107). The management of these symptoms is complex, requiring a structured approach using a range of therapeutic interventions (Sampson, 2010). In particular the impaired communication experienced by the person with advanced dementia may potentially inhibit palliative care interventions (Johnson et al., 2009).

4. Communication skills in the provision of care with advanced dementia and their families

4.1 The need for effective communication

One of the goals in palliative care is to encourage open communication which leads to a positive attitude to death and dying. Effective communication in this context must address the cultural, social, psychological and spiritual aspects of a person and their family, so that their needs are met. Achieving this goal assists in reducing a person's suffering and managing their symptoms that leads to improved quality of care (Johnson et al., 2009).

4.2 Knowledge about dementia among family caregivers

International studies highlight an inadequacy in the quality and quantity of dementia information which is given to people with dementia and their family members particularly in the latter stages of dementia (Birch & Draper, 2008; Sampson, 2010). In many instances they might feel uncomfortable in asking questions of health professionals (Chang et al., 2010).

4.3 Complexity of knowledge and skills provision that impacts on communication

Communicating with the family is one of the greatest challenges faced by health professionals. There is the need to frequently discuss end of life issues directly with the family in the absence of the person with advanced dementia because of the cognitive decline associated with dementia that ultimately results in impaired communication.

The authors conducted a study with key professional providers of care to examine the challenges with caring for people with advanced dementia. The study was informed by a qualitative framework based on action research. Action research collects information from key stakeholders and provides ongoing feedback to participants, thereby facilitating change that improves practice (Kemmis & McTaggart, 1988). Data collection was through five focus groups and 20 individual in-depth interviews. Participants were drawn from the key groups of professional providers of care in an outlying urban area of Sydney, Australia, which includes three local government areas having a total population of 320,000. The five focus group included general practitioners, palliative care speciality staff, palliative care volunteer managers and volunteers, aged or dementia specialist health care professionals and residential aged care facility staff. The data attest to the complexity of caring for people with advanced dementia living in residential aged care facilities, and the associated challenges for key professional carers. The main areas of challenge identified were: knowledge and skills in the direct provision of care, knowledge relating to dementia as a disorder, and knowledge relating to palliation. Participants in this study emphasized the need for improvements in knowledge and skills, and the need for policy changes (Chang, et al., 2009, p.42). From this study, it was recommended that professionals of care need to have skills in assessment, pain, and symptom management, and negotiation of care with the family. Advance care plans and directives will assist clinical decision -making when an individual can no longer communicate. Negotiations between family members and the multidisciplinary care team to achieve consensus about the goals of care might improve resident comfort by ensuring that symptoms are controlled without unnecessary, burdensome interventions (Chang, et al., 2009 p.46).

4.4 Advance care planning

Advanced care planning involves the assessment of the person and family needs and to identify and discuss care options across the illness trajectory in the context of the person's preferences (Mariano, 2007). In the context of people with advanced dementia, they experience progressively declining cognitive function which impedes their capacity to make decisions about their care (Sampson, 2010). Therefore it is advocated that advance care planning for this group of people occur early on in the disease trajectory as compared to other diseases (Sampson, 2010). Importantly this will allow for the personal characteristics and behaviour of the individual to be understood and to tailor the interventions to support the person's symptoms, behaviour and coping mechanisms of the person and their family in the palliative context. The person with advanced dementia is progressing towards the terminal phase when death will occur. The problems described in this section usually require the *person responsible* (lawful substituted decision maker) to make decisions about treatments including whether or not to use certain life prolonging medical treatments. It may be considered that certain life prolonging treatments (Mitchell et al., 2009) may not add to the comfort or quality of life of the person with advanced dementia (Palliative Care Dementia Interface: Enhancing Community Capacity Project, 2011).

At a community level, people generally do not understand dementia well and negative attitudes can exist. In the face of this, family caregivers of someone diagnosed with dementia face many challenges in both itself and informing a realistic picture of what to expect and the nature of dementia, especially in the advanced stages. Responding to a highlighted need by family care givers to be given basic information about dementia progression (Chang et al., 2006), the authors developed a booklet entitled, Information for Families and Friends of People with Severe and End Stage Dementia (Palliative Care Dementia Interface: Enhancing Community Capacity Project, 1st edition, 2006), in consultation with dementia and aged care experts. This 41 page booklet provided information about what to expect as dementia progresses, including cognitive ability, functional ability (sleep cycle, walking, incontinence, eating and swallowing), behaviours and emotions, physical symptoms (pain, weight loss, infections, changes in limb movements), end of life issues and palliative care options that can be discussed with health professionals, the dying process, what to expect at the time of death and where to obtain ongoing support (Chang et al., 2009.) More recently the 3rd edition of this booklet included important aspects of advanced care planning (Palliative Care Dementia Interface: Enhancing Community Capacity Project, 2011) in response to acknowledging advanced dementia as a terminal illness. Clearly, improved knowledge, gained by the provision of additional information relevant to the family caregiver, has a role to play in improving this situation.

4.5 The importance of the family carer role in planning care for the person with advanced dementia

Advance care planning is all about talking about the future care of the person with advanced dementia. The point of talking about future care for a person living with advanced dementia is that medical care for both expected and unexpected health issues can be considered well before a crisis. In this way, decisions can be made calmly, based on what the person with dementia's wishes would be if they could talk for themselves. Misunderstandings and possible areas of conflict can be dealt with so everyone comes to a clear and agreed understanding about the care to be given to the person with dementia.

Usually a number of advance care planning discussions are needed. Key times when discussion might be held are when the person with dementia is diagnosed with a new medical condition that will impact on their health, after a hospital admission, or on admission to a residential care facility. Topics that might be discussed, depending on the circumstances, include:

- The values, wishes, beliefs and expectations of the person with dementia regarding what quality of life means to them. The *person responsible* and other family and friends contribute by recalling conversations and events where the person with dementia indicated their beliefs.
- The role and importance of the *person responsible* as a substitute decision maker. This person needs to "put themselves in the shoes of the person in dementia" and make decisions from the person's viewpoint.
- The understanding of everyone involved about the dementia diagnosis, and what will happen in the future.
- The benefits and risks of any treatment options.
- The goal of care, so the person with dementia will have the best possible quality of life, with their wishes respected.
- The person with dementia's preferences for end of life care.

Making decisions about another person's care and treatment options is a major responsibility. Some families prefer more than one person to help with the decision making. However, the *person responsible* is the person who legally can consent to, or refuse consent for, any treatment, so that the person has the final say. By involving other family members in advance care planning discussions, the *person responsible* can make sure everyone concerned understands the issues and the reasons for decisions. (Chang et al., 2009). The more the *person responsible* and family members know about dementia and the changes that occur over time, the more likely it is that the person with dementia will receive care that respects their wishes and improves comfort and quality of life. Further involvement of family members at key decision points assists them to understand about the multiple losses they have experienced in relation to the person with dementia and the anxiety their care causes for them (Hennings, Froggatt & Keady, 2010). The person that is responsible for care needs to be encouraged to ask questions and discuss with their health professional. Ideally, advanced care planning should be encouraged in the earlier stages of dementia when a person is still competent to make decisions about what is important to them communicate and their preferences (Sampson, 2010).

5. Conclusion

Advanced dementia brings numerous somatic, affective and behavioural symptoms, impairments and co-morbidities. Diagnosing and managing pain and symptoms in people with advanced dementia is often made difficult by communicative difficulties of a person with dementia. Adopting a systematic and holistic approach to assessment and management of pain and other symptoms means that people with advanced dementia are more likely to receive appropriate care. These challenges point to the professional development and training needs for dementia care staff, so that patients/residents with dementia and their carers' expectations are met. Advanced care directives expressing the resident's prospective care preferences would give clinicians' clearer guidelines for responding to patients, and would assist in negotiating care decisions with family members.

There is also a pressing need for investing in research which explores various models of care for people with advanced dementia, from the health professional and caregivers' perspectives, in relation to their cost effectiveness and suitability for practice. Only by investing in research and providing the evidence can governments and health care services improve the lives of people with dementia and those who care for them. Implementing palliative care for people with dementia makes an important contribution to their comfort and promotes healthy grieving in family members while at the same time attempting to minimise the impact of stress for all concerned.

6. References

Access Economics. (2009). *Keeping dementia front of mind: Incidence and prevalence 2009-2050.* Retrieved from http://www.alzheimers.org.au/research-publications/access-economics-reports.asp April 7th 2011.

Albinsson, L. & Strang, P. (2002). A palliative approach to existential issues and death in end-stage dementia care. *Journal of Palliative Care,* 18(3), pp. 168-175.

Alzheimer's Association (2010). *Changing the trajectory of Alzheimer's disease: A national imperative.* Alzheimer's Association: Chicago

Alzheimer's Association. (2011). 2011 *Alzheimer's disease facts and figures report.* Retrieved from http://www.alz.org/alzheimers_disease_facts_andfigures.asp on 7th April 2011.

Alzheimer's Disease International (2010). World Alzheimer Report 2010 The Global Economic Impact of Dementia, Alzheimer's Disease International accessed via www.alz.co.uk on 7th April 2011.

Australian Institute of Health and Welfare (2010a). *Australia's Health 2010.* AIHW: Canberra

Australian Institute of Health and Welfare (2010b). *Residential aged are in Australia 2008 – 2009 a statistical overview.* Aged care statistics series no. 31 Cat no Age 62, AIHW: Canberra

Banerjee, S. & Owen, J. (2009). *Living well with dementia. A national dementia strategy.* London: Department of Health

Bidewell, J. Chang, E., (2010). Managing dementia agitation in residential aged care. *Dementia 2011,* 10(3), pp. 299-315

Birch, D. & Stokoe, D. (2010). Caring for people with end-stage dementia. *Nursing Older People,* pp. 22(2) 31-36

Birch, D. & Draper, J. A. (2008). A critical literature review exploring the challenges of delivering effective palliative care to older people with dementia. *Journal of Clinical Nursing,* 9, pp.1144-1163

Burns, A., Jacoby, R., Luthert, P. et al. (1990). Cause of death in Alzheimer's disease. *Age Ageing,* 19, pp. 341-4

Chang, E., Easterbrook, S., Hancock, K., Johnson, A., & Davidson, P. (2010). Evaluation of an information booklet for caregivers of people with dementia: An Australian perspective. *Nursing and Health Sciences,* 12, pp.45-51

Chang, E. M., Daly, J., Johnson, A., Harrison, K., Easterbrook, S., Bidewell, J., Stewart, H., Noel, M., Hancock, K. (2009). Challenges for professional care of advanced dementia. *International Journal of Nursing Practice,* 15(1), pp.41-47.

Chang, E., Johnson, A., Easterbrook, S., Harrison, K. & Luhr, M. (2008). Dementias. In: Chang, E. & Johnson, A. (Eds.). *Chronic Illness and Disability: Principles for Nursing Practice.* Elsevier: Sydney

Chang, E., Hancock, K., Harrison, K., Daly, J., Johnson, A., Easterbrook, S., Noel, M., Luhr-Taylor, M., Davidson, P.M. (2005). Palliative care for end-stage dementia: A discussion of the implications for education of health professionals. *Nurse Education Today*, pp. 25(4),pp. 326-332

Chang, A. & Walter, L.C. (2010). Recognizing dementia as a terminal illness in nursing home residents. *Archives of Internal Medicine*, 170(13), pp. 1107-1109

Emre, M. (2009). Classification and diagnosis of dementia: a mechanism-based approach. *European Journal of Neurology*, 16, pp. 168-173

Erickson, H.L. (2007). Philosophy and theory of holism. *Nursing Clinics of North America*, 42(2), 139-163

Evans, C. & Goodman, C. (2009). Changing practice in dementia care for people in care homes towards end of life. *Dementia*, 8, pp. 424-431

Fulton, A.T., Rhodes-Kropf, J., Cocoran, A.M., Chau, D. & Castillo, E.H. (2011). Palliative care for patients with dementia in long-term care. *Clinical Geriatric Medicine*, 27, pp. 153-170

Hancock, K., Chang, E., Johnson, A., Harrison, K., Daly, J., Easterbrook, S., Noel, M., Davidson, P. (2006) Palliative care for people with advance dementia: the need for a collaborative evidence-based approach. *Alzheimers's Care Quarterly*, 7(1), pp. 49-57.

Haley, C. & Daley, J. (2008). Palliation in chronic illness. In: A. Johnson & E. Chang (Eds.). *Chronic illness and disability. Principles for nursing practice.* Elsevier: Chatswood, pp. 168-184.

Hallberg, I.R. (2006). Palliative care as a framework for older people's long term care. *International Journal of Palliative Nursing*, 12, 5, pp. 224-229

Hennings, J., Froggatt, K. & keady, J. (2010). Approaching the end of life and dying with dementia in care homes: the accounts of family carers. *Reviews in Clinical Gerontology*, 20, pp. 114-127

Johnson, A. (2012). Working with Families. In M. O'Connor, S. Aranchia & S. Lee (eds.). *Palliative Care: A guide to Practice.* Victoria: Ausmed

Johnson, A., Chang, E., Daly, J., Harrison, K., Noel, M., Hancock, K., Easterbrook, S. (2009).The communication challenges faced in adopting a palliative care approach in advance dementia. *International Journal of Nursing Practice*, 15, pp. 467- 474

Johnson, A., Harrison, K., Currow, D., Luhr-Taylor, M., & Johnson, R. (2006). Chapter 17: *Palliative Care and Health Breakdown.* In E. Chang, J. Daly & D. Elliot (Eds.), Pathophysiology Applied to Nursing Practice, pp. 448-471 Elsevier: Sydney:

Johnson, C., Girgis, A., Paul, C., Currow, D.C., Adams, J. & Aranda, S. (2011). Australian palliative care providers' perceptions and experiences of the barriers and facilitators to palliative care provision. *Support Cancer Care*, 19, pp. 343-352

Kemmis, S. & McTaggert, R. (1988). *The action research planner* (3rd edn.). Geelong, Victoria: Deakin University Press

McCarthy, M., Addington-Hall, J., & Altman, D. (1997). The experience of dying with dementia: A retrospective study. *International Journal of Geriatric Psychiatry*, 12, pp. 404-409

McKeel. D.W., Burns, J.M, Meuser, T.M. 7 Morris, J.C. (2007). *An atlas of investigation and diagnosis. Dementia.* Clinical publishing: United Kingdom

Maher , D. & Hemmings, L. (2005). Understanding patient and family: holistic assessment in palliative care. British *Journal of Community Nursing*. 10(7), pp. 318-322

Marinano, C. (2007). Holistic nursing as a specialty: Holistic nursing – scope and standards for practice. *Nursing Clinics of North America*, 42(2), pp. 165-188

Mitchell, S.L., Teno, J.M., Kiely, D.K. (2009). The clinical course of advanced dementia. *New England Journal of Medicine*, 361(16), pp. 1529-1538

Moss, M., Braunschweig, H., & Rubinstein, R. (2002). Terminal care for nursing home residents with dementia (ethics). *Alzheimer's Care Quarterly*, 3(3), pp. 233-249

Old, J.L. & Swagerty, D.L. (2007). *A practical guide to palliative care.* Lippincott Williams & Wilkins: Philadelphia

Palliative Care Australia (2008). *Strategic plan 2008-2011.* Palliative Care Australia: Deakin, ACT

Palliative Care Australia (2011). *Caring for older Australians: Productivity Commission Draft Report.* Palliative Care Australia: Deakin, ACT

O'Brien King, M. & Gates, M.F. (2007). Teaching holistic nursing: The legacy of nightingale. *Nursing Clinics of North America*, 42(2), pp. 309-333

Palliative Care Dementia Interface: Enhancing Community Capacity Project, (2006). *Information for families and friends of people with severe and end stage dementia,* University of Western Sydney: Sydney

Palliative Care Dementia Interface: Enhancing Community Capacity Project. (2011) *Information for families and friends of people with severe and end stage dementia* (3rd edn.). University of Western Sydney: Sydney ISBN 0957756836

Panke, J.A. & Volicer, L. (2002). Caring for persons with dementia: A palliative approach. *Journal of Hospice and palliative Nursing*, 4(3), pp. 143-149

Pautex, S., Hermann, F.R., Le, L.P., Ghedira, M., Zulian, G.B., MIchon, A., & Gold, G. (2007). Symptom relief in the last week of life: is dementia always a limiting factor? *Journal of American Geriatric Society*, 55, pp. 1316-1317

Sampson, E. (2010). Pallliative care for people with dementia. *British Medical Bulletin*, 96,1, pp. 159-174

Sampson, E., Blanchard, M., Jones, L., Tookman, A. & King, M. (2009). Dementia in the acute-hospital: prospective cohort study of prevalence and mortality. *British Journal of Psychiatry*, 195, pp. 61-66

Shuster, J. (2000). Palliative care for advanced dementia. *Clinical Geriatric Medicine*, 17, pp. 377-391

van der Steen, J. (2010). Dying with dementia: What we know after more than a decade of research. *Journal of Alzheimer's Disease*, 22, pp. 37-55.

Williams, C.S., Zimmerman, S., Sloane, P.D., & Reed, P.S. (2005). Characteristics associated with pain in long-term care residents with dementia. *Gerontologist*, 45, Spec no1, pp. 68-73

World Health Organisation (2005). *Definition of palliative care.* World Health Organisation: Geneva

Zwakhalen, S.M., Koopmans, R.T., Geels, P.J., Berger, M.P., & Hamers, J.P. (2009). The prevalence of pain in nursing home residents with dementia measured using observational pain scale. *European Journal of Pain*, 13, pp. 89-93

11

The Changing Landscape – Palliative Care in the Heart Failure Patient Population

Michael Slawnych[1], Jessica Simon[1] and Jonathan Howlett[2]
[1]*Division of Palliative Medicine,*
[2]*Department of Cardiac Sciences, University of Calgary, Canada*

1. Introduction

The practice of cardiovascular medicine has changed dramatically over the course of the last several decades (Figure 1). Heart failure (HF), a condition characterized by damaged myocardium, abnormal ventricular filling and/or ejection, and symptoms of vascular congestion or poor cardiac output, was once deemed a terminal illness with few good therapeutic options. However, advances in treatment have led to significant increases in life expectancy and quality of life. Patients with HF now have numerous medication options available. In select patient subsets, these medications are associated with greater than 80% reductions in mortality. Current clinical guidelines support the implantation of implantable cardioverter defibrillators (ICDs) for both primary and secondary prevention indications. Cardiac resynchronization therapy (CRT) extends the efficacy of these devices in specific patient subgroups. External mechanical support devices, previously considered as a temporizing measure, are now being used as at as permanent therapy. Trans-catheter aortic valve implantation (TAVI) has not only been shown to be vastly superior to medical therapy in non-operative patients with severe aortic stenosis, but is also being considered as an alternative to cardiac surgery in lower risk groups.

As a result of all of these advances, there has been a shift in the cardiac patient demographic. Current patients with HF are older, have more co-morbidities, and take more medications than in the past (Wong et al. 2011). This trend is likely to continue, as the proportion of elderly individuals is projected to increase for some time (Foot et al. 2000).

As early as the 1960's it was recognized that HF was associated with significant levels of mental and physical distress, with this distress sometimes exceeding that observed in other populations such as cancer (Hinton 1963). The progress of medical and technological developments that prolong life may initially appear to have made palliative care appear irrelevant for the cardiac patient population. Ironically though, nearly all of our treatment advances for such patients are not in fact, cures. Thus patients will eventually become refractory to even these treatment modalities, which will necessitate complex symptom management. In this setting, care deliver by a multidisciplinary team that includes palliative care is needed. Patients with HF continue to suffer mortality rates greater than 40% over 5 years (Lloyd-Jones et al. 2010). Lessons can be taken from the cancer literature that shows that the early introduction of palliative care as an adjunct to disease-focused treatment not only improves quality of life, but can increase longevity as well (Temel et al. 2010).

While palliative care is now incorporated into several HF guidelines, implementation is still lacking. This is likely a reflection of several barriers (Selman, Harding, and Beynon 2007) not the least of which is the physician and patient comfort in focusing on life-prolonging therapies and a reluctance to acknowledge or plan for death as an outcome of advancing disease. This tension is amplified by the inherent difficulty in estimating prognosis in this patient population, given the highly variable course of advanced HF. While there are now several models that provide prognostic guidance, they are most useful for estimating outcomes in patient populations as opposed to individual patients (McKelvie et al. 2011). In this chapter, we highlight opportunities for incorporating palliative care to the HF population, despite the uncertain prognosis.

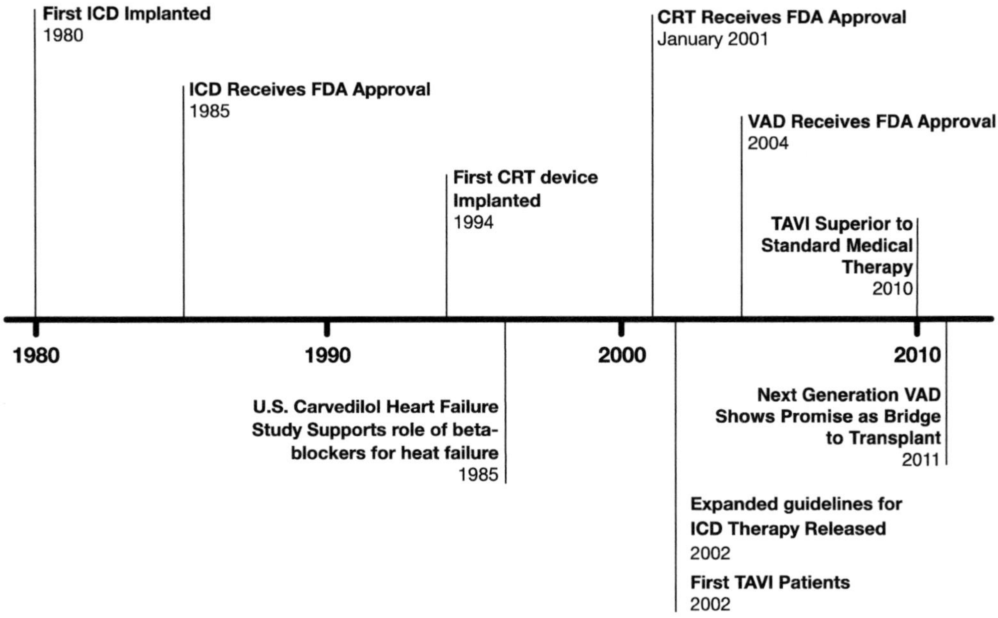

Fig. 1. Treatment advances in cardiology (1980 - present).

2. Heart failure – Some basic facts

Heart failure is common. There are close to six million Americans living with HF, with 670,000 new cases diagnosed annually (Lloyd-Jones et al. 2010). The prevalence of HF increases significantly with age, and is noted to be greater than 20% in patients greater than 80 years of age (Lloyd-Jones et al. 2010). As a result, HF has become a significant health care burden, particularly in developed countries (Braunschweig, Cowie, and Auricchio 2011). With the expected doubling of the number of Americans older than 65 years during the next few decades, an marked increase in the number of patients with HF (Abouezzeddine and Redfield 2011) will occur.

There are many causes of heart failure, including ischemia, hypertension, valvular heart disease, arrhythmias and primary cardiomyopathies. The typical symptoms associated with

HF include dyspnea, fatigue, and reduced exercise tolerance, but many other symptoms including pain and psycho-social suffering are associated with advanced disease (Scott A Murray et al. 2002; Nordgren and Sörensen 2003).

HF is the leading cause of hospital admissions in patients greater than 65 years of age. Hospitalization is an independent risk factor for shortened survival in patients with chronic HF, and is associated with an average life expectancy of approximately two years (Howlett 2011), which is less than that of many cancers. Even as the national death rate decreased by 2% from 1994 to 2004, deaths due to heart failure increased by 28% (Adler et al. 2009).

The severity of heart failure is commonly assessed using the well-known New York Heart Association (NYHA) classification scheme, which categorizes patients on the basis of limitation of physical activity (Table 1). In 2001, the American College of Cardiology (ACC) and the American Heart Association (AHA) developed a complementary classification scheme for HF, which progressively categorizes patients on the basis of the presence of cardiac risk factors, cardiac structural impairment, symptoms of heart failure, and then culminating in refractory disease (Figure 2). This classification scheme emphasizes evidence-based treatment for each stage, as well as disease prevention. Specifically, the first stage can be viewed as "pre-heart failure" where risk factor intervention can potentially prevent progression to overt symptoms. Of note, this first stage does not have a corresponding NYHA class.

Class I - No limitation of physical activity • Ordinary physical activity not associated with symptoms (fatigue, palpitation, or dyspnea).
Class II - Slight limitation of physical activity • Comfortable at rest, but ordinary physical activity results symptoms.
Class III - Moderate limitation of physical activity • Comfortable at rest, but less than ordinary activity causes symptoms.
Class IV - Severe limitation of physical activity • Unable to carry out any physical activity without discomfort. Symptoms at rest.

Table 1. NYHA classification scheme.

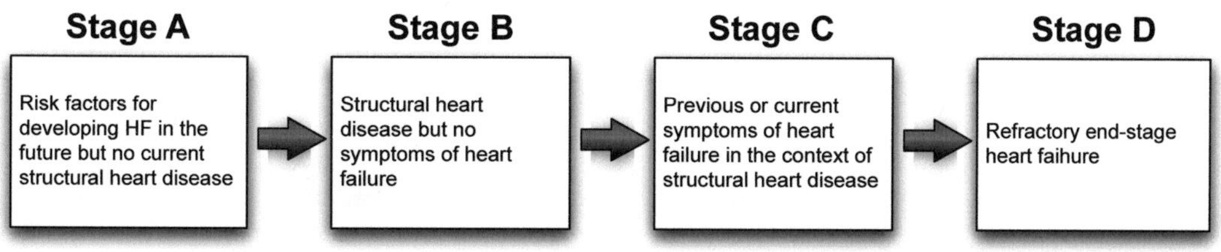

Fig. 2. ACC/AHA heart failure classification scheme.

While the disease trajectory of each individual HF patient is unique (Gott pall med 2007), there is a general overall theme (Murray et al. 2007; Murray and Skeikh 2008; Goodlin 2009). Typically, several episodes of acute "decompensation" are observed on a background of gradual decline, subsequently progressing to "end-stage" HF (Figure 3). Some patients, such as those with large anterior myocardial infarctions, will go through these transitions very quickly. For other patients, these transitions can take decades.

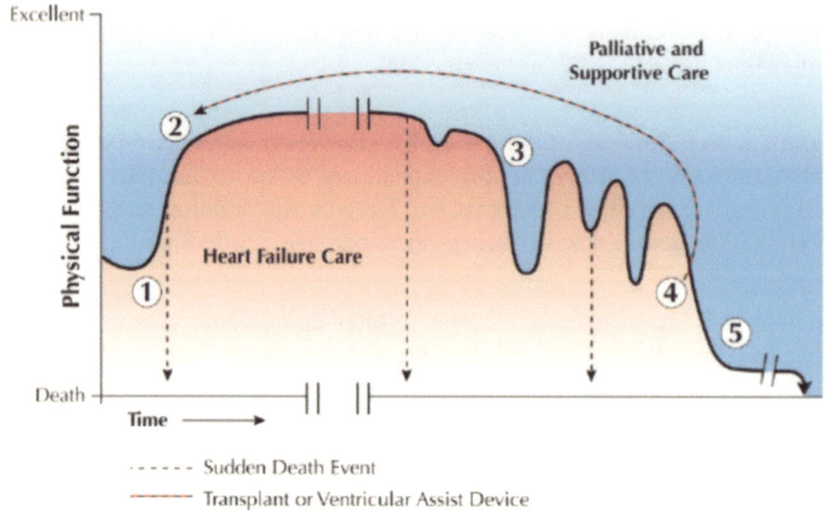

Fig. 3. Heart failure disease trajectory (from Goodlin 2009).

While there is no universally accepted definition of "end-stage" HF, it typically refers to ACC/AHA Stage D patients who have refractory symptoms despite maximal medical therapy (Murthy and Lipman 2011). Some of these "end-stage" patients may be candidates for advance treatment modalities such as transplant or self-contained mechanical support (i.e. LVAD), thus resetting the disease trajectory. However there is a limited availability of donor hearts, and most patients with HF will not benefit from advanced HF therapies such a mechanical support LVAD implantation, leaving many patients without these options.

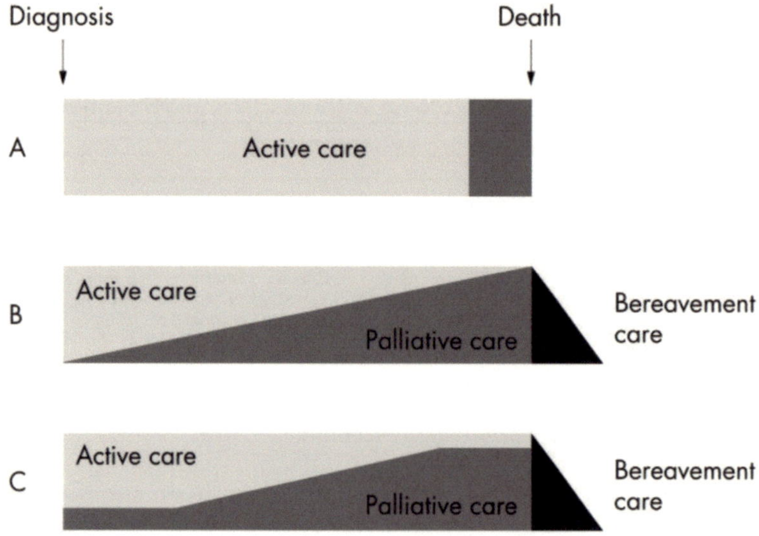

Figure 2 Models showing involvement of palliative care in cancer (A and B) and a proposed model for heart failure (C).

Fig. 4. Model of palliative care for HF (from Gibbs et al. 2002).

As HF progresses and patients deteriorate to a poorer functional status, hospitalization rates increase. Health care resource utilization is particularly high in the last few months of life. A recent study of 30,000 Canadian patients who died with HF showed that more than 75% were hospitalized during the last 6 months of life and > 50% died while in hospital (Kaul et al. 2011). In this context, Murray and colleagues developed a HF classification scheme that recognizes the three different treatment phases that most patients with HF will go through (Table 2). What sets this scheme apart from the more commonly employed NYHA and ACC/AHA classifications is that for the first time, all stages of heart failure are related to the World Health Organization (WHO) definition of palliative care. This classification scheme forms an integral component of the European position statement on palliative care in heart failure (Jaarsma et al. 2009). It should be noted that the idea of early introduction of palliative care to the HF patient population is not unique. Gibbs and colleagues (Gibbs et al. 2002) proposed a model of HF management in which palliative care plays a prominent role throughout all stages of treatment (figure 4).

Stage 1: Chronic disease management phase (NYHA I–III)

- The goals of care include active monitoring, effective therapy to prolong survival, symptom control, patient and carer education, and supported
- self-management.
- Patients are given a clear explanation of their condition including its name, aetiology, treatment, and prognosis.
- Regular monitoring and appropriate review according to national guidelines and local protocols

Stage 2: Supportive and palliative care phase: (NYHA III–IV)

- Admissions to hospital may herald this phase.
- A key professional is identified in the community to co-ordinate care and liaise with specialist heart failure, palliative care, and other services.
- The goal of care shifts to maintaining optimal symptom control and quality of life.
- A holistic, multidisciplinary assessment of patient and carer needs takes place.
- Opportunities to discuss prognosis and the likely course of the illness in more detail are provided by professionals, including recommendation for completing an advance care plan.
- Out-of-hours services are documented in care plans in the event of acute deterioration

Stage 3: Terminal care phase

- Clinical indicators include, despite maximal treatment, renal impairment, hypotension, persistent oedema, fatigue, anorexia
- Heart failure treatment for symptom control is continued and resuscitation status clarified, documented, and communicated to all care providers
- An integrated care pathway for the dying may be introduced to structure care planning
- Increased practical and emotional support for carers is provided, continuing to bereavement support
- Provision of and access to the same levels of generalist and specialist care for patients in all care settings according to their needs

Table 2. Characteristics of the three stages in progressive heart failure (from Jaarsma et al., 2009)

3. Incorporation of palliative care to the heart failure patient population

Historically, palliative care has been associated primarily with cancer patients. In this regard, there is now a significant body of literature that shows that the incorporation of palliative care has resulted in better symptom control for these patients. Patients and families also benefit from other factors such as improved psychological support and patient advocacy. There is also new literature showing that the early introduction of palliative care in this patient population can increase longevity as well (Temel et al. 2010).

Canadian Cardiovascular Society (McKelvie et al. 2011) • "We recommend that the provision of palliative care to patients with HF should be based on a thorough assessment of needs and symptoms, rather than on individual estimate of remaining life expectancy " • "We recommend that the presence of persistent advanced HF symptoms (NYHA III-IV) despite optimal therapy be confirmed, ideally by an interdisciplinary team with expertise in HF management, to ensure appropriate HF management strategies have been considered and optimized, in the context of patient goals and comorbidities" • "We recommend an interdisciplinary chronic care model for the organization and delivery of palliative care to patients with advanced HF"
ACC/AHA (Jessup et al. 2009) • " ... palliative care for patients with chronic HF should be addressed as an ongoing key component of their plan of care, especially when hospitalized with acute decompensation"
European Society of Cardiology (Dickstein et al. 2008; Jaarsma et al. 2009) • "A palliative care approach is applicable to patients with HF and is particularly relevant to those with advanced disease." • "Palliative care should be integrated as part of a team approach to comprehensive HF care and should not be reserved for those who are expected to die within days or weeks." • " ... clinicians should prepare for a 'change in gear' from a chronic stable disease management approach, to enhancement of the supportive and palliative care elements at times of crisis, and then to terminal care when death is imminent"

Table 3. Summary of recommendations of the various guideline agencies.

Conversely, it has only been over the last decade that the palliative needs of the HF population have started to be addressed. As recently as the late 1990's, the number of cancer patients in the United Kingdom (UK) receiving specialist palliative care services was more the 50-fold higher than the number of patients with heart disease receiving this care, despite an actual preponderance of deaths due to cardiovascular disease (Gibbs et al. 2002). Many potential barriers to the involvement of palliative care in this patient population have been identified, including the perceived unwillingness of cardiovascular specialists to seek palliative assistance, as this may be viewed as "giving up". While many treatments for cancer are associated with upfront side effects and difficulty, treatments for HF typically improve symptoms with relatively few side effects. There is also the perceived inability of palliative care specialists to manage complex cardiac patients (Gibbs et al. 2002). However as stated earlier, the main barrier is the inherent difficulty in estimating prognosis in this patient population, given the highly variable disease course. Despite these potential barriers, many cardiovascular associations now include palliative care provisions in their guideline documents (Table 3). The European guidelines also provide a general stepwise framework to facilitate the introduction of palliative care (Table 4). The most recent Canadian guidelines (McKelvie et al. 2011) contain practical tips in terms of carrying out many of these steps.

Patient features • 1 of more episodes of decompensation per 6 months despite optimal tolerated therapy • Need for frequent or continual IV support • Chronic poor quality of life with NYHA IV symptoms • Signs of cardiac cachexia • Clinically judged to be close to the end of life
Confirm diagnosis • Essential to ensure optimal treatment
Patient education • Principles of self-care maintenance and management of HF
Establish an Advanced Care Plan • Designed with the patient and a family member. • Reviewed regularly and includes the patients' preferences for future treatment options (must involve provider(s) with knowledge and experience in care of HF)
Services should be organised • The patients' care within the multidisciplinary team, to ensure optimal pharmacological treatment, self-care management and to facilitate access to supportive services.
Symptom Management • Requires regular and frequent assessment of patients' physical, psychological, social and spiritual needs. • Patients frequently have multiple co-morbidities that need to be identified.
Identifying end-stage heart failure • Confirmation of end-stage HF is advisable to ensure that all appropriate treatment options have been explored a plan for the terminal stage of illness should be agreed upon.
Breaking bad news to the patient and family • Explaining disease progression and a change in treatment emphasis is a sensitive issue and must be approached with care.
Establishing new goals of care • End-of-life care should include avoidance of circumstances that may detract from a peaceful death. • All current pharmacological treatment and device programmes should be considered. • Resuscitation orders should be clear.

Table 4. Goals and steps in the process of providing palliative care in patients with heart failure (modified from the 2008 European Heart Failure Guidelines).

3.1 The Importance of effective communication

A critical component in the management of heart failure is communication. Given the progressive nature of HF, discussions should be carried out with patients and their family members in regards to advanced care-planning issues (Table 5). Ideally, these discussions should take place early in the course of the disease process, as patients with HF are not only at risk of dying from progressive heart failure, but sudden cardiac death as well. While the mortality rate increases as a function of NYHA class, the majority of deaths for patients with lesser NYHA class symptoms are due to sudden cardiac death (Hjalmarson and Goldstein 1999). Early discussion with subsequent updates as clinical condition changes also helps minimize any possible misunderstanding of prognosis. In one study of bereaved family members of heart failure patients with non-sudden cardiac deaths, only 8% of patients and 44% of family members were informed by a physician that time was limited (McCarthy and Hall 1997). It is worthwhile noting that in patients with end-stage refractory heart failure, discussing end-of-life plans and the option of turning off an ICD is a class I recommendation according to the ACC/AHA heart failure guidelines (Jessup et al. 2009). The 2011 Canadian heart failure update provides practical assistance in terms of how to conduct advanced care-planning discussions (McKelvie et al. 2011).

• Identification of a surrogate decision-maker.
• Introduction to "goals of care" designations, and establishing preferences for cardiopulmonary resuscitation and advanced life support.
• Encourage Living Wills and Advanced Directives.
• Exploration of non-traditional symptoms of heart failure in the physical, social, functional or psychological domains.
• The potential role and impact of other comorbidities and frailty in shaping or altering the patient's prognosis.
• Circumstances for discontinuing or turning off an invasive therapy, such as an ICD or other cardiac devices, hemodialysis, laboratory testing.
• Reassurance that periodic re-evaluation of preferences and treatment goals will occur.
• Potential treatment plan for sudden increase in symptoms while at home.

Table 5. Topics of discussion for advanced care planning (modified from (Howlett 2011)).

3.2 Symptom management

Patients with chronic HF experience a multitude of symptoms that have significant impact on their overall sense of wellbeing. The majority of these symptoms are the same as those experienced by cancer patients (Table 6). Unfortunately, non-cardiac symptoms are not commonly addressed in the context of a cardiovascular care setting (Boyd et al. 2004; Solano, Gomes, and Higginson 2006). Patients with HF are more likely to be admitted to hospital, more likely to be admitted to an intensive care unit once hospitalized, more likely to undergo invasive treatments, and more likely to die in an acute care setting (Setoguchi and Stevenson 2009). By ignoring non-cardiac symptoms, patients with HF are sub-optimally treated, leading to the potential of inappropriately aggressive care (Howlett 2011).

Similar to Cancer		Different from Cancer
• Pain	• Anxiety	• More edema
• Dyspnea	• Depression	• More renal dysfunction
• Anorexia	• Fatigue	• More signs of poor perfusion
• Cachexia		
• Postural Hypotension		

Table 6. Common symptoms experienced by heart failure and cancer patients.

3.2.1 Dyspnea, fatigue, and exercise Impairment

Dyspnea is the classic symptom of heart failure. Population studies have shown the incidence to range between 60 to 88% (Solano, Gomes, and Higginson 2006). Severe dyspnea is observed in 35% of patients in the last 3 to 6 months of life (Krumholz et al. 1998). Both fatigue and exercise impairment are also commonly observed in association with dyspnea, with similar prevalence rates (Solano, Gomes, and Higginson 2006). All of these symptoms impact the ability of patients with HF to perform basic activities required for normal daily life, and thus have important implications in terms of their independence and quality of life. These symptoms also contribute to social isolation.

Nitrates and diuretics are the mainstay of treatment for dyspnea. Opioids have also been previously shown to be efficacious (Johnson et al. 2002). However, a recent placebo-controlled study of two different oral opioids (morphine and oxycodone) in patients with CHF was not able to demonstrate any benefit (Oxberry et al. 2011). Similarly, a Cochrane review failed to demonstrate the benefit of benzodiazepines for the relief of dyspnea (Simon et al. 2010), however it is worthwhile point out that this result is based on a total of only 64 patients from 4 different studies. Conversely, regular exercise training has been shown to have beneficial effects in terms of improvement in functional capacity, symptoms, and quality of life (Downing and Balady 2011; Crimi, Ignarro, and Cacciatore 2009). In addition, there also appears to be a modest reduction in repeat hospitalization and mortality (O'Connor et al. 2009). Lastly, alternative care models such as day hospice programs have been shown to be beneficial (Daley, Matthews, and Williams 2009).

3.2.2 Pain

Pain is the second most common symptom experienced by patients with end-stage HF, surpassed only by dyspnea (Nordgren and Sörensen 2003). Anti-anginals are the mainstay for anginal pain. Nonsteroidal anti-inflammatory drugs should be avoided, as they are associated with sodium retention and peripheral vasoconstriction, and can also attenuate the efficacy of diuretics and ACE inhibitors. Although both physicians and patients tend to be wary of opioids, addiction is rare in the terminal patient population (Kanner 2001). For moderate to severe pain, opioids should be used as first-line agents (Adler et al. 2009).

3.2.3 Depression and anxiety

Depression and anxiety are also common symptoms, with prevalences on the order of 20 to 48% and 18 to 45%, respectively (Haworth and Moniz-Cook 2005). The prevalence of both of these symptoms is correlated with HF severity, with lower rates being observed in stable outpatient populations, and higher rates noted in patients with NYHA class IV symptoms. It is interesting to note that some HF therapies such as ICDs can increase anxiety and depression in certain patient subsets, particularly younger patients (Freedenberg, Thomas, and Friedmann 2011).

Patients with depression tend to do poorer than their non-depressed cohorts, in that they have increased rates of cardiac events and hospitalization (Rutledge et al. 2006). Death rates are also noted to be higher in depressed patients with HF (Rutledge et al. 2006). Many studies also show that higher anxiety and depression levels are related to an increased likelihood of ICD shocks (Freedenberg, Thomas, and Friedmann 2011).

Unfortunately, as with other symptoms in HF, large well-designed clinical trails have not been carried out to address optimal management in this patient population (Adler et al. 2009). An important component of managing depression and anxiety is the management of other symptoms, such as dyspnea and pain. While anti-depressants are commonly employed in the general patient population with depression, a recent observational study showed that the use of selective serotonin reuptake inhibitors (SSRIs) or tricyclic antidepressants (TCAs) in the HF patient population was associated with an increased risk of death (Fosbøl et al. 2009). In terms of SSRIs, this study showed that risk was further potentiated when they were co-administered with beta-blockers. Conversely, other studies such as the SAD Heart trial showed improved symptoms with no increase in mortality, although there was a trend for increased CV events in women (O'Connor, Jiang, and Kuchibhalta 2010). More research is required to help clarify this issue. From a non-pharmacologic perspective, cognitive behavioural therapy appears to be beneficial for reducing psychological distress in both the general HF population as well as patients with ICDs (Lewin et al. 2009; Dekker 2011).

3.2.4 Sleep-disordered breathing

Sleep-disordered breathing is common in patients with HF, with prevalence rates ranging up to 50 to 80% (Herrscher et al. 2011). Both central and obstructive etiologies have been observed in this patient population. Central sleep apnea (CSA) results from withdrawal of central drive to the respiratory muscles, whereas obstructive sleep apnea (OSA) results from complete or partial collapse of the pharynx. CSA appears to be a sign of more severe HF (Oldenburg et al. 2007). Both forms of sleep-disordered breathing have been associated with HF symptom progression, as well a poorer overall prognosis compared to patients with HF without sleep-disordered breathing (Javaheri, Shukla, and Zeigler 2007; Wang et al. 2007). Patients suspected of having sleep disordered breathing should be referred on to specialized sleep physicians for formal diagnosis and review of treatment options.

3.2.5 Cardiac cachexia

While cachexia is commonly associated with cancer, it is also observed in the advanced stages of other chronic illnesses including HF. Cardiac cachexia is a complex syndrome and is associated with poor clinical outcomes (Haehling et al. 2009). While anorexia contributes to cardiac cachexia, there are also profound metabolic and inflammatory changes that are observed in this syndrome (Haehling et al. 2009). Unfortunately, treatments targeted at the inflammatory pathways have not been successful. As with the other non-cardiac symptoms, more research is required to help establish optimal therapy, as even optimal nutritional recommendations are unknown at the current time (Haehling et al. 2009).

4. Discontinuation of therapy

In general terms, the initiation of various therapies for patients with HF is relatively straightforward. In many instances, there are consensus documents or formal guidelines published by the various cardiovascular governing agencies (e.g. ACC, AHA, CCS, ESC) to help guide appropriate therapy. Conversely, discontinuation of therapy does not have the same wealth of supporting evidence. In many instances, clinicians are left to make decisions on a patient-by-patient basis, particularly with the discontinuation of medications.

4.1 Medications

As stated at the beginning of this chapter, current patients with HF are older, have more co-morbidities, and take more medications than in the past (Wong et al. 2011). During the time period of 2003 to 2008, patients with HF were taking an average of 6.4 prescription cardiac medications, with 10% of these patients taking more than an average of 11 cardiac medications (Wong et al. 2011). There are suggested methods (Steinman and Hanlon 2010; Bain, Holmes, and Beers 2008) but no guideline documents specific to HF to assist in the process of discontinuing medications for patients who may no longer be benefiting from them as they approach end of life. There does not even appear to be a consensus for medications such as statins whose benefits are achieved mainly with long term use (Vollrath, Sinclair, and Hallenbeck 2005; Davis 2006; Vollrath and Sinclair 2006). In many instances, practical constraints such as hypotension and renal dysfunction come into play. Additionally, patients may reach a point at which pill burden is a source of suffering or they are no longer able to swallow oral medications.

4.2 Devices

Over the course of the last several decades, medical devices have gained an increasingly significant role in the management of many patients with poor left ventricular ejection fraction. Current device options include ICDs, CRT-ICDs, and VADs. In 2008, more than 127,000 ICDs were implanted in the United States (Hammill et al. 2009). As indications for these devices continue to expand, a commensurate increase in the number of patients with these devices will likely be seen (Hammill et al. 2009). In addition, with an aging population, there will be an increasing number of patients with cardiac disease requiring advanced care including device therapy (Groarke et al. 2010).

While the implantation of these devices is directed by well-defined consensus guidelines that have been published by the various cardiovascular governing agencies (e.g. ACC, AHA, CCS, ESC), it has only been in the last year that formal deactivation policies have been published, with the support of other specialty agencies including palliative care (Lampert et al. 2010; Padeletti et al. 2010).

4.2.1 ICDs and CRT devices

As HF worsens, patients are likely to receive more frequent shocks, which cause significant pain and anxiety. This leads to not only patient distress, but also distress of their families and supporting health care team (Goldstein et al. 2004). Discontinuation of ICD therapy is an option for eliminating this distress. Ideally, conversations about when ICD therapy discontinuation would be warranted should be initiated at the time of implantation (Lampert et al. 2010). Not surprisingly, these early conversations occur infrequently (Goldstein, Mehta, and Siddiqui 2008).

Patients must be informed that most ICDs and CRT devices have multiple functions, including tachy-arrhythmia therapies (shock, anti-tachycardia pacing), brady-arrhythmia therapies (conventional pacing), and cardiac resynchronization therapies (bi-ventricular pacing). In this regard, a decision must be made in terms of which functions will be discontinued. The input of a cardiovascular specialist is essential in this regard, as the benefits and burdens of each individual therapy can be reviewed. The majority of patients and their care providers typically elect to only suspend the tachy-arrhythmia therapies (shock, anti-tachycardia pacing), keeping the brady-arrhythmia and cardiac resynchronization therapies (if applicable) in place.

The recent consensus statement published by the Heart Rhythm Society (HRS) states that device deactivation requires a written order from the responsible physician (in emergent situations, a verbal order can be used, followed by written documentation within 24 hours). The ordering physician does not necessarily have to be a cardiologist or cardiac electrophysiologist, but can be the patient's primary care physician, or a hospitalist or palliative care specialist. The written order must address a number of points, as summarized in Table 7.

• Confirmation that the patient (or legal surrogate) has requested device deactivation.
• Capacity of the patient to make the decision, or identification of the appropriate surrogate.
• Confirmation that alternative therapies have been discussed if relevant.
• Confirmation that consequences of deactivation have been discussed.
• The specific device therapies to be deactivated.
• Notification of family, if appropriate.

Table 7. Points for discussion and documentation for device discontinuation (modified from Lampert et al, 2010).

4.2.2 VADs

Left ventricular assist devices have only recently been approved for use as "destination therapy"(Boilson et al. 2010), a term which refers to long term mechanical circulatory support in patients with end-stage heart failure (Boilson et al. 2010). Unlike ICDs and CRT devices, the implantation of a VAD requires open-heart surgery, and as such is associated with all of the associated peri-operative risks. At the present time, the surgical mortality rate is on the order of 5 to 10% (Lund, Jennifer Matthews, and Aaronson 2010). Many patients with significant comorbid conditions will not be suitable for this kind of support. Post implantation, patients are left with a number of on-going medical risks including infection, bleeding, and stroke. Even with a VAD in place, two-year mortality is on the order of 40 – 50%.

VADs impose a psychosocial strain on both patients and their caregivers (Swetz et al. 2011). In recognition of the unique medical and the psychosocial needs of VAD patients, Petrucci and colleagues have developed a framework that addresses the ethical and psychosocial issues that should be discussed with these patients (Petrucci et al. 2011). This framework is provided in Table 8.

Phase I: Initial Information (Understanding Consent)
• Surgical intervention: physical events leading up to this type of surgical intervention including elective vs. emergency consideration.
• Device technology: current device technology including risks, benefits, and outcomes with possible future surgical revisions. VAD as a therapy and rescue device rather than a "cure," with mortality and morbidity remaining high as per recent trials. Review realistic vs. idealistic expectations for recovery.
• Expected recovery: reasons and length of time for expected hospital course and usual recovery after heart surgery.
• Changing plans: the notions that "care plans" can change at any time based on physical, hemodynamic, or neurologic needs. Discuss unexpected events such as machine withdrawal, technical failure, and pump replacement.
Phase II: Pre-implant Preparation (Future Directions)
• Care planning: necessity of advance directives and care planning specific to BTT/DT before implant.
• Appointing a decision maker: appoint a spokesperson, with possible need for capacity determination, neurologic or psychiatric evaluations, and involvement of the institution's risk management group.
• Cultural preference: consider possible cultural and religious preferences.
• Conflict resolution: involve institution's ethics committee when conflicts persist beyond advance care planning between family expectations and patient's progress.
Phase III: VAD-Specific End-of-Life Issues (Withdrawing Care)
• Palliative plan: defining and discussion of ECMO, DNR, and DNI orders, and removal of life support in light of mechanical support. Discuss palliative or comfort care in hospital, home, or other facility.
• Acceptable withdrawal: develop an acceptable device withdrawal process for patient and family.
Abbreviations:
• BTT, bridge to transplant; DNI, do not intubate; DNR, do not resuscitate; DT, destination therapy; ECMO, extracorporeal membrane oxygenation;

Table 8. A framework for ethical and psychosocial issues associated VADS (modified from Petrucci et al., 2011).

5. Conclusion

Heart failure is a progressive disease responsible for significant morbidity and mortality throughout the world. There is no question that advances in medical therapy have improved the prognosis of this patient population. But with these advances, other elements in the care of these patients have been neglected. Specifically, patients with HF commonly have a poor overall sense of well-being. Optimal therapy in this regard remains unknown but it is unlikely that medical and technology advances alone will improve well-being (O'Leary and Murphy 2009). In addition, unique issues arise, including the indications and timing for discontinuation of these therapies at end-of-life. Evolution of HF care in the future will incorporate elements of palliative care (sensitive communication, attention to patient's goals, family and caregiver support assessment and attending to all a persons' needs) with the medical model of "cardiac optimization", throughout all phases of the disease trajectory. Working across disciplines to translate guidelines from various cardiovascular governing bodies into practice may help to facilitate this approach.

6. References

Abouezzeddine, Omar F, and Margaret M Redfield. 2011. "Who has advanced heart failure? Definition and epidemiology." *Congestive heart failure (Greenwich, Conn.)* 17 (4) 160–168.

Adler, E D, J Z Goldfinger, J Kalman, M E Park, and D E Meier. 2009. "Palliative Care in the Treatment of Advanced Heart Failure." *Circulation* 120 (25) 2597–2606.

Bain, KT, HM Holmes, and MH Beers. 2008. "Discontinuing Medications: A Novel Approach for Revising the Prescribing Stage of the Medication-Use Process." *Jurnal of the American Geriatrics Society* 56(10): 1946-52.

Boilson, Barry A, Eugenia Raichlin, Soon J Park, and Sudhir S Kushwaha. 2010. "Device therapy and cardiac transplantation for end-stage heart failure." *Current problems in cardiology* 35 (1) 8–64.

Boyd, Kirsty J, Scott A Murray, Marilyn Kendall, Allison Worth, T Frederick Benton, and Hans Clausen. 2004. "Living with advanced heart failure: a prospective, community based study of patients and their carers.." *European journal of heart failure* 6 (5) 585–591.

Braunschweig, Frieder, Martin R Cowie, and Angelo Auricchio. 2011. "What are the costs of heart failure?." *Europace* 13 Suppl 2 ii13–7.

Crimi, E, LJ Ignarro, and F Cacciatore. 2009. "Mechanisms by which exercise training benefits patients with heart failure." *Nature Reviews Cardiology*. 6(4): 292-300.

Daley, Andrew, Christine Matthews, and Anne Williams. 2006. "Heart failure and palliative care services working in partnership: report of a new model of care.." *Palliative medicine* 20 (6) 593–601.

Davis, George F. 2006. "Discontinuing Lipid-Lowering Agents." *Journal of palliative medicine* 9 (3) 619–619.

Dekker, Rebecca L. 2011. "Cognitive Therapy for Depression in Patients with Heart Failure: A Critical Review." *Heart failure clinics* 7 (1) 127–141.

Dickstein, K, A Cohen-Solal, G Filippatos, J J V McMurray, P Ponikowski, P A Poole-Wilson, A Stromberg, et al. 2008. "ESC Guidelines for the diagnosis and treatment of acute and chronic heart failure 2008: The Task Force for the Diagnosis and Treatment of Acute and Chronic Heart Failure 2008 of the European Society of Cardiology. Developed in collaboration with the Heart Failure Association of the ESC (HFA) and endorsed by the European Society of Intensive Care Medicine (ESICM)." *European Heart Journal* 29 (19) 2388–2442.

Downing, Jill, and Gary J Balady. 2011. "The role of exercise training in heart failure.." *Journal of the American College of Cardiology* 58 (6) 561–569.

Foot, D K, R P Lewis, T A Pearson, and G A Beller. 2000. "Demographics and cardiology, 1950-2050.." *Journal of the American College of Cardiology* 35 (5 Suppl B) (April): 66B–80B.

Fosbøl, Emil Loldrup, Gunnar H Gislason, Henrik Enghusen Poulsen, Morten Lock Hansen, Fredrik Folke, Tina Ken Schramm, Jonas Bjerring Olesen, et al. 2009. "Prognosis in heart failure and the value of {beta}-blockers are altered by the use of antidepressants and depend on the type of antidepressants used.." *Circulation: Heart Failure* 2 (6) 582–590.

Freedenberg, Vicki, Sue A Thomas, and Erika Friedmann. 2011. "Anxiety and depression in implanted cardioverter-defibrillator recipients and heart failure: a review.." *Heart failure clinics* 7 (1) 59–68.

Gibbs, J S R, A S M McCoy, L M E Gibbs, A E Rogers, and J M Addington-Hall. 2002. "Living with and dying from heart failure: the role of palliative care." *Heart (British Cardiac Society)* 88 Suppl 2 ii36–9.

Goldstein, Nathan E, Rachel Lampert, Elizabeth Bradley, Joanne Lynn, and Harlan M Krumholz. 2004. "Management of implantable cardioverter defibrillators in end-of-life care.." *Annals of internal medicine* 141 (11) 835–838.

Goldstein, NE, D Mehta, and S Siddiqui. 2008. ""That"s Like an Act of Suicide" Patients" Attitudes Toward Deactivation of Implantable Defibrillators." *Journal of general internal medicine.* 23 Suppl 1: 7-12.

Goodlin, Sarah J. 2009. "Palliative care in congestive heart failure.." *Journal of the American College of Cardiology* 54 (5) 386–396.

Groarke, J D, G Blake, H McCann, D Sugrue, and N Mahon. 2010. "Increasing cardiac interventions among the aged.." *Irish medical journal* 103 (10) (October): 308–310.

Haehling, von, Stephan, Mitja Lainscak, Jochen Springer, and Stefan D Anker. 2009. "Cardiac cachexia: A systematic overview." *Pharmacology & Therapeutics* 121 (3) 227–252.

Hammill, Stephen C, Mark S Kremers, Alan H Kadish, Lynne Warner Stevenson, Paul A Heidenreich, Bruce D Lindsay, Michael J Mirro, et al. 2009. "Review of the ICD Registry's third year, expansion to include lead data and pediatric ICD procedures, and role for measuring performance.." *Heart rhythm : the official journal of the Heart Rhythm Society* 6 (9) 1397–1401.

Haworth, JE, and E Moniz-Cook. 2005. "Prevalence and predictors of anxiety and depression in a sample of chronic heart failure patients with left ventricular systolic dysfunction." *European journal of heart failure* 7(5):803-8.

Herrscher, Tobias E, Harriet Akre, Britt Øverland, Leiv Sandvik, and Arne S Westheim. 2011. "High Prevalence of Sleep Apnea in Heart Failure Outpatients: Even in Patients With Preserved Systolic Function." *Journal of cardiac failure* 17 (5) 420–425.

Hinton, JM. 1963. "The physical and mental distress of the dying.." *The Quarterly journal of medicine* 32:1-21.

Hjalmarson, Å, and USA) B Fagerberg secretary Sweden H Wedel biostatistician Sweden F Waagstein Sweden J Kjekshus Norway J Wikstrand senior medical advisor Astra Hässle Sweden G Westergren project leader Astra Hässle Sweden S Goldstein cochairman. 1999. "Effect of metoprolol CR/XL in chronic heart failure: Metoprolol CR/XL Randomised Intervention Trial in Congestive Heart Failure (MERIT-HF)." *The Lancet* 353 (9169) 2001–2007.

Howlett, Jonathan G. 2011. "Palliative care in heart failure: addressing the largest care gap.." *Current opinion in cardiology* 26 (2) 144–148.

Jaarsma, T, J M Beattie, M Ryder, F H Rutten, T McDonagh, P Mohacsi, S A Murray, et al. 2009. "Palliative care in heart failure: a position statement from the palliative care workshop of the Heart Failure Association of the European Society of Cardiology." *European journal of heart failure* 11 (5) 433–443.

Javaheri, S, R Shukla, and H Zeigler. 2007. "ScienceDirect - Journal of the American College of Cardiology: Central Sleep Apnea, Right Ventricular Dysfunction, and Low Diastolic Blood Pressure Are Predictors of Mortality in Systolic Heart Failure." *Journal of the American College of Cardiology* 49(20): 2028-34.

Jessup, M, W T Abraham, D E Casey, A M Feldman, G S Francis, T G Ganiats, M A Konstam, et al. 2009. "2009 Focused Update: ACCF/AHA Guidelines for the Diagnosis and Management of Heart Failure in Adults: A Report of the American College of Cardiology Foundation/American Heart Association Task Force on Practice Guidelines: Developed in Collaboration With the International Society for Heart and Lung Transplantation." *Circulation* 119 (14) 1977–2016.

Johnson, M J, T A McDonagh, A Harkness, S E McKay, and H J Dargie. 2002. "Morphine for the relief of breathlessness in patients with chronic heart failure--a pilot study.." *European journal of heart failure* 4 (6) 753–756.

Kanner, R M. 2001. "Opioids for severe pain: little change over 15 years.." *Journal of pain and symptom management* 21 (1) 3.

Kaul, P, F A McAlister, J A Ezekowitz, J A Bakal, L H Curtis, H Quan, M L Knudtson, and P W Armstrong. 2011. "Resource Use in the Last 6 Months of Life Among Patients With Heart Failure in Canada." *Archives of internal medicine* 171 (3) 211–217.

Krumholz, HM, RS Phillips, MB Hamel, and JM Teno. 1998. "Resuscitation preferences among patients with severe congestive heart failure: results from the SUPPORT project." *Circulation* 98(7): 648-55.

Lampert, Rachel, David L Hayes, George J Annas, Margaret A Farley, Nathan E Goldstein, Robert M Hamilton, G Neal Kay, et al. 2010. HRS Expert Consensus Statement on the Management of Cardiovascular Implantable Electronic Devices (CIEDs) in patients nearing end of life or requesting withdrawal of therapy. In *Heart rhythm : the official journal of the Heart Rhythm Society*, 7:1008–1026. July.

Lewin, R J, S Coulton, D J Frizelle, G Kaye, and H Cox. 2009. "A brief cognitive behavioural preimplantation and rehabilitation programme for patients receiving an implantable cardioverter-defibrillator improves physical health and reduces psychological morbidity and unplanned readmissions.." *Heart (British Cardiac Society)* 95 (1) 63–69.

Lloyd-Jones, Donald, Robert J Adams, Todd M Brown, Mercedes Carnethon, Shifan Dai, Giovanni de Simone, T Bruce Ferguson, et al. 2010. "Executive summary: heart disease and stroke statistics--2010 update: a report from the American Heart Association."*Circulation* 121 (7) 948–954.

Lund, Lars H, Jennifer Matthews, and Keith Aaronson. 2010. "Patient selection for left ventricular assist devices.." *European journal of heart failure* 12 (5) 434–443.

McCarthy, M, and JA Hall. 1997. "Communication and choice in dying from heart disease.." *Journal of the Royal Society of Medicine* 90(3):128-31.

McKelvie, Robert S, Gordon W Moe, Anson Cheung, Jeannine Costigan, Anique Ducharme, Estrellita Estrella-Holder, Justin A Ezekowitz, et al. 2011. "The 2011 Canadian Cardiovascular Society heart failure management guidelines update: focus on sleep apnea, renal dysfunction, mechanical circulatory support, and palliative care.." *The Canadian journal of cardiology* 27 (3) 319–338.

Murray, Sa, A Worth, K Boyd, M Kendall, and J Hockley. 2007. *Patients', carers' and professionals' experiences of diagnosis, treatment and end-of-life care in heart failure: a prospective, qualitative interview study*. British Heart Foundation.

Murray, Scott A, K Boyd, M Kendall, A Worth, and TF Benton. 2002. "Dying of lung cancer or cardiac failure: prospective qualitative interview study of patients and their carers in the community." British Medical Jurnal 325:924.

Murray, Scott A, and Aziz Sheikh. 2008. "Palliative Care Beyond Cancer: Care for all at the end of life.." *BMJ (Clinical research ed.)* 336 (7650) 958–959.

Murthy, Sandhya, and Hannah I Lipman. 2011. "Management of end-stage heart failure.." *Primary care* 38 (2) 265–76, viii.

Nordgren, Lena, and Stefan Sörensen. 2003. "Symptoms experienced in the last six months of life in patients with end-stage heart failure.." *European journal of cardiovascular nursing : journal of the Working Group on Cardiovascular Nursing of the European Society of Cardiology* 2 (3) 213–217.

O'Connor, Christopher M, David J Whellan, Kerry L Lee, Steven J Keteyian, Lawton S Cooper, Stephen J Ellis, Eric S Leifer, et al. 2009. "Efficacy and safety of exercise training in patients with chronic heart failure: HF-ACTION randomized controlled trial.." *JAMA : the journal of the American Medical Association* 301 (14) 1439–1450.

O'Connor, CM, W Jiang, and M Kuchibhatla. 2010. "Safety and Efficacy of Sertraline for Depression in Patients With Heart Failure:: Results of the SADHART-CHF (Sertraline Against Depression and Heart Disease in Chronik Heart Failure "*Journal of the American College of Cardiology* 56(9):692-9.

O'Leary, N, and NF Murphy. 2009. "A comparative study of the palliative care needs of heart failure and cancer patients." *European Journal of heart failure* 11(4):406-12.

Oldenburg, O, B Lamp, L Faber, H TESCHLER, D HORSTKOTTE, and V TOPFER. 2007. "Sleep-disordered breathing in patients with symptomatic heart failureA contemporary study of prevalence in and characteristics of 700 patients." *European journal of heart failure* 9 (3) 251–257.

Oxberry, Stephen G, David J Torgerson, J Martin Bland, Andrew L Clark, John G F Cleland, and Miriam J Johnson. 2011. "Short-term opioids for breathlessness in stable chronic heart failure: a randomized controlled trial.." *European journal of heart failure* 13(9):1006-12.

Padeletti, L, D O Arnar, L Boncinelli, J Brachman, J A Camm, J C Daubert, S Kassam, et al. 2010. "EHRA Expert Consensus Statement on the management of cardiovascular implantable electronic devices in patients nearing end of life or requesting withdrawal of therapy." *Europace* 12 (10) 1480–1489.

Petrucci, Ralph J, Lynne A Benish, Barbara L Carrow, Lisa Prato, Shelley R Hankins, Howard J Eisen, and John W Entwistle. 2011. "Ethical considerations for ventricular assist device support: a 10-point model.." *ASAIO journal (American Society for Artificial Internal Organs: 1992)* 57 (4) 268–273.

Rutledge, Thomas, Veronica A Reis, Sarah E Linke, Barry H Greenberg, and Paul J Mills. 2006. "Depression in Heart Failure." *Journal of the American College of Cardiology* 48 (8) 1527–1537.

Selman, L, R Harding, and T Beynon. 2007. "Modelling services to meet the palliative care needs of chronic heart failure patients and their families: current practice in the UK." *Palliative Medicine* 21(5):385-90.

Setoguchi, Soko, and Lynne Warner Stevenson. 2009. "Hospitalizations in patients with heart failure: who and why.." *Journal of the American College of Cardiology* 54 (18) 1703–1705.

Simon, Steffen T, Irene J Higginson, Sara Booth, Richard Harding, and Claudia Bausewein. 2011. "Benzodiazepines for the relief of breathlessness in advanced malignant and non-malignant diseases in adults.." *Cochrane database of systematic reviews.*

Solano, Joao Paulo, Barbara Gomes, and Irene J Higginson. 2006. "A comparison of symptom prevalence in far advanced cancer, AIDS, heart disease, chronic obstructive pulmonary disease and renal disease.." *Journal of pain and symptom management* 31 (1) 58–69.

Steinman, M A, and J T Hanlon. 2010. "Managing Medications in Clinically Complex Elders: 'There's Got to Be a Happy Medium'." *JAMA : the journal of the American Medical Association* 304 (14) 1592–1601.

Swetz, Keith M, Abigale L Ottenberg, Monica R Freeman, and Paul S Mueller. 2011. "Palliative Care and End-of-Life Issues in Patients Treated with Left Ventricular Assist Devices as Destination Therapy." *Current heart failure reports* (May 3).

Temel, Jennifer S, Joseph A Greer, Alona Muzikansky, Emily R Gallagher, Sonal Admane, Vicki A Jackson, Constance M Dahlin, et al. 2010. "Early palliative care for patients with metastatic non-small-cell lung cancer." *The New England journal of medicine* 363 (8) 733–742.

Vollrath, AM, and C Sinclair. 2006. "Lipid-Lowering Agents: The Authors' Response." *Journal of Palliative Medicine* 8(4):876-81

Vollrath, Annette M, Christian Sinclair, and James Hallenbeck. 2005. "Discontinuing Cardiovascular Medications at the End of Life: Lipid-Lowering Agents." *Journal of palliative medicine* 8 (4) 876–881.

Wang, H, JD Parker, GE Newton, and JS Floras. 2007. "Influence of obstructive sleep apnea on mortality in patients with heart failure." *Journal of the American College of Cardiology* 49(15):1625-31.

Wong, C Y, S I Chaudhry, M M Desai, and H M Krumholz. 2011. "Trends in Comorbidity, Disability, and Polypharmacy in Heart Failure." *AJM* 124 (2) 136–143.

Part 3

Models of Care

12

A Framework for Policy-Based Data Integration in Palliative Health Care

Benjamin Eze
University of Ottawa,
Canada

1. Introduction

Electronic Health (e-Health) processes are data-focused, event-driven, and dynamic. Palliative Health care presents a challenge of caring for patients from home by doctors, nurses and other patient providers that operate in domains and organizations that do not share common collaboration technologies. Integrating data across these providers is often difficult or impossible because of incompatible applications, as well as security and privacy concerns. In addition, these exchanges need to be systematically monitored for compliance with legislation, privacy, accreditation guidelines, and quality of care protocols.

To address these specific requirements for e-Health processes especially as it relates to Palliative healthcare, we extend traditional SOA infrastructure with policy-based processing of streaming event data based on a general publish/subscribe model in a business-to-business (B2B) healthcare domain. This entails the use of a policy-based message broker to execute subscription policies on streaming event messages. This approach provides great flexibility to the distribution and integration of data within a B2B network. Applying this framework to palliative healthcare provides a dynamic data sharing model for real-time monitoring of a patient health status, medical records, reports and other necessary information with healthcare providers operating in disparate domains.

2. Background

In palliative health care, patients are catered for from their homes and this brings with it added complexity in terms of who has the permissions to access patient medical records, under what conditions and what time span. Most importantly, there is also the need to have real-time monitoring of patient health status and the ability to provide timely and accurate interventions when emergencies occur. Using a common collaboration portal is often not appropriate. Portals provide a common port of call for information but fail to address the dynamic nature of the patient relationship as well as rules of association with their healthcare providers.

Recent initiatives advocate that healthcare should be delivered as integrated services that make data accessible within distributed processes across different contexts (Coiera and Hovenga, 2007). Community care, especially at-home care, usually requires the integration of care processes across several providers and organizations in a business-to-business (B2B) network.

We also recognize that effective and efficient collaboration for applications in a B2B depends on the ease of information flow between parties. Collaboration must cut across all the communications strata: software applications, databases, server processes, mobile devices and low level sensors (Foster et. al, 2002).

Service Oriented Architecture (SOA) (Huhns & Singh, 2005) has emerged as the standard framework for an extensible machine-to-machine interaction using the Internet as a veritable communication platform. SOA enables applications to exchange data across organization domains and firewall. As depicted in Figure 1, clients discover a service address from a registry and need to subsequently pool this service broker for data in a request/response style interaction. As a result many implementations of SOA entail unnecessary procedural interaction and data polling that could limit flexible data integration (Eze et al., 2010). This is particularly true with processes that run within a B2B network as opposed to a single enterprise (Doshi& Peyton, 2008).

Unlike SOA, event-driven systems (Niblet & Graham, 2005) are characterized by their ability to decouple service providers and consumers through messages (Etzion et. al, 2006) or data being exchanged. Event-driven Architectures (EDA) contextually decouple data producers and consumers only by their data exchanges and not through procedural calls (Eugster et. al, 2003).

The Publish/subscribe framework follows the EDA model but allows many data consumers to subscribe to data sources, and have event data sent to them as messages, as they become available. A combination of SOA with EDA publish/subscribe type interaction provides a more robust interaction. Service providers and consumers are totally decoupled by a central middleware, the message broker.

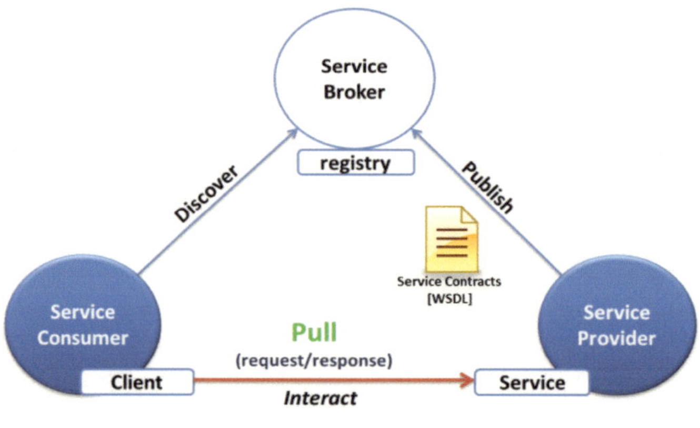

Fig. 1. Service Oriented Architecture Illustrated.

Data consumers indicate interest to data through subscriptions and data publishers only publish data to the broker as they become available. Clients do not poll data; they simply present an interface for a broker to push data to as they are made available from other publishers or data sources.

Figure 2 present a combined SOA and publish-subscribe style interaction. We can see that both SOA and event-driven architecture provide communication and data sharing flexibilities that are complimentary for efficient data sharing and enterprise collaboration. However, they still do not address fully the information management requirements of e-

Health monitoring processes. In particular, both frameworks lack support for a common data model across a B2B network to support data integration (Eze et al., 2010).

In an e-Health network that supports Palliative Healthcare, there may be many different types of data from many different organizational sources that must be integrated to provide a single consistent view of the information flow. Such complex data exchanges also need robust privacy (Peyton et. al, 2007) considerations and enforcement. As well, policy compliance is an issue with respect to privacy legislation, hospital guidelines, and procedures that dictate under what circumstances individuals can view data.

To support such flexibility, rules-based policies are used to govern system behaviour by providing reactive functionalities (Harrocks et. al, 2003). Executed through policy engines, rule-based policies are very adaptable to a wide range of applications, such as adapting composite services with constantly changing business processes. Rules languages in the form of event-condition-action tuples, when presented in XML (Bailey and Wood, 2003), become powerful tools for expressing both attribute and role-based access control policies. eXtensible Access Control Markup Language (XACML) (OASIS eXtensible Access Control Markup Language [OASIS], 2011)is a standardized common security-policy language that "allows the enterprise to manage the enforcement of all the elements of its security policy in all the components of its information systems".

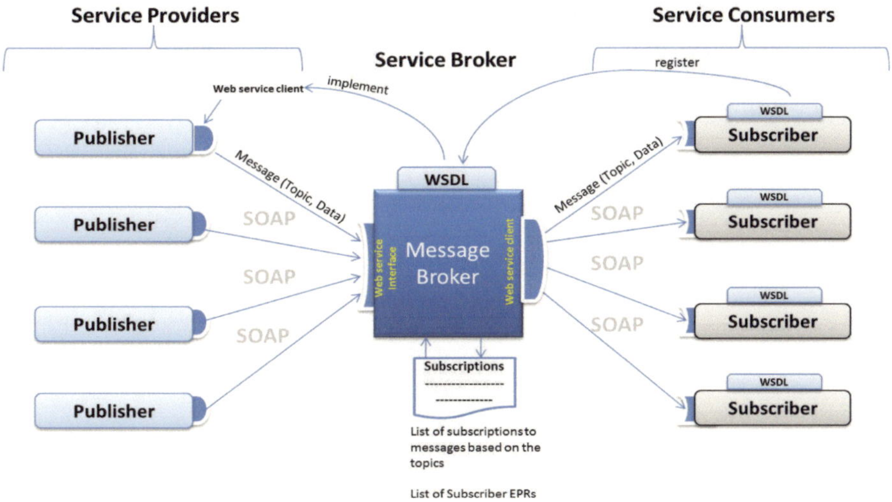

Fig. 2. SOA Publish/Subscribe Style Interaction.

It has been applied to compliance, including data sharing, as determined by the message context (Barth et. al, 2006).

In this chapter, our focus is to find the right fit of technologies and methodologies to support dynamic data sharing and collaboration as required with Palliative Healthcare. We present a framework that is designed to achieve this flexibly. This framework provides dynamic interaction and data sharing by extending the traditional SOA publish/Subscribe framework to support a common communication model through dynamic policies that can flexibly reflect dynamic changing rules of exchange as well as privacy and security considerations. Our framework supports policy-based processing of streaming event data using a general publish/subscribe model. This model provides good flexibility in the distribution and integration of data within a B2B network.

3. Palliative severe pain management scenario

Let us start with a Palliative Severe Pain Management Scenario. Palliative Severe Pain Management addresses one of the application areas of Palliative Care: Severe Pain Management (SPM). Severe pain is a pain score of 8 and above on a 10-point numeric rating scale (Kuziemsky et. al, 2008).

In discussing this scenario (Figure 3), we make the following assumptions:

- A patient is admitted into Palliative Care and starts receiving medical care from home. This patient is able to check and post periodic Pain Scores using the home PC, PDA or through automatic sensors.
- A patient assigned nurse automatically cumulates and analyses these pain scores to determine how the effective pain medications are on the patient.
- If the nurse's pain reports indicate severe pain above the acceptable threshold, the nurse sends a Pain alert to the patient physician for action. It should be noted that this nurse doesn't necessarily know the physician that will act on the alert.
- The patient physician then pulls historical reports to determine if the patient needs a new prescription. If required, the physician sends a new pain relief prescription back to the nurse who then administers the new prescription on the patient.
- The entire interaction is captured by the Palliative Care Portal (PCP) for reporting, non-repudiation and legal compliance.

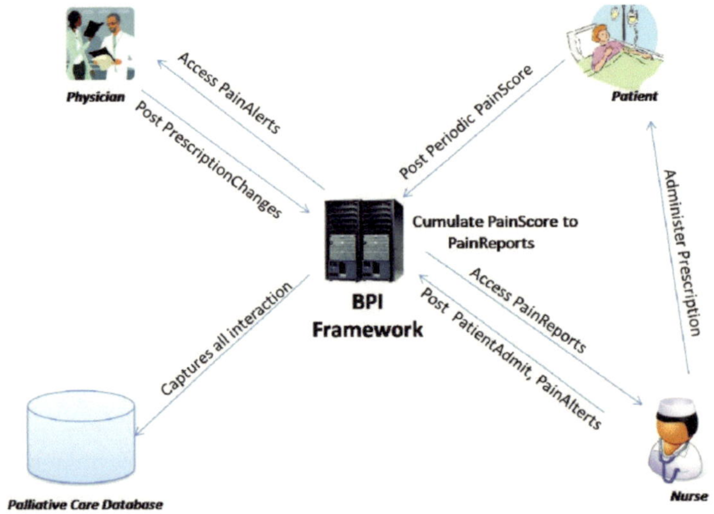

Fig. 3. Palliative SPM Scenario.

Palliative SPM Scenario described above requires an appropriate BPI framework for coordinating the data-sharing between the patient, nurse, doctor and the database infrastructure. Subsequent sections describe different approaches to solving the problems presented in this scenario and how our framework provides the most flexible architecture for achieving flexible data sharing and collaboration for all the players described in this scenario.

4. Web portal based approach

Web Portals are the most popular collaboration technology available on the Internet today. They are popular because they are easy to setup, central and easy to manage and control. It sells well when the participants belong to the same organization or union and agree to use a common collaboration portal. In addition, it must be operated by humans in real-time and all the data belongs to the portal custodian or host.

See Figure 4, the Web Portal connects the clinical management, patient care, and SPM applications as well as a number data sources into one application portal. Patients are admitted into Palliative Care when nurses create profiles for them. Patients are likely setup to use their home PC to periodically enter their *PainScore* to the portal through the Patient interface. The nurse periodically runs *PainReports* on each of the patient to analyze and determine the performance of their prescriptions. When anomalies are detected, a doctor is notified to advice on the next line of action.

In this approach, all parties: patients, nurses, and physicians are required to have access to the Web application portal in order to participate in Palliative Care. This doesn't reflect a true B2B interaction since it provides no mechanism for automatically integrating external but already existing clinical and hospital management systems.

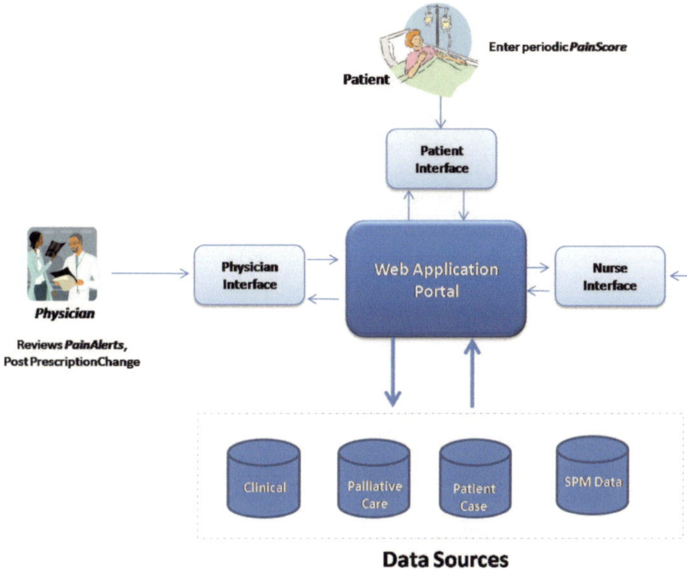

Fig. 4. Web Portal Based Approach to SPM.

The Web Portal based approach is not data-driven but interface-driven because interfaces define data and they are not easily modified to meet new requirements across the organizations using them.

Finally, the data sources are statically linked and represent a strong coupling. Rules of data exchanges are embedded in low-level business rules stuck in complex database views, stored procedures, applications methods and objects. They are usually not dynamic enough to capture new requirements. This is essentially a monolithic framework with static processes, interfaces, roles and permissions.

5. Traditional SOA Publish/Subscribe approach

SOA Publish/Subscribe approaches this problem by describing interactions as a network of events. Participating parties are seen as producers and consumers of event messages. This is very similar to the way emails are exchanged between various application domains. However in SOA publish/subscribe, these messages are application messages. Each event results in some data being communicated from an event source to an event destination.

In SOA publish/subscribe, the Palliative Sever Pain Management scenario described above is broken down into a set of *Topics* representing data exchanges. Figure 5 provides an architectural representation of this interaction. All communication amongst the partners uses HTTP/SOAP as the transport protocol.

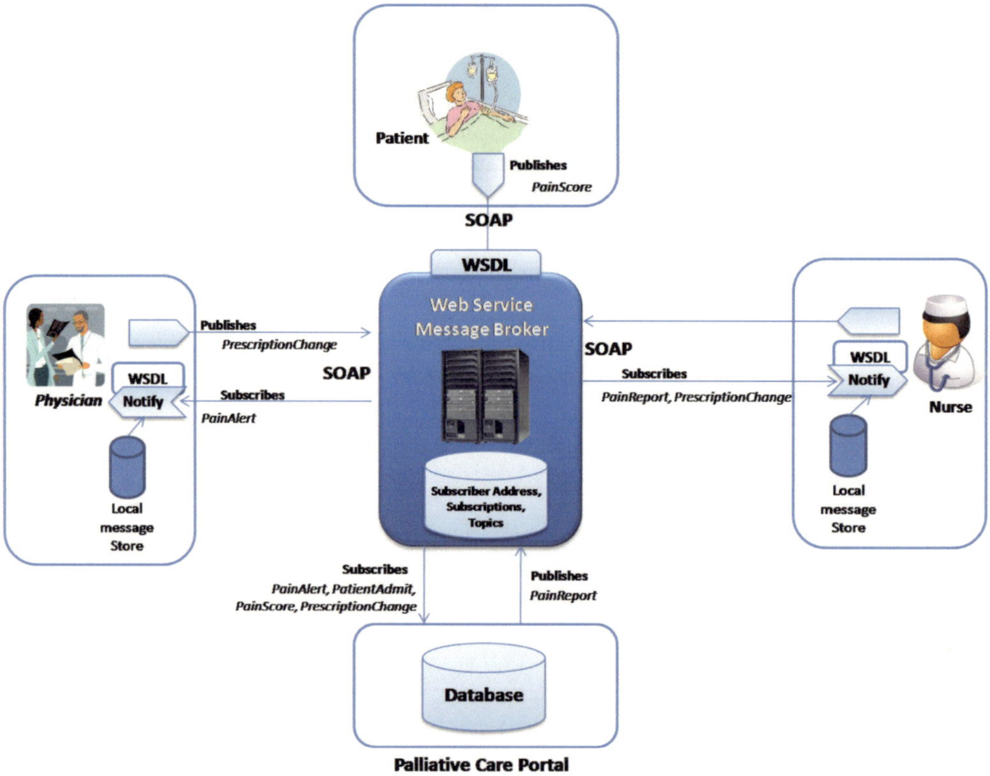

Fig. 5. SPM using SOA Publish/Subscribe Architecture.

This is realized by implementing a Partner Service Component for each collaborating party. This tool helps a participating party to push and receive data from the B2B network. Then there is a message broker that creates the virtual message pathway for message distribution. A Partner Service component implements a generic web service *notify()* interface that the message broker pushes messages to as well as a web service client that is used internally for publishing messages meant for other parties in the B2B network, through the same message broker.

The message broker plays the role of a message router. It receives all communication and routes them to the destination subscribers. In addition, the message broker maintains a list of all participating partners through a registration process for both publishers and subscribers. It also keeps a list of subscribers' topic subscriptions. Table 1 summarizes the roles played by the Partners in this scenario.

In this approach data sources need to publish data to the message broker while data consumers are required to have registered and active subscriptions to the topic of interest with the message broker.

For example the nurse plays the role of a publisher of *PatientAdmit and PainAlert* data, as well as a subscriber to *PainReport and PrescriptionChange.* Since the topics are pre-defined, the Palliative Care Portal subscribes to all the topics. This way, it is able to receive all the messages sent on these topics. We assume these messages are simple data blobs, with no support for content filtering.

Node/Service	Role	Topic of messages published	Message Topic Subscriptions
Broker	Message Broker	None	None
Nurse	Publisher/Subscriber	PatientAdmit PainAlert	PainReport PrescriptionChange
Patient	Publisher	PainScore	None
Physician	Publisher/Subscriber	PrescriptionChange	PainAlert
Palliative Care Portal	Publisher/Subscriber	PainReport	PatientAdmit PainAlert PainScore PrescriptionChange

Table 1. Palliative SPM Management in a Publish/Subscribe Topology.

The SOA publish/subscribe implementation described in this section supports our Palliative SPM scenario by decomposing complex BPI problems into multiple atomic events with multiple interactions using publish/subscribe. Unlike the Web Application portal approach, the definition is not statically tied to a B2B. Rather they are dynamically defined as run-time attributes to the framework.

However, despite the flexibilities introduced by this approach, it still utilizes publish/subscribe broadcast type interaction. Topic advertisement from arbitrary publishers is not a secure way of decomposing processes. It fails to define a mechanism for defining more flexible subscriptions that filters message contents for specific patterns, support message transformation and describe how and when the notification should be delivered.

6. Policy-based SOA Publish/Subscribe data sharing model

This architecture is functionally similar to the SOA publish/subscribe described in the previous section but with additional components for dynamic BPI using a policy model.

Consider the data sharing model in Figure 6, where data is being published and subscribed to by applications, devices and in some cases business processes. This approach tries to marry topic-based Publish/subscribe with content-based filtering. Self-describing topics identified by a name, and set of attribute value pairs, describe the published messages. The topic registrar is a service that defines as well as describes topics to the message broker.

In addition, the registrar could optionally define policies that restrict message publishers to defined topics. Subscriptions on the other hand describe interest to messages. Like topics and messages, policies are used to describe this interest flexibly, as well define attributes for message transformation, aggregation, and delivery Quality of Service.

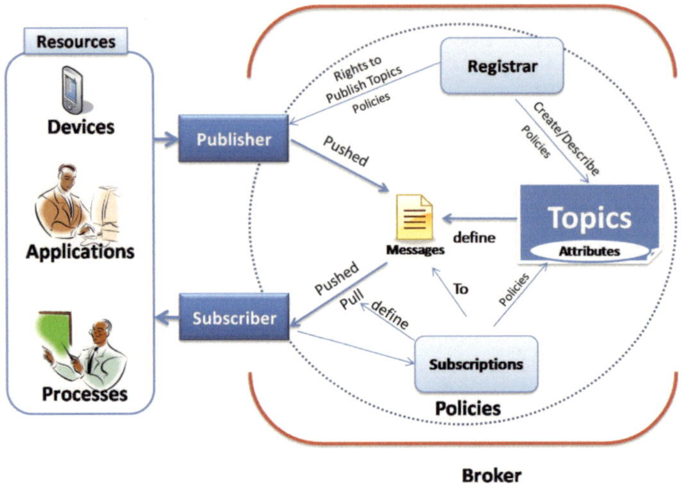

Fig. 6. Policy-based Pub/sub data sharing model.

6.1 Policy types

The policy framework described above is to extend an SOA publish/subscribe with added flexibilities and functionalities. As described in Figure 7, our framework supports four types of policies:

1. **Topic Policy**: Topics describe a message to the message broker. A *Topic Policy* provides a means of controlling "who has access to publish what". Topic creation can be controlled by delegating this responsibility to select publishers called *Topic Registrars*.

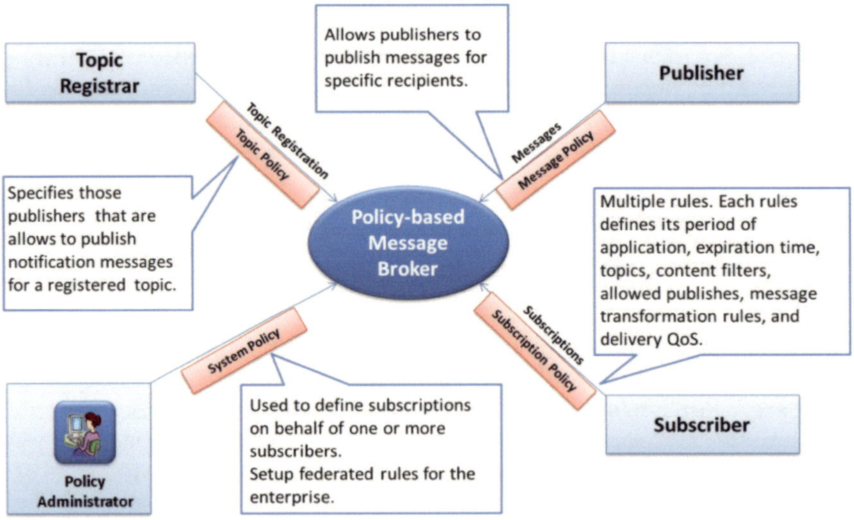

Fig. 7. Policy Types.

2. **Message Policy:** In publish/subscribe, messages are sent off from publishers to be routed to subscribers based on their subscriptions. In this approach, publishers of messages have no mechanism for controlling the recipients. Messages are simply broadcast to subscribers based on their subscriptions to a topic. In B2B, it is often required that certain communication be restricted to select parties. Message policies describe a means of achieving this flexibility in publish/subscribe. They define intended recipients to a message, thus allowing us to support various variants of broadcast type messaging as well as one-to-one messaging using publish/subscribe.
3. **Subscription Policy:** Simply stated, subscriptions are used by subscribers to indicate interests to a type of message usually by the topic or other meta-data as seen in content-based subscription. Our framework extends subscription through declarative policies to support scheduling, a more efficient combination of topic and content filtering, context-based message transformation and delivery QoS.
4. **System Policy:** It is often not appropriate security wise or in terms of management of data-driven rules of association to rely on applications/users to describe their interest to data appropriately. System policies are subscriptions done on behalf of subscribers by a policy administrator. System policies help define federated rules for data sharing with an enterprise view to its application. They can be automated and tied to an organization security policy and operations.

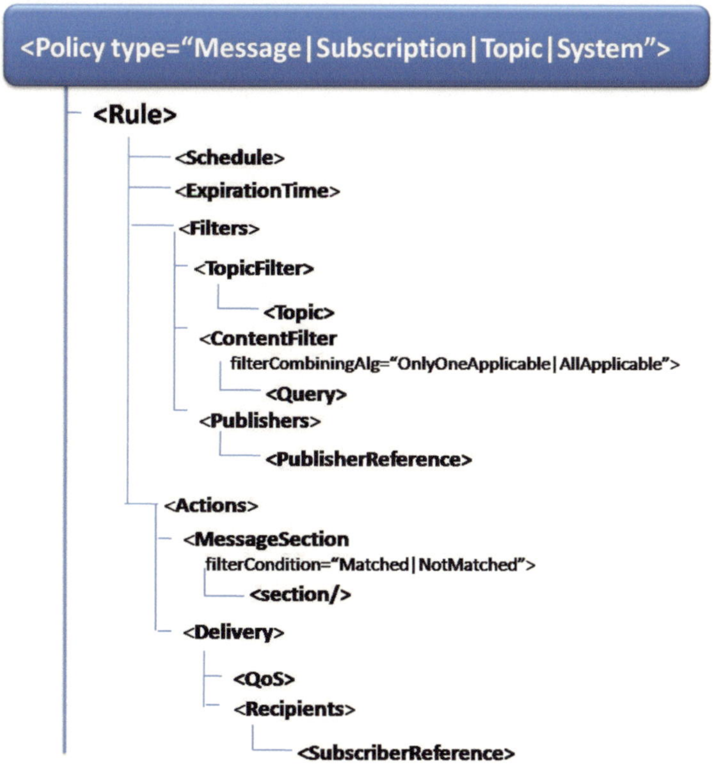

Fig. 8. Policy Representation.

Figure 8 shows a tree representation depicting a policy as a set of rules that describe a message. Notice that:

1. The <*TopicFilter*> element contains one or more <*Topic*>elements that define the topics for messages that it applies to.
2. <*ContentFilter*> element contains one or more XPath queries defined in <*Query*> elements and can be combined on the basis of the filter combining algorithm.
3. <*Publisher*> elements contain a list of allowed publishers described by the <*PublisherReference*> elements
4. <*Actions*> describe message transformation and rules for message delivery. Message transformation depends on the result of the result of filter execution.
5. <*Delivery*> element defines message delivery QoS. The <QoS> element values can be set as "BestEfforts", "Reliable" or batched/queued "Pullpoints".

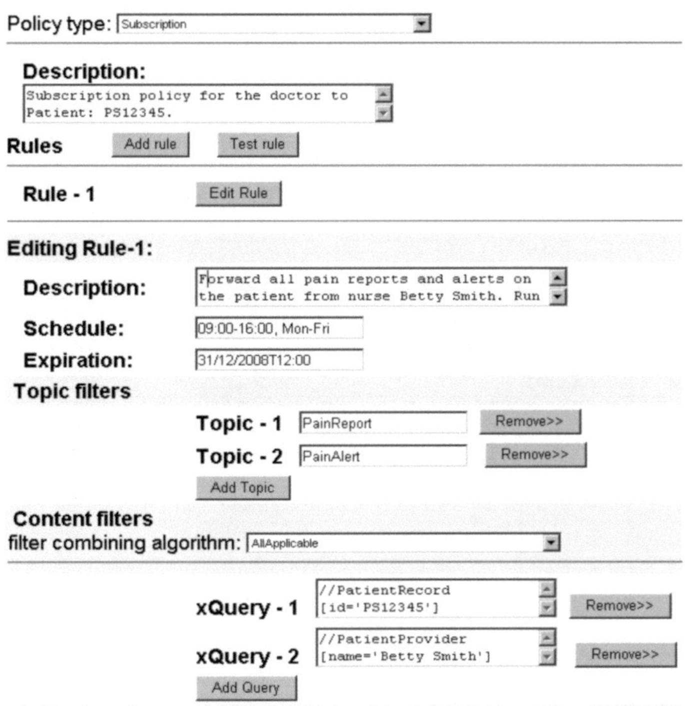

Policy type: Subscription
Description:
Subscription policy for the doctor to Patient: PS12345.
Rules
Add rule
Test rule
Rule - 1
Edit Rule
Editing Rule-1:
Description:
Forward all pain reports and alerts on the patient from nurse Betty Smith. Run
Schedule:
09:00-16:00, Mon-Fri
Expiration:
31/12/2008T12:00
Topic filters
Topic - 1
PainReport
Remove>>
Topic - 2
PainAlert
Remove>>
Add Topic
Content filters
filter combining algorithm: AllApplicable
xQuery - 1
//PatientRecord [id='PS12345']
Remove>>
xQuery - 2
//PatientProvider [name='Betty Smith']
Remove>>
Add Query

Fig. 9. Describing Policies.

Figure 9 shows a sample subscription policy that will send Patient (PS12345) Pain Reports and Pain Alerts from the nurse Betty Smith to a doctor. This will only be sent from 09:00 – 16:00, Monday to Friday and expires on the 31st of December, 2008.

6.2 Policy-based partner service component

People, devices and sensors, surveillance infrastructure share real-time data in adhoc B2B networks using an SOA publish/subscribe model. Because of differences in technology, capacities and running platforms, a special component (Partner Service Component) interacts with these applications through an application message *inbox/outbox* type interface. This component is both a publishers and a subscriber to a policy-based SOA message broker. It also handles those publish/subscribe administrative details on behalf of these B2B resources using policy-based declarative subscriptions.

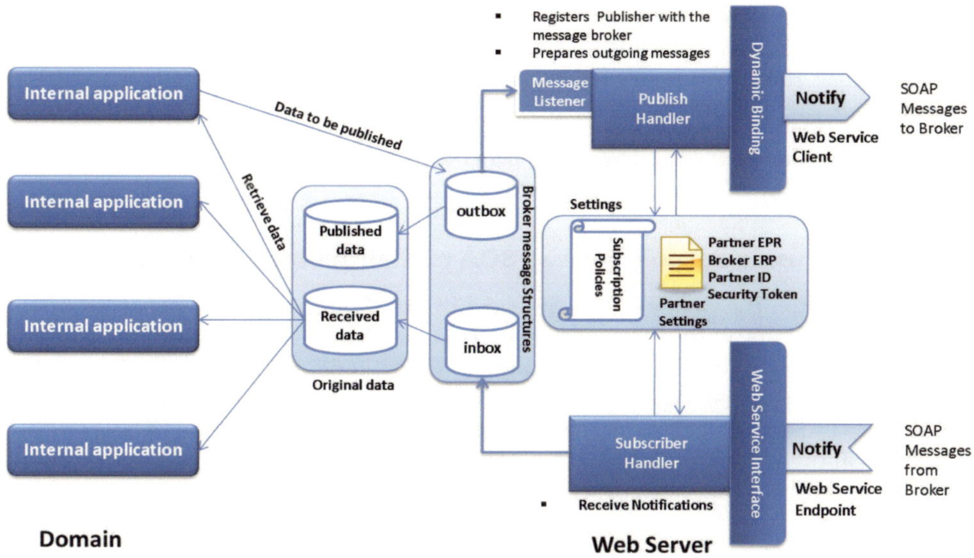

Fig. 10. Extended Partner Service Component.

In this framework, we extend the traditional SOA Message broker to support declarative policies. We also extend the PS component to support policy-based subscriptions and publishing (Figure 10). We use a partner service (PS) component as an adapter interface between the policy-based message broker and the application or process that publishes or subscribes to data. For example, a patient "John Smith" using a monitoring device attached to his wrist sends a *painscore* periodically. This device communicates locally to drop this *painscore* data structures into the *message outbox* of the partner service component. The Patient's PS component could be hosted on the patient home computer or a specially issued PDA from the hospital. It can also be in the form of a smart-phone application.

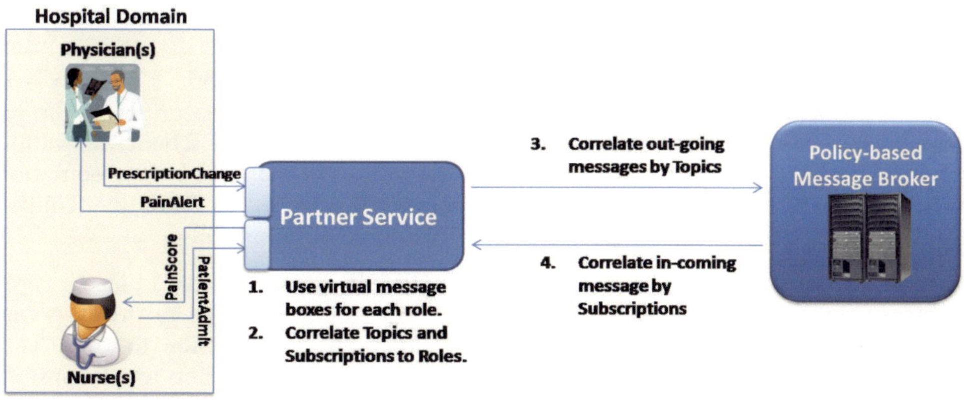

Fig. 11. Supporting multiple groups and roles in a Partner Service Component.

The PS component is then pre-configured to dynamically bind and forward this data to the policy-based message broker. The component correlates messages by their topics and subscriptions. For example, since "NurseBetty" subscribes to *PainReport* and

PrescriptionChange, it stores these subscriptions and correlates them to outbound and in-bound messages. This way, it is able to manage data for multiple applications. It could even sit as a message proxy in a domain environment, ensuring that various parties and processes receive the appropriate messages.

In Figure 11, we illustrate how the same PS component correlates nurses and physician subscriptions in a hospital domain environment.

6.3 SPM scenario using the policy-based SOA publish/subscribe approach

Putting it all together, the policy-based message broker (Figure 12) is our core middleware. It manages interactions with all the participating parties Partner Server components on behalf of collaborating applications through a Policy engine and the policy database. Community-care appointed Policy administrators use a special tool to deploy subscription policies to the broker on behalf of collaborating partners. In addition it supports both synchronous and asynchronous data exchanges, self-describing topics since topic registration includes schemas that describe data published on the topic.

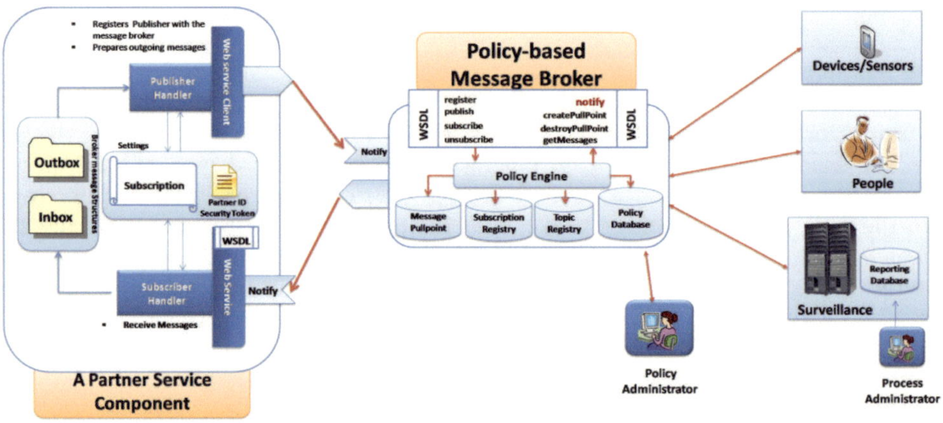

Fig. 12. Policy-based Message Broker.

Figure 13 shows the architectural represented of the interaction. Notice a special surveillance infrastructure hosted by the Palliative Care Portal. It subscribes to the policy message broker internal topic creation event and is able to receive the schema definition for each new topic. It subsequently uses this schema to create automatic table representation for capturing the event data. It then subscribes to messages attached to this topic. Unlike the SOA publish/subscribe, all these operations are performed automatically.

The Palliative Care Portal performs the surveillance role in our framework. Since it captures all messages published by data publishers, this infrastructure is able to provide various reports on the data exchanges. Various parties are able to subscribe to these reports automatically. In addition it is able to provide complete non repudiation for the entire B2B and perform automatic report generation based on threshold incidences and pattern triggers on data. These potentials are investigated in greater details in (Middleton et. al, 2009).

The entire infrastructure uses HTTP/SOAP as the communication protocol and therefore supports uninhibited communication on Internet. The policy-based message broker and all the interacting PS components are Web services endpoints.

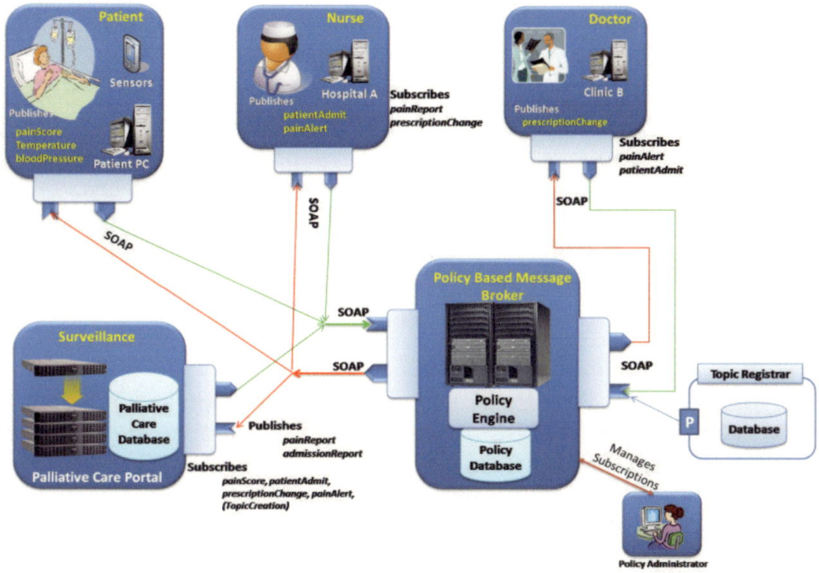

Fig. 13. Policy-based SOA Publish/subscribe Architecture.

7. Conclusions

Palliative Healthcare presents a unique challenge of caring for patients from home. Doctors, nurses, and other patient providers usually operate from domains and organizations that do not share common collaboration technologies. In this chapter, we have presented a scenario that describes a dynamic data sharing relationship between patients, nurses, and doctors from various domains with Palliative Care Portal acting a central database for the streaming events in the B2B network.

We have reviewed how the Policy-based SOA publish/subscribe was used to extend the basic Palliative Severe Pain Management scenario to support the requirements for data-driven interaction described in this chapter.

1. Data is dynamically defined at run-time using a combination of topic name and data attributes, thus providing an automatic connection between the management and logging of streaming data to reporting and historical information.
2. Data topics are not advertised by any arbitrary publisher as it is with classic SOA publish/subscribe. Rather, the Topic Registrar defines event topics alongside policies that control the rights to publish on the topics. For example, by publishing the *PatientAdmit* topic creation event, we automatically have the surveillance infrastructure create logging table for the topic and subscribe to data from the topic publishers.
3. All communication and data exchanges on this framework are received by the policy-based message broker (or a network of brokers) using a similar generic interface. Messages representing management operations are handled similarly like notification messages. Various handlers tie to the message context handler to process various types of message. This makes it very convenient to handle authentication, synchronous and asynchronous communication for all interactions.
4. The Partner Service components provide a great tool for easily integrating applications participating in SOA publish/subscribe. We have demonstrated its use as a local

middleware for publishing, subscribing, receiving and correlating messages for applications and users.

Most importantly, this framework demonstrates through the scenarios described in this chapter, the flexibility of defining XACML-based subscription policies on a streaming data model. Policy-based subscriptions provide the means of defining interest to data through topic and content filtering, message transformation and delivery QoS. Data queries provide access to stateful as well as historical data and reports to customers. Message policies provide a means of performing directed point-to-point notification using a publish/subscribe infrastructure.

8. References

BaileyJ., PoulovassilisA., and WoodP. (2003). An event-condition-action language for XML, In Proceedings of the 11th International Conference on World Wide Web, Honolulu, Hawaii, USA, pp. 486-495.

BarthA., DattaA., MitchellJ., and Nissenbaum H. (2006). Privacy and contextual integrity: Framework and applications, in IEEE Symposium on Security and Privacy,pp. 184-198.

CoieraE., and HovengaE. J. S. (2007), Building a sustainable health system, IMIA Yearbook of Medical Informatics 2007, vol. 2, no. 1, pp. 11-8.

DoshiC., PeytonL. (2008) Trusted information process in B2B networks, in Proceedings of the 10th International Conference on Enterprise Information Systems, Barcelona, Spain.

EtzionO., ChandyM., AmmonR.V., and Schulte R. (2006).Event-driven architectures and complex event processing, IEEE International Conference on Services Computing, Chicago, 2006, p. 30.

EugsterP. T., FelberP. A., GuerraouiR., and KermarrecA. (2003). The many faces of publish/subscribe. ACM Computing Surveys, vol. 35, no. 2, pp. 114-131.

Eze, B., KuziemskyC., PeytonL., MiddletonG., MoutthamA. (April 2010).,A Framework for Continuous Compliance Monitoring of eHealth Processes in Journal of theoretical and applied electronic commerce research, vol5/issue 1 p 56-70.

FosterI., KesselmanC., NickJ., and TueckeS. (2002). Grid services for distributed system integration, Computer, vol. 35, no. 6, pp. 37-46.

HarrocksI., AngeleJ., DeckerS., KiferM., GrosofB., and WagnerG. (2003), What are the rules? IEEE Intelligent Systems, vol. 18, no. 5, pp. 76-83.

HuhnsM. N. and SinghM. P. (2005), Service-oriented computing: Key concepts and principles. Internet Computing, IEEE.Vol. 0/issue 1, p 75-81.

KuziemskyC. E, Weber-JahnkeJ., Lau F., Downing G.M. (2008). "An Interdisciplinary Computer-based Information Tool for Palliative Severe Pain Management." Journal of the American Medical Informatics Association15(3): 375-382.

NiblettP. and GrahamS. (2005).Events and service-oriented architecture: The OASIS web services notification specifications, IBM Systems Journal, vol. 44, no. 4.

PeytonL., HuJ., DoshiC., and SeguinP. (2007). Addressing privacy in a federated identity management network for e-health, in 8th World Congress on the Management of eBusiness, Toronto, 2007. Internet Computing, vol. 9, no. 1, pp. 75-81.

MiddletonG., PeytonL., KuziemskyC., EzeB. (2009). "A Framework for Continuous Compliance Monitoring of eHealth Processes", World Congress on Privacy, Security, Trust and Management of eBusiness.

Information Needs in Palliative Care: Patient and Family Perspectives

Yaël Tibi-Lévy and Martine Bungener
National Centre for Scientific Research (CNRS), France

1. Introduction

The development of palliative care in France is relatively recent compared to English-speaking countries. The first French Palliative Care Unit opened its doors in Paris in 1987 (following "the Laroque circular" of August 26, 1986 that defined palliative care and support), but it was only twelve years later that a specific law was passed, the law of June 9, 1999. This law is important because it aims at "guaranteeing the right of access to palliative care for all citizens who are in need of it" (article 1). Consequently, palliative care became a national health priority and the object of ministerial programmes[1] for development at the level of the home as well as at the institutional level.

- First, in the home, two types of structures were set up to ensure that people wishing to remain at home could do so: on the one hand, Home Hospitalisation services (that depend on a hospital), and on the other hand, palliative care networks, which coordinate a range of private practitioners providing home care to patients while maintaining links with hospitals, should rehospitalisation becomes necessary.
- In France, the Anglo-American notion of "hospice" does not exist. From the beginning, the clearly stated policy choice was for palliative care to be integrated into hospitals (rather than existing outside them). Three types of hospital structures facilitating the provision of graduated care were thus created: Palliative Care Units (PCUs), Identified Palliative Care Beds (IPCBs), and Mobile Palliative Care Teams (MPCTs). While PCUs are small units with a dozen beds reserved for the most complex cases, the IPCBs are beds located directly inside acute care services. The latter are of recent creation (2004) and permit patients to stay hospitalised in their regular department, thus reducing risks related to the separation to which they have already been exposed by entering into palliative care. In contrast to the PCUs and IPCBs, the MPCTs have no beds. These are teams that intervene across the hospital at the request of acute care services to give support in caring for their patients at the end of life. On December 31, 2010, there were estimated to be in France 107 PCUs (1.176 beds), 353 mobile teams and 4.826 IPCBs (spread over 784 care institutions) (Aubry, 2011). At the same time, all hospital caregivers confronted with death are requested to "progressively integrate palliative care into their practice", whether or not they practice as a palliative care team (circular

[1] 1999-2002, 2002-2005, 2008-2012

dated February 19, 2002). In order to do this, "a guide to best practice in the palliative approach" was written up and the diffusion of "the palliative culture" in all departments is strongly encouraged (circular dated June 9, 2004).

2. Major issues involved in the provision of information in Palliative Care

2.1 Information/communication: a fundamental need at the end of life

Faced with a crisis in medical care (worsening working conditions for nurses, loss of trust in caregivers, the disclosure of judicial cases, etc.) and searching for legitimacy, patients in the 21st century have become authentic consumers of the health care system. Armed with rights they intend to have respected, concerned with transparency and able to make informed decisions, they now appear to be fully participating actors in their own care. In this context, they are increasingly inclined to develop their own standards for what constitutes quality of care (Falls, 2008). While this quality encompasses several dimensions (physical comfort, psychological care, configuration of the care facilities etc.), one topic – that of information and, more broadly, communication with the care team – is found to recur frequently in the literature, as it constitutes a potentially important source of conflict with caregivers. It is this dimension, not specific to the end of life but rather exacerbated in this context, that we have chosen to address in this article.

Many studies underline the extent to which information transmission and communication between patients, families and caregivers represent major issues in care given to persons at the end of life. While some authors describe as "extremely important" the quality of communication in the special context of palliative care (de Haes & Teunissen, 2005), others insist on "the decisive importance" that information, communication and attitudes of professionals have on these patients' families (Andershed, 2006). It is also argued that providing information (together with the possibility to make choices) is one of three principal needs in palliative care, the other two being social and psychological support on the one hand and attention to financial concerns on the other (McIlfatrick et al., 2007).

However, while communication is thus important, it is particularly difficult in the context of the end of life. Indeed, not only must one know how to announce bad news, but also be able to sensitively discuss treatments, establish good relationships with the families and be ready to listen to patients and those close to them (Buckman, 2000). Despite of the importance of the need for information, it is clear that defects in communication are frequent at the end of life (Mangan et al., 2003; Rainbird et al., 2009). This lack of communication is especially common in situations of treatment cessation, the unmet communication needs being due both to a lack of listening and of information (its timeliness, honesty and clarity) (Norton et al., 2003). In this context, it seems particularly important that physicians are aware of these conflicts (even if they are infrequent) and that they investigate them. This would enable them to reduce both the frequency of conflicts that may occur as well as the stress they cause (Norton et al., 2003). While the lack of communication among caregivers, patients and families is often mentioned, a second problem (equally important) is also emphasized: the lack of communication within medical teams themselves (Fassier, 2005; Faulkner, 1998). Thus, the development of palliative care and multidisciplinary care is described as an "urgent need" (especially in Europe) and as an effective way of promoting end of life care in intensive care units (Fassier, 2005). In this context, because of their enhanced communication skills, the potential impact of palliative care teams on hospitals is stressed (Jack et al., 2004).

2.2 Information as the founding principle of Palliative Care

Generally speaking, and aside from any context of palliative care, information for patients and their families has become both a right and a duty in several countries, including France (National Assembly, 2002; National Agency for Accreditation and Evaluation in Health, 2000; National Council of the Order of Physicians, 1995), where the content as well as the form of this information are the subject of recommendations. As concerns the content, it is stipulated that the duty to inform should include information on the state of patients' health (diagnosis, prognosis), their treatment (its nature, effectiveness, urgency and risks) as well as the potential consequences of refusing treatment (National Assembly, 2002). As concerns the form taken by information to be communicated, caregivers are asked that it be provided to patients "honestly, clearly and appropriately" (the doctor should "take account of the patient's personality in his explanations and ensure they are understood" (National Council of the Order of Physicians, 1995), that it be conveyed in a "progressive and adapted" way (National Agency for Accreditation and Evaluation in Health, 2002) and that "the wish of someone to be kept in ignorance of a diagnosis or prognosis" be respected (except if there is a risk of transmission to others) (National Assembly, 2002). A difficult question, and one widely discussed in official texts and the literature, faces those persons responsible for communicating the information. This concerns the disclosure of the truth, which may be defined as the act of giving truthful information to family members of a patient or to the patient him or herself, even when it is liable to be psychologically painful or unpleasant. Should the truth always be stated, in its entirety, and to whom, when and in what manner?

For French palliative care professionals, informing patients and their families, and more generally "communication", constitutes one of eight fundamental principles of care, on the same level as respecting patients' comfort, evaluating their overall pain, or preparation for bereavement (National Agency for Accreditation and Evaluation in Health, 2002). If properly done, effective communication may enable not only "the evaluation of the psychological and social suffering" of the patient and his or her family, but also an understanding of their needs and expectations concerning the care team, in order to better respond to them (National Agency for Accreditation and Evaluation in Health, 2002). In this end of life context, it is often suggested that to tell the truth is not only necessary, but also desirable for patients themselves as well as for their families, the premise being that the latter need this information, especially for saying their goodbyes. But whereas giving information is considered a basic principal, for some authors, the act of informing can become a source of uneasiness for caregivers, especially if they have not been well prepared for it. "The bad news, regardless of all the definitions one might have, is the narrative of an impending death announcement and the 'don't say anything' finds a place, or at least the 'don't say anything about the future', since it is so difficult to express but also because it is often associated with a 'fear of speaking ill'" (Julian-Reynier, 2007).

This trend, aimed at establishing recommendations for communicating information to persons at the end of their life and to their families, is part of a much larger context than the one described above. Thus, professional guidelines on best practice in palliative care are regularly put in place at an international level, each country defining its own standards (National

Hospice and Palliative Care Organization, 2008). In this context, the Council of Europe has defined the main principles concerning communication of caregivers with patients and families. In particular, it is recommended that: 1) care be delivered in an atmosphere encouraging clarity of information delivered to patients and their families, which implies an appropriate attitude on the part of care personnel; 2) professionals communicate openly with patients desiring to be informed about their situation, with particular attention to cultural differences; 3) doctors adapt their imparting of information to the emotional or cognitive barriers often associated with a progressive and incurable illness (Council of Europe, 2003).

2.3 Study objectives

Within this context of disseminating best practice, it is important to define "best" palliative care, not from a professional point of view, but from that (less well-known) of patients and their families. Going beyond the general rules established over time and their resulting recommendations, the objective of this article is to answer a central question: how is this flow of information perceived by those receiving it (patients benefiting from palliative care and families)? Within a policy framework promoting palliative care, two further questions arise: 1) what aspects of information are most appreciated by patients and their families? 2) what are the main sources of their dissatisfaction in this respect, or of tensions with caregivers? Attempting to answer these questions will draw attention to techniques and improvements that should be encouraged.

3. Methodology

Data used here are part of a larger research project on needs and expectations of individuals and their families at the end of life (Tibi-Levy, 2007; Tibi-Lévy & de Pouvourville, 2007, 2009). Although the delivery of information is only one dimension of patient and family satisfaction regarding care given, our work shows the central place it occupies in the perceived quality of care. Indeed, not only is the question of information brought up repeatedly, but it constitutes an important potential source of friction with caregivers as well.

This study was carried out exclusively in Palliative Care Units (PCUs). All together, 5 PCUs participated (3 in the Paris region and 2 in cities outside this region). They were located in public hospitals and had from 8 to 15 beds. They were chosen on the basis of size, level of staff supervision, and location. We had no prior information or assumptions concerning the reputations of these units. In each PCU, five patients and five families were selected to participate in the study, for a total of 50 persons. The patients studied were recruited according to their clinical status (those patients too tired, confused, disoriented or having difficulty communicating were excluded) and the time between their admission and the interview (recent admissions were excluded). Average age was 63 years (35-88 years) and two-thirds were women (64%). All had cancer and had been hospitalised for an average of two weeks (standard deviation = 14 days) and their average Karnofsky score was close to 40% ("disabled patient, requires special care and assistance, relatively autonomous with limited ability to move about"). In most cases (and to the extent possible) families in the study were those of the patients studied (18 patient-family duos). Out of the 25 families studied, the spouse was the person met with in half the cases (48%), the children in a third of cases (32%) and the parents and brothers/sisters in close to 10% of cases. In seven out of ten cases, these were women (68%).

This qualitative study is based on individual semi-directed interviews with 25 patients and 25 families. These persons were interviewed by a sociologist from outside the hospital, using an interview guide specifically focused on the way the care team took into consideration their needs and expectations generally speaking (cf. Interview guide below) (Tibi-Levy & de Pouvourville, 2007, 2009). The same guide was used for patients and families, with certain variations being occasionally introduced. Interviews lasted 40 minutes on average. Out of the 50 interviews, 42 were recorded (with the agreement of the interviewees) and completely transcribed, representing more than 500 single-spaced pages of discourse. Handwritten notes taken for the eight others (4 "patients" and 4 "families") were also transcribed. After having extracted them from the main body of discourse, we carried out a content analysis on those passages relating to information and communication with the care team. Narratives were submitted to a vertical and horizontal thematic analysis, with the screening tool used identifying two topic areas: 1) those aspects of the information they received that the interviewees found satisfying and that they emphasized; 2) those aspects causing dissatisfaction or even tension with the care team.

INTERVIEW GUIDE

I - Relationship of the patient with the unit

Can you tell me about your first contact with this unit?
What happened? **What information were you given at that time?***
What questions did they ask you at that time?* Did some things capture your attention more than others?
How did you feel about this first contact?

What happened when you arrived here? (admission)
What information were you given at that time?* What questions did they ask you at that time?* Did some things capture your attention more than others?
How did you feel about this contact?

How is your hospitalisation here going overall?
How are your relationships with the doctors? And with the rest of the team? **What kind of questions do they ask you?* Do they give you enough information?*** (example)
Do you **feel you are being listened to enough*** in this unit. By whom? (example)

What do you think about the environment in the unit (your room and the common rooms)?

II - Attention to the needs and expectations of the patient by the care team

What aspects of care do you think are especially important today? (important aspects)

Do the team doctors pay sufficient attention to these aspects? And does the rest of the team? (example)
OR What do you think is especially important today in the way this unit takes care of you?
Do the doctors pay sufficient attention to this? And does the rest of the team?
What would you like the staff in this unit to do for you?

What aspects of your care would you like to see improved? (example)
OR What improvements would you like to see in the way this unit takes care of you? (example)

III. - Former situation

Could you tell me a little about your situation before you arrived in this unit? Where were you? How did that go? Were you satisfied with service where you were? (medical care and relationships with caregivers)

Did you personally choose to come to this unit? Why?
IF NOT: Who directed you to this unit? **What reasons were you given at that time?***

*** Underlined questions: questions related to information provided**

4. Results

Table 1 displays the main findings described below, identifying those aspects appreciated by patients and families on the one hand (to promote and disseminate) and potential sources of dissatisfaction on the other hand (to be resolved).

4.1 Factors related to satisfaction with the information received

4.1.1 Aspects of satisfaction

Eighty percent of patients and families interviewed said they were completely satisfied with the quality of information given by caregivers, because of a combination of five of its aspects:

- its accessibility: "If there is a lack of information, I can ask a question. Anyone, depending on their competence." (n°22, male, 62 years old, PCU5); "When we ask questions, we get all the answers we want." (n°34, patient's sister, PCU2).
- its completeness: "Every time I ask a question, I have a complete answer." (n°22, male, 62 years old, PCU5), "They explain everything. They don't do anything without telling the patient and us (n°45, spouse of a patient, PCU4).
- the frankness with which the explanations are given (no "taboos", "evasiveness", "lies", or "little secrets"). "Here, the doctors don't hide behind their white coats to avoid giving an answer. And that is very important." (n°22, male, 62 years old, PCU5); "They favour openness. They don't beat around the bush, you see. Whereas where we were before, the doctors kept passing the buck to each other. In the end, I didn't know any more than before. But here, everything's perfectly clear." (n°47, spouse of a patient, PCU5).
- its appropriateness : «When my mother asks you a question, answer her question. But, it's not your role to get ahead of things [by telling her everything] because the patient doesn't need to know everything» (n°38, daughter of a patient, PCU3).
- its comprehensibleness (clearness): "Some doctors are still difficult to understand. Then I understood what they anticipated for me. And for me, that was tremendous. I started to come out of the fog I was in." (n°21, female, 71 years old, PCU5).

Those things most appreciated by patients and families (to disseminate)		Things causing dissatisfaction (to resolve)	
Factors giving satisfaction according to the kind of information given		**From "too much" to… "not enough" information**	
- Accessibility - Completeness - Frankness - Appropriateness - Comprehensibleness (clearness)		**Too much information**	**Not enough information**
		Too "blunt": - People who say they "know what to expect" and therefore prefer not to ask questions - Idea that one must not "provoke misfortune"	- Physicians that "don't visit rooms enough" - "Unanswered" questions Sometimes: a feeling of a lack of information (idea that it's the physician's role to seek out the family, and not the opposite)
Interpersonal skills of caregivers: - "Availability, openness" - "Get on people's level" - "Real understanding, real dialogue, real interest"		+ Situations resulting from the way persons experienced the announcement of a transfer to a USP (lack of information, elusive attitudes from caregivers, lack of tact)	
Techniques identified for delivering information		**Desires to filter information for families**	
Patients	**Families**	- Worries about "protecting" their ill family member from what he or she could learn. As a result: 1/ apprehension in these families; 2/ the impression that caregivers "lack consideration" for their family culture - A desire to withold information generally well respected by the teams, however, without abandoning their duty to inform (sharp reminders to families that their family member should know the truth) - Families that revised upwards their jugement concerning caregivers, during the hospitalisation	
- Availability of caregivers - The consultations-conversations - Attention given to the non-verbal - Fact that caregivers regularly ask questions	- To be "taken aside" - The fact that caregivers ask them questions (especially, how they are experiencing things) - To be told if there is a problem - The booklets "with all the telephone numbers"		
The positive impact of using these techniques			
Patients	**Families**		
- Establishes confidence - Helps to progress	- Reduces drama - Helps in coping - Helps give support to their ill family member		
Calming words and attitudes		**Upsetting words and attitudes**	
- Enables patients to cope with the shock of the announcement - "Beneficial" hospitalisations		- Repeated calls to take courage…that are discouraging - Overly sympathetic behaviours	
… knowing that their are situations where the patients and families will never be satisfied, regardless of caregiver communication skills (especially when patients are waiting for an "effective treatment")			

Table 1. Providing information in Palliative Care

The quality of information goes hand in hand with the interpersonal skills of the caregivers. Many people emphasized these skills ("availability, openness, real understanding, real dialogue, real interest"), and interpret them as a sign of attention and of "professionalism", that lead them to believe the caregivers are "truly" interested in them, as these two excerpts demonstrate: 1) "I have the impression the doctors really want to communicate with me, to discover any progress, to discuss what I do or do not want to do, to inform themselves clearly on what's happening to me, to the extent I ask for it, with no holding back of information, and not at all with a desire to use doctor talk, but a good explanation of things. That's striking." (n°6, female, 48 years old, PCU2); 2) "The doctor made a good impression on me from the beginning because he seemed to be a professional who knew what he was talking about. I think a current passed between us and that he is going to try and do what he can." (n°4, male, 80 years old, PCU1). In this context, the ability of caregivers to "put themselves at the level" of the patients is highly appreciated, as this patient describes: "Here, the caregivers feel like they are on the same level as we are; a doctor and a worker, it's like that [they're the same]." (n°17, male, 58 years old, PCU4).

4.1.2 Techniques for delivering information

Techniques and attitudes used by caregivers for informing patients and families are pointed out by some and they often compare their present hospitalisation in a PCU with what they observed in other types of facilities throughout the course of their stay.

Patients highlight four positions adopted by caregivers, reproduced here in the context of the diffusion of palliative culture:

- the availability of caregivers and their ability to "take their time": "The doctor really took her time to explain to me the sequence of events from A to Z. It wasn't just an interview: your last name, first name, motivations. It was the time that she devoted to me. Somehow, that made me feel better, especially since in the hospital where it's usually a factory, where there's no tendency to devote time to you. Therefore, when you have this illness, sometimes you have a tendency of wanting to be listened to." (n°8, male, 35 years old, PCU2).
- the fact that medical visits "are like conversations": "The doctor sits on the table or a chair. You're on the bed or sitting there. And then, the visit is carried on like a conversation, which is most probably focused by the practitioner on particular topics that you don't always notice in the conversation, but that are certainly aimed at particular questions." (n°25, male, 82 years old, PCU5).
- the fact that caregivers show an interest in what is non-verbal as well (facial expressions and body language), an interest that suggests to them the team "is concerned about them": "From the nurse's aid to the nurse, they don't hesitate to talk a couple of minutes, to say: 'oh, you're looking sad today, what's the matter, do you have some bad news, what's wrong?' They see it in your expression." (n°19, female, 63 years old, PCU4).
- the fact that caregivers regularly ask them questions about their needs and expectations: "We get information practically daily when we are in the unit. They ask you questions: 'are you alright madam, do you have any questions, you can ask questions, do you need anything, would you like something?' They ask me if I slept badly for example or if I have some bad news, is there a reason why I'm in this state." (n°19, female, 63 years old, PCU4).

For their part, families evoke four techniques used by caregivers in their role to inform:

- to be "taken aside" by caregivers at admission to evaluate what the patient knows: "When we got here, the doctor took me aside and asked me if mama realised what type of service she had 'landed in'." (n°32, daughter of a patient, PCU2).
- to be questioned by caregivers on the health status of their ill family member, as well as on how they personally experience the events, as a family: "What struck me was the professionalism because they asked questions on her status, on how we felt about things." (n°32, daughter of a patient, PCU2).
- to be informed by the care team as soon as there are problems: "In some hospitals, they tell you: yes, everything's fine, everything's fine. And then when you arrive, things aren't fine at all. Whereas here, they telephone you and tell you: things aren't going well today. There. They let you know." (n°34, sister of a patient, PCU2).
- the giving family members "booklets with all the telephone numbers of the team", and insisting on the fact they can call them at any time: "Above all, which is pretty rare, they say: you can call us whenever you wish, day or night, there's no need to take an appointment." (n°32, daughter of a patient, PCU2).

4.1.3 Reasons for satisfaction

These ways of giving out information, based on communication techniques, have the effect, on the one hand, of "gaining the patient's trust" ("All this makes you trust them." (n°8, male, 35 years old, PCU2)) and on the other hand, helps them to move forward ("It was important that I understand what was in store for me, what I could expect. He was very explicit. For me he's a doctor who knew how to use the words that helped me." (n°21, female, 71 years old, PCU5)). In addition, some families emphasized this process of gaining trust with relief ("They were able to get my mother to trust them. That means they have considerable powers of persuasion, but through human warmth, through gentleness I think. And I find that brilliant because a lady like my mother, the fact she was able to find calm here…that's wonderful!" (n°33, daughter of a patient, PCU2)). These families say they also feel comfortable reaching out to caregivers and stress how important it is for them "to be able to talk to them without fear of being rebuffed or told lies" (n°34, sister of a patient, PCU2).

The question concerning the truth is evoked more by the families than by the patients. Some of them explain that, in their case, knowing the truth is preferable for two reasons. On the one hand, they can avoid "over dramatising the situation" ("We make a lot of assumptions that are generally wrong. We always think its worse, worse than it is." (n°47, spouse of a patient, PCU5)). On the other hand, it helps them cope and give support to those close to them ("When we are faced with the facts, we can react differently, both me and my husband. He can react differently, given the state of his illness, since he is very much of a fighter as well, and say to himself: well no, I'm not going to let myself sink, I'm going to give it a go. And from our side, we can carry on and encourage him to fight." (n°47, spouse of a patient, PCU5)).

4.2 Friction with the Palliative Care teams about information provided

Discourse analysis brings out three potential sources of dissatisfaction: inappropriateness in the amount of information given by caregivers, fear within some families that the patient will "learn the truth", and disturbing attitudes or words.

4.2.1 From "too much" to ..."not enough" information

While three people feel there is too much information given, four others think that, on the contrary, there isn't enough. These feelings of over-abundance or insufficiency are sometimes found in the same care unit and are essentially related to the announcement, or not, of the approaching end of life; should it be announced or not, and to whom?

As concerns the perception of too much information, the arguments used by patients and families are similar. It is felt the caregivers are "too blunt", as explained by a patient and her daughter, interviewed separately: "They were less considerate with me than where I was hospitalised before. It doesn't bother them to talk to you about your illness." (n°13, female, 48 years old, PCU3); "Its not for the doctors to take the initiative. I don't see the point of going into a room and telling someone: 'you know, you have tumours in the stomach, ok, if you have a blockage, you could have one, if you have one, we wouldn't be able to operate on you." (n°38, daughter of a patient, PCU3). The information can also appear redundant: "Ok, I know it now, let's not talk about it anymore. It's no use going on and on about it." (n°23, female, 48 years old, PCU5). In this context, some people prefer not to ask questions, either "to not know the answers" (n°13, female, 60 years old PCU3), or in order "not to bring on bad luck" (n°22, male, 62 years old, PCU5):

- *The interviewer:* When you arrived here, the team may have talked to you about this term "palliative care"; may have said something to you?
- *The patient:* Oh no, no, no. Nobody talks about that here.
- *The interviewer*: And didn't you ask any questions?
- *The patient:* No. There are taboo questions that I really avoid asking. No, I'm not going to go looking, I'm not going to bring on bad luck.

As for observations concerning a lack of information, these are often accompanied by a felt difficulty in obtaining answers to questions, to the extent these questions can even be formulated. These patients are disappointed that the doctors don't visit their rooms enough on the one hand ("You don't see the doctors every day. They could stop by to ask if your better, for example" (n°24, female, 56 years old, PCU5)) and that some of their questions are not answered on the other hand ("The doctors are not especially talkative. Sometimes, when you want an answer, you have to pester them several times with the question." (n°24, female, 56 years old)). Taken to the extreme, this feeling of lack of information can give the impression of being abandoned, as noted by this gentleman waiting for a "cure": "Uh, they [the doctors] don't come very often, they hardly ever come. Here I haven't got anything [any cure]! They just put me there like a guard dog..." (n°16, male, 64 years old, PCU4), or this bewildered sister: "The patients don't know why they are here, beginning with my sister. What I think is that they are at the end of life and there are people that die. And they know this, they even see them go by their room. So when a patient asks questions, like my sister's question: 'is this a place to die'? Yes, I think it's the last place you go and you leave from. It's not really completely clear. As for me, the doctor doesn't contact me. I don't have any report on anything. No explanation whatsoever. I come every day, I just don't know. Ok, I can guess why she's here. But no one told me anything at all, at all." (n°40, sister of a patient, PCU3). But from this woman's point of view, normally, it's not for the families to go towards the doctors... but the opposite: "They should be the ones to make contact, for the simple reason that every time they come to see my sister, I'm always in the room. And I can't talk in front of her, ask the questions I want answers to. So I wait. But apparently, it's when there's nothing more that can be done that they contact you." (n°40, sister of a patient, PCU3).

These perceptions of having too much or too little information are felt to be even more negative by these patients and their families because the announcements of a transfer to a PCU by the traditional hospital departments were considered unsatisfactory, for at least one of the following three reasons, mentioned by the daughter of a patient (n°32, daughter of a patient, PCU2) and reiterated less strongly by six other people (three patients and three families): 1) an unsatisfied need for supplemental information ("I wanted to know a little more. And then I told myself: ok, I'll get more information at the place."); 2) attitudes of avoidance on the part of referring physicians ("It wasn't her doctor who told her: 'you're going into palliative care'. And that was someone who had followed her for nine years and who didn't have the courage to tell her to her face! It was the young departmental intern where she was who told her. And I find that absurd."; 3) a feeling of a lack of tact in the announcement of the transfer ("One evening, I call my mother and she says to me: 'they just told me that I'm being transferred to palliative care'. Then, I really got mad. I called the nurse and said: 'give me a doctor'. Impossible to talk to a doctor. And the head nurse tells me: 'oh yeah, we're transferring her to hospital Y'. And I told her: 'you have no tact at all, my mother is in tears now, you just announce it to her like that'. And she answers: 'yes, but you know, we explained to her that it would be good for her and in any case, I'm telling you, she's not going to die right away'."

4.2.2 A desire by the families to filter information

The issue of imparting unpleasant information directly to patients was brought up by two families in particular, who desired that the information should go through them first, or at least, that it be communicated to their loved ones less bluntly. Their reason is a desire to protect them: 1) "My husband doesn't know he has cancer. I never wanted him to know. He would have rapidly let himself die. Whereas now, he's eating again, he's walking. If he knew he had cancer, he wouldn't do all that anymore, he'd really let himself go." (n°50, spouse of a patient, PCU5); 2) "If they tell you everything, they douse whatever little spark of life force you have left." (n°38, daughter of a patient, PCU3).

These people regret the present tendency of wanting to tell everything to patients out of principle, and are afraid their loved ones will end up being informed of their critical state ("I'm always worried, because I'm afraid they'll tell things to my husband too directly. Nowadays, it's true they say things to patients a little too directly" (n°46, spouse of a patient, PCU5)). Aside from these concerns, these families perceive the failure of caregivers to comply with their wishes as a lack of consideration for their family culture, as clearly expressed by the daughter of a patient: "What I didn't like was that they didn't take the family into consideration enough, the family structure, the reasons why you hide things from your family. Why? Because you know your family better than anyone. We're really close to one another, very, very close, really close. Now, when you have doctors who tell you after five minutes that they understand your family structure, your family, and that they understand it better than you do…" (n°38, daughter of a patient, PCU3).

However, in spite of this dissatisfaction, the study shows that the desire to withhold information is generally well respected by the caregivers. Thus, some patients don't know what kind of unit they are hospitalised in (two think they are in a rest home[2], one thinks he's in a pain unit[3] and two others say they don't know where they are[4]) and others talk about getting better, like this woman who died a month later: "Most people see palliative care as the end of life. But these services also have the objective of compensating for problems, so you can get back on your feet. Palliative care is also a place where you can recover." (n°6, female, 48 years old, PCU2). In addition, attitudes are not fixed and the teams adjust their behaviour during a hospitalisation, as this woman emphasises: "Here, they hide nothing, they tell the truth. I told them: 'I'm not asking you to lie to her, I'm just asking you not to tell her anything'. Now, things are a lot better. But in the beginning, I really felt bad." (n°38, daughter of a patient, PCU3).

4.2.3 Words and attitudes of caregivers in their role to inform

The study underlines the importance of caregivers' attitudes and words in the way the information delivered is perceived by patients and their families. They are alternately described as destructive or as an important source of comfort.

In the first instance, some people express dismay in regard to some caregivers, because of their words or their behaviours. Two factors are felt to be responsible:

- repeated calls to "take courage" that are… discouraging ("I noticed that each person told me to take courage, things like that. And that weakened me more than anything else because I don't need that plus the rest. I felt like they were driving the point home even more, telling me: 'you're almost there'. I come here to be with my husband, to have some good moments with him and not to be crying all the time. He doesn't need to see me like that either, because that makes it worse for him. I told the doctor, I made him understand that I should be talked to in a normal way, that I had to hold up for my husband and I absolutely shouldn't break down, because of my husband. Since then, it's a lot better." (n°29, spouse of a patient, PCU1).
- exaggeratedly sympathetic behaviours (compassionate looks and smiles, excessive niceness and gentleness, decorations that are not typical for a traditional hospital department) ("I noticed that sometimes, when my mother was going to say something, they would look at her with a smile, give her a little caress. She said to me: 'did you see, they look at me that way, I really feel like it's the end, that I'm finished'." (n°38, daughter of a patient, PCU3); "It's nice here. I mean there are flowers. It's like the friendliness, it's nice… but then right after you say to yourself it's because…" (n°37, daughter of a patient, PCU3)).

Similar attitudes can, on the contrary, prove soothing (and that is the second instance), such as for this patient: "It's true that, in the beginning, palliative care was horrible. I was really

[2] "I wasn't strong enough to stand that new operation. That's why they put me in a convalescent home, two or three weeks, to be able to rest in a calm place, to eat well, to pay attention to what I eat." (N°15, female, 45 years old, USP3)

[3] "My doctor decided to hospitalise me here, in a pain unit, in a department specialising in pain." (n°25, male, 82 years old, USP5)

[4] "My lung specialist told me they are well-known here, so she preferred to send me directly here. She said: 'it's very, very good'. That's all. Because it has a good reputation." (n°10, female, 47 years old, USP2)

afraid. I imagined that someone was dying in every room. Now, it's better. I see that you can live and continue your life. I feel good in my room. I mean, I feel just as good as if I were at home. Here, I am reassured by the team. It changed the way I see this kind of place." (n°7, female, 52 years old, PCU2). Another patient explains how beneficial the hospitalisation has been for her because of the attitude the team has taken concerning her: "I like simplicity. And I have been lucky for that as well. These are people that are flexible, who love life and give it to you. They share this with you. Its funny, but I would never have thought that one day I would stay so long in hospitals and that it would bring me so much." (n°23, female, 48 years old, PCU2). Some patients nevertheless have other expectations, not always possible to meet: "I'm looking for efficiency; I'm looking for a cure, not words. I think it's normal for a hospital to look for a cure!" (n°16, male, 64 years old, PCU4)).

5. Discussion

These results highlight two topics for discussion, central to the way patients and families perceive the information activities of caregivers: 1) the team's communication and interpersonal skills; 2) the ability of the caregivers to manage unique situations by adapting the information they deliver according to the needs and expectations of each person. The discussion is based in particular on a review of literature covering the past ten years (2001-2011) via Medline (key words: "palliative care, "information", and "communication").

5.1 Providing information: knowing how to communicate

5.1.1 Communication skills: contours and visibility

Discourse recorded among patients and families confirms the substantial overlapping of the activities of informing and communicating in the context of palliative care and approaching death (Faulkner, 1998; Kirk et al., 2004). To inform is to know above all how to communicate. This means making the information accessible, providing complete answers, being frank and expressing oneself in a comprehensible way (cf. Table I). These four elements are associated with a fifth, more overarching one: the availability of caregivers, which is a special skill for opening up to those they care for, putting themselves in their place and making time available to them. Kirk et al. underlined the special attention to be given to these aspects and stressed in particular three of them: fairness on the part of caregivers, the clarity of their discourse and their ability to take time with patients (Kirk et al., 2004). It's what one of the interviewed patients in our study called "a good explanation of things, and not just doctor talk" (n°6, female, 48 years old, PCU2). But communicating is more than delivering information; it's a two-way relationship that gives patients and their families the impression that caregivers are "really" at their side ("real listening", "real dialogue", "real understanding", "real interest", "real desire to communicate", etc.). It appears then that "what the patient wants is a truthful relationship rather than just a medical truth" (Ruszniewski, 2004). The issue is not whether one should tell the truth, to whom, how and about what, but rather whether the relationship caregivers have with patients and families is "real", that is, whether caregivers are able put themselves in a position to listen.

In this context, one of the contributions of our work is to have shown that the efforts expended on communication in a PCU are highly visible to patients and families:

- First, it shows that techniques used by caregivers to inform are seen not only for what they are (consultations-conversations, frequent and regular questions, booklets with all the telephone numbers, etc.), but also in contrast to their experience in acute care facilities (e.g., a feeling of being listened to, the possibility of talking to caregivers without fear of bothering them, a perception that doctors have time for them and that they communicate on the patient's level, etc.). This contrast, mentioned spontaneously[5], is confirmed when we compare these results with those of studies carried out in acute care facilities. The latter scenario has the doctors on one side who "don't say anything" and on the other side, the patients who "don't dare to ask questions" and who feel they've "lost possession of their bodies", or are even "not involved in the consultation" (Fainzang, 2006). In particular, our work highlights two things to be given priority in traditional hospitalisations: on the one hand, increased use of protocols in announcing the transfer to a PCU (timing and place of the announcement, the caregiver who should do it, the words to be used, the attitude to adopt) and on the other hand, the integration into these departments of relationship techniques used in PCUs.
- Secondly, some patients and families underline the strong impression the caregivers' communication skills have on them: confidence building, not overdramatising the situation, helping to fight, etc. Some family members emphasise in particular the positive effect the attitude of the caregivers has on their sick relative ("calming") and explain that this pleasant attitude encourages them to approach the caregivers more easily than they would have spontaneously (absence of "fear of being rebuffed or told lies" (n°34, sister of a patient, PCU2)). Efforts by team members to adapt their actions to be more in line with actual needs and expectations of patients and families are also reported by some. The perception of these efforts is actually reflected in the positive changes in the way they see their hospitalisation (e.g. "I explained [such and such] to the caregivers. Now, things are a lot better").

5.1.2 Interpersonal skills: associating patients and families with the information process

Communication skills are related to a larger concept, that of caregivers' interpersonal skills. Two sensitive points are mentioned in the interviews, underlining the desire of many people to be truly associated with the informational process that concerns them most: the announcement of diagnoses and prognoses on the one hand, and the importance of maintaining hope on the other.

- On the first point, recent work has found that a significant proportion of patients in palliative care do not know their diagnosis and/or their prognosis. This information was not given to them by the physicians in their department, in spite of all the professional recommendations published on the topic. In this respect, silence is judged by caregivers to be more effective than an intrusive announcement in aiding patients to face death with dignity (Giardini et al., 2011), while some families complain about the lack of information they are given on prognosis (Yoshida et al., 2011) and many patients leave the hospital with false hopes (Gott et al., 2011). This censuring of information by physicians is based on what may appear to be a legitimate concern, that of protecting

[5] That is, without a precise question about this being asked during the interview.

the patient from potentially upsetting, depressing or bad news (Fallowfield et al., 2002). Sometimes, it's the families themselves[6] who withhold information. Indeed, it is not rare that they explicitly request the caregivers (sometimes in an insistent manner) to not tell the truth to their ill family member (Fainzang, 2006; Faulkner, 1998), whether this person is in palliative care or not. In fact, many patients and some families are kept in ignorance and uncertainty about their condition, as our study has shown. While this may suit some of them (in spite of their right to information and transparency), others explain on the contrary that being left in the dark is worse for them than knowing the truth, even if it is serious. Knowing would in fact allow them not to overdramatise the situation, while giving them more strength to "fight" and "give support" to each other. More than silence or the blunt truth (two extreme attitudes commonly observed in hospitals in the end of life context), some authors affirm that a third position, deceit, is even more damaging because it prevents patients and families from reorganising their lives accordingly and from doing what can be done at that moment in time (Fallowfield et al., 2002). In this respect, our study clearly shows that, contrary to what has often been noted in traditional hospital departments (Fainzang, 2006), caregivers in PCUs do not attempt to avoid their responsibility of transmitting information, on the pretext that the family doesn't want the patient to know the truth. Starting from the premise that patients should be informed about their critical condition, they regularly attempt to increase the families' awareness of patients' need for information, at the risk of being in disagreement with them. (e.g., "I told the doctors: 'listen, it's not necessary to tell my mother everything'. And they told me: 'yes, but you understand, it's necessary to tell them the truth'." (n°38, daughter of a patient, PCU3)). Because of this, the desire on the part of families to withhold information probably constitutes a greater source of friction in a PCU than in other types of units, where caregivers more frequently renounce giving information.

- Maintaining hope clearly emerges as a fundamental component in patient and especially family satisfaction concerning information, a result also found in the literature (Innes & Payne, 2009; de Haes & Teunissen, 2005). Even when all appears lost, many people still want to believe in a "miracle" (Kirk et al., 2004). Although physicians have the duty and responsibility to inform patients and families about the past, the present and the coming situation (Hippocratic Oath), they must do it while respecting the need for ambiguity about the future, among patients who desire this (Innes & Payne, 2009). While telling the "blunt truth" is sometimes called "criminal" (Serryn, 2008, as cited in Roy, 1988,), giving false hope is equally open to criticism (Gott et al., 2011; Ngo-Metzger et al., 2008). In this respect, the "truth step by step" model seems to be a good alternative to either a "headlong rush" (consisting of "telling everything", under the pretence of honesty and frankness) and a "paternalistic attitude" (in which the physician "says nothing") (Ruszniewski, 2004). This model consists in disclosing information in a gradual way and to "qualify one's statements", which implies that caregivers let themselves be guided by the patients and families, and that leaves a place in the practice for "an absence of rules" on the matter. Sometimes, what patients and families want is not to be told things, but to be listened to, as explained by a young patient in our study: "When you have this illness, sometimes you have a tendency of

[6] When they have been informed.

wanting to be listened to." (n°8, male, 35 years old, PCU2). The debate about the truth moves from the question of announcements (announce what, when and how?) to that of listening (how does one listen?). More generally, the confidence patients and families have in caregivers is a major factor in building a solid caring relationship (de Haes & Teunissen, 2005), as is the degree of empathy found in that relationship (Schaefer & Block, 2009). Other factors should also be encouraged here, such as talking to patients fairly early about palliative care (when the illness is not too far advanced and they still feel well) or the prioritising of key points to discuss with them (Ngo-Metzger et al., 2008).

If it's necessary to inform "without giving the blunt truth" (Roy, 1988) and to be honest while "maintaining hope" (Innes & Payne, 2009), "there aren't any [miraculous] recipes" for doing that (Ruszniewski, 2004). On the other hand, caregivers' interpersonal skills can be noticeably improved by gaining a minimum of knowledge in this area. To this end, recommendations for best practice in palliative care have been developed in several countries (National Hospice and Palliative Care Organization, 2008; National Agency for Accreditation and Evaluation in Health, 2002) and disseminated in health facilities. In particular, the announcement of bad news, the notification of transfer to palliative care, as well as the disclosure of medical errors should be given special attention (Hatem et al., 2008). In addition, programmes of study on special topics exist almost everywhere, within the context of initial training of caregivers (medical schools, nursing schools) as well as in continuing education programmes. Their goal is to teach health professionals to be more vigilant concerning the content of what they are going to say, the way they say it and the circumstances surrounding the delivery of information. The people we interviewed spontaneously cited some of the important points, such as the fact that caregivers make themselves available, sit down next to them and regularly ask them questions about their health. There is a rich literature concerning this training (Hatem et al., 2008; Miyashita et al., 2008; Ferrell et al., 2007; Alexander et al., 2006; McFarland & Rhoades, 2006; Clayton et al., 2005), which is aimed at increasing the communication skills of caregivers, or at least making them aware of these issues. It is none the less necessary that their aspirations and actual conditions of work on a daily basis make possible the desired improvements.

5.2 Giving more attention to the needs and expectations of each person

5.2.1 Recognising a two-fold heterogeneity

This study shows the extent of subjectivity in the perception of good informational activity by each patient or family member, due to a two-fold heterogeneity that must be taken into account:

- While the place and role of families is largely recognised and developed in palliative care, their needs and expectations regarding care teams are not necessarily similar to those of the patients themselves. For example, our study shows that the patients don't always ask for diagnostic and prognostic details, contrary to families, who expressed no reservations on this point and would sometimes like to know even more (especially on the time left to live). These results confirm those of Kirk et al. in particular, showing that informational needs of patients and families diverge as the illness progresses, with patients not wanting to have details, especially concerning their prognosis, while families wish to have that information (Kirk et al., 2004). Because of this, many families take up a position of defending the interests and well-being of their loved one, evoking the importance, from their perspective, that caregivers "don't say anything" so that the patient doesn't lose hope (e.g.: "If my husband knew he had cancer, he'd have let himself die in a short time" (n°50, spouse of a patient, PCU5)). Therefore, and for each hospitalisation, caregivers should bear in mind and evaluate these two levels of needs (patients, families), that are sometimes opposed to each other.

- The second type of heterogeneity is more complex since it is conditioned by the uniqueness of the needs and expectations of each person concerning care and information. This infinitely variable uniqueness depends not only on clinical characteristics of patients (pathology[7], symptoms, disparities linked to age[8], etc.), but also to specificities in the broader sense of each individual (nationality[9], culture[10], personality, experience, family circle, social status, etc.). In addition, all these components can fluctuate over time because of the extreme variability of this population. Thus, aside from the heterogeneity of the illness and of the people affected, the question for each caregiver of what information to deliver (quantity, content) depends on the person it is intended for. And the perception of each patient or family concerning the information received varies according to his or her own expectations (this is especially obvious in situations of over and under information described above). What suits some does not necessarily suit others, as expressed a patient's wife concerning the repeated statements to "take courage" addressed to her by several members of the team: "That's the way I am. Maybe it would be okay for other people, but not for me." (n°29, spouse of a patient, PCU1). In spite of their desire to "do the right thing", caregivers can then find themselves in an awkward situation, even in latent or open conflict with some patients and/or families. Even in PCUs, where the interpersonal skills of caretakers are well developed, increased attention should be given to deciphering the real needs and expectations of those under care, which requires even more attention to the personality of each one, to their personal experiences, and, as underlined by the daughter of a patient, to their "family culture" (n°38, daughter of a patient, PCU3).

5.2.2 Manage uniqueness by better adapting information to be communicated

The diversity of patient situations found in care facilities highlights a fundamental aspect of satisfaction for patients and their families: the importance (as suggested in the interview results) of caregivers further adapting the way they disclose information. This means individualising it to the extent possible, according to the unique needs and expectations of each person. Personalisation implies adapting norms of professional conduct and attitudes on a case by case basis. This requires a special skill, that of managing the uniqueness of

[7] Cancer (Rainbird, 2009; Parker et al., 2009; Nanton et al., 2009; Mills, 2009), cardio-respiratory illnesses (Exley et al., 2005), renal diseases (Kurella Tamura & Cohen, 2010), intellectual disabilities (Tuffrey-Wijne & McEnhill, 2008), etc.

[8] Paediatrics (Hsiao, 2007; Meyer, 2006), the elderly (Just et al., 2010)

[9] Differences according to country (Cartwright et al., 2007)

[10] Aborigines (Decourtney et al., 2010), African-Americans (Jenkins, 2005), etc.

situations as they occur daily. In order to meet the need for further adaptation of the information process (Kirk et al., 2004), discussions should be held (in PCUs as well as in acute care facilities) on methods and techniques to be put in place for evaluating what patients and families know, what they would like to know (or not) and what they find satisfying (or not) in terms of the quantity and quality of the information received.

The first type of strategy is based on the establishment of an open and direct dialogue with patients and families. In this respect, several authors emphasize the benefit of family conferences in PCUs (Yennurajalingam et al., 2008), as well as in intensive care units (Curtis, 2005 et al.; Lautrette et al., 2006). This involves formal and structured meetings between caregivers and families. These are the occasion for taking the opportunity to create a space for dialogue, for listening to families, answering their questions and sharing their feelings, while respecting key principles of medical ethics and palliative care (consideration of patient preferences, explanation prior to taking decisions, reassurance of non-abandonment) (Curtis et al., 2005). To do this, such conferences should consider the needs of families (to reassure them, for example, of the proper management of their relative's symptoms), be the place to deliver clear explanations concerning decision-making, and give continuous and compassionate attention to the needs of the patient, until his or her death (Lautrette et al., 2006). Therefore, these conferences are considered by some authors as an opportunity to considerably improve the quality of care for palliative care patients (Hudson et al., 2008), even the "keystone" around which care at the end of life should be built (Lautrette et al., 2006). From this perspective, recommendations on the preparation, conduct and evaluation of these meetings with families have been made (Hudson et al., 2008). More generally, the international literature highlights the importance of testing structured approaches to disseminating information, to determine the most appropriate attitude to adopt for each unique situation (Hudson et al., Aranda & Kristjanson, 2004). In addition, some authors underline the importance of promoting advanced directives in order to facilitate communication between caregivers and patients concerning the end of life (Pautex et al., 2008). This concerns written instructions given in advance by competent adults, in the event they are no longer able to express their wishes when a decision to stop treatment is envisaged. While this scheme is relatively new in France (law of 22 April 2005 on patients' rights and end of life), it would significantly reduce the degree of anxiety and depression of those involved, thus improving their overall satisfaction with regard to the care they receive (Pautex et al., 2008).

The second type of strategy appears even more structured. This entails several tools which caregivers can use either for evaluating the needs and expectations of each person in the initial stages (often not disclosed by the latter), or for evaluating *a posteriori* the quality of care from the patients' and families' points of view. In this respect, information and communication constitute one dimension among others of the quality of care given, and evaluations are generally done using a scale (Casarett et al., 2008) or questionnaires (Mystakidou et al., 2002). The results of our study can contribute to initiating such an approach by identifying attributes of "good" information transfer from the patients' and families' viewpoint (on five basic dimensions: the accessibility of information, its appropriateness, its frankness, its completeness and its comprehensibleness). In addition and along with these tools that have become traditional in the area of care, others are beginning to appear. New technologies[11] have the potential of markedly improving

[11] for example, electronic patient reported outcome collection, web-based tools, cyber infrastructure, etc.

communication in palliative care, not only between patients and caregivers, but between caregivers themselves (Dy et al., 2011; Madhavan et al., 2011; Kallen et al., 2011). As an example, we can cite schemes put in place in the context of hospice programmes (to achieve proactive patient management) and including e-mail alert systems, based on answers by patients to various aspects of care (for example, their uncontrolled symptoms or their medication needs) (Dy et al., 2011). But whereas all these standardised tools (scales, questionnaires, new technologies) appear especially interesting for significantly improving patient and family satisfaction concerning the provision of information, they should not replace caregivers' interpersonal skills, nor their communication skills. In other words, communication aids should not be a substitute for communication.

6. Conclusion

One of the contributions of this study, carried out in 5 PCUs among 50 patients and families, was to underline what they like and what they regret about the communication of information, in terms of its form as well as its content. While identified factors leading to satisfaction should be encouraged and broadened with a goal of disseminating best practice in palliative care, factors leading to dissatisfaction can be considered as levers for improvement. Indeed, further adjustment efforts should target these aspects. Three elements in particular have been emphasised: 1) the broad overlapping in palliative care of information skills, communication skills and interpersonal skills; 2) the high visibility, to those interviewed, of communication efforts made by the team, which suggests the presence of a special savoir-faire in PCUs (this point is supported by numerous comparisons made spontaneously by interviewees between their present hospitalisation and what they observed in acute care facilities); 3) the difficulties inherent in the coexistence of opposing viewpoints, which express the considerable heterogeneity of the needs and expectations of each person in terms of information, and thus the need to further adapt this information to particular personalities and family cultures.

Within a national and international context of promoting palliative care, these reflections on what information should be provided constitute an important issue, especially if we highlight the positive impact that techniques and attitudes of caregivers have had on many of the patients and families interviewed in this study. Beyond simply knowing the degree of patient and family satisfaction with respect to information communicated, the development and use of specific evaluation tools may help to effectively implement the necessary corrective actions (in Palliative Care Units as well as in acute care facilities) and to meet as nearly as possible the unique needs and expectations of each person. However, while these new modes of communication are promising, they must be envisaged as a way of better understanding and meeting the needs and expectations of patients and their families, and not as a substitute for the interpersonal skills of caregivers.

7. Acknowledgment

We would like to thank those in charge of the five Palliative Care Units in which this study was carried out, as well as the patients and families who accepted to give us some of their time. We would also like to thank the French National Authority for Health for its financial support, and Sylvie Amsellem for carrying out the interviews.

8. References

Alexander S.C., Keitz S.A., Sloane R & Tulsky J.A. (2006), A controlled trial of a short course to improve residents' communication with patients at the end of life, *Academic Medicine*, Vol.81, No.11, (November 2006), pp. 1008-1012, ISSN 1040-2446

Andershed B. (2006), Relatives in end-of-life care - part 1: a systematic review of the literature the five last years, January 1999-February 2004, *Journal of Clinical Nursing*, Vol.15, No.9, (September 2006), pp. 1158-1169, ISSN 0962-1067

Aubry R. (2011), *Etat des lieux du développement des soins palliatifs en France en 2010*, Rapport à M. le Président de la République et à M. le Premier Ministre, April 2011

Buckman R. (2000), Communication in Palliative Care: a practical guide (Chapter 26), In *Death, dying and bereavement*, Dickenson D., Johnson M. & Katz J. (Eds), pp. 146-173, Second Edition, ISBN 0761968563, SAGE Publications, London, United-Kingdom

Cartwright C., Onwuteaka-Philipsen B.D., Williams G., Faisst K., Mortier F., Nilstun T., Norup M., van der Heide A. & Miccinesi G. (2007), Physician discussions with terminally ill patients: a cross-national comparison, *Palliative Medicine*, Vol.21, No.4, (June 2007), pp. 295-303, ISSN 0269-2163

Casarett D., Pickard A., Bailey F.A., Ritchie C.S., Furman C.D., Rosenfeld K., Shreve S. & Shea J. (2008), A nationwide VA palliative care quality measure: the family assessment of treatment at the end of life, *Journal of Palliative Medicine*, Vol.11, No.1, (January-February 2008), pp. 68-75, ISSN 1096-6218

Clayton J.M., Butow P.N. & Tattersall M.H. (2005), When and how to initiate discussion about prognosis and end-of-life issues with terminally ill patients, *Journal of Pain and Symptom Management*, Vol.30, No.2, (August 2005), pp. 132-144, ISSN 0885-3924

Council of Europe (2003), *Recommendation Rec 24 of the Committee of Ministers to member states on the organisation of palliative care*, adopted by the Committee of Ministers' Deputies on 12 November 2003 at the 860th meeting of the Ministers' Deputies, (November 2003)

Curtis J.R. (2005), Engelberg RA, Wenrich MD, Shannon SE, Treece PD & Rubenfeld GD, Missed opportunities during family conferences about end-of-life care in the intensive care unit, *American Journal of Respiratory and Critical Care Medicine*, Vol.171, No.8, (April 2005), pp. 844-849, ISSN 1073-449X

De Haes H. & Teunissen S. (2005), Communication in palliative care: a review of recent literature, *Current Opinion in Oncology*, Vol.17, No.4, (July 2005), pp. 345-350, ISSN 1040-8746

Decourtney C.A., Branch P.K. & Morgan K.M. (2010), Gathering information to develop palliative care programs for Alaska's Aboriginal peoples, *Journal of Palliative Care*, Vol.26, No.1, (Spring 2010), pp. 22-31, ISSN 0825-8597

Dy S.M., Roy J., Ott G.E., McHale M., Kennedy C., Kutner J.S. & Tien A. (2011), Tell Us™: A Web-Based Tool for Improving Communication Among Patients, Families, and Providers in Hospice and Palliative Care Through Systematic Data Specification, Collection, and Use, *Journal of Pain and Symptom Management*, doi:10.1016/j.jpainsymman.2010.12.006, (March 2011), ISSN 0885-3924

Exley C., Field D., Jones L. & Stokes T. (2005), Palliative care in the community for cancer and end-stage cardiorespiratory disease: the views of patients, lay-carers and health care professionals, *Palliative Medicine*, Vol.19, No.1, (January 2005), pp. 76-83, ISSN 0269-2163

Fainzang S. (2006), *La relation médecins-malades: information et mensonge*, PUF (Eds), Collection Ethnologies, 2006, 160 p, ISBN 2130558283, Paris, France

Fallowfield L.J., Jenkins V.A. & Beveridge HA. (2002), Truth may hurt but deceit hurts more: communication in palliative care, *Palliative Medicine*, Vol.16, No.4, (July 2002), pp. 297-303, ISSN 0269-2163

Falls C.E. (2008), Palliative healthcare: cost reduction and quality enhancement using end-of-life survey methodology, *Journal of Gerontological Social Work*, Vol.51, No.1-2, (2008), pp. 53-76, ISSN 0163-4372

Fassier T., Lautrette A., Ciroldi M. & Azoulay E. (2005), Care at the end of life in critically ill patients: the European perspective, *Current Opinion in Critical Care*, Vol.11, No.6, (December 2005), pp. 616-623, ISSN 1070-5295

Faulkner A. (1998), ABC of palliative care: Communication with patients, families and other professionals, *British Medical Journal*, Vol.316, No.7125, (January 1998), pp. 130-132, ISSN 0959-8138

Ferrell B.R., Dahlin C., Campbell M.L., Paice J.A., Malloy P. & Virani R. (2007), End-of-life Nursing Education Consortium (ELNEC) Training Program: improving palliative care in critical care, *Critical Care Nursing Quaterly.*, Vol.30, No.3, (July-September 2007), pp. 206-212, ISSN 0887-9303

Giardini A., Giorgi I., Sguazzin C., Callegari S., Ferrari P., Preti P. & Miotti D. (2011), Knowledge and expectations of patients in palliative care: issues regarding communication with people affected by life-threatening diseases, *Giornale Italiano di Medicina del Lavoro ed Ergonomia*, Vol.33, No.1 Suppl A, (January-March 2011), pp. A41-A46, ISSN 1592-7830

Gott M., Ingleton C., Bennett M.I. & Gardiner C. (2011), Transitions to palliative care in acute hospitals in England: qualitative study, *British Medical Journal*, Vol.342:d1773, doi: 10.1136/bmj.d1773, (March 2011), ISSN 0959-8138

Hatem D., Mazor K., Fischer M., Philbin M. & Quirk M. (2008), Applying patient perspectives on caring to curriculum development, *Patient Education and Counseling*, Vol.72, No.3, (September 2008), pp. 367-373, ISSN 0738-3991

Hsiao J.L., Evan E.E. & Zeltzer L.K. (2007), Parent and child perspectives on physician communication in pediatric palliative care, *Palliative & Supportive Care*, Vol.5, No.4, (December 2007), pp. 355-365, ISSN 1478-9515

Hudson P., Aranda S., Kristjanson L. & Linda J. (2004), Information provision for palliative care families, *European Journal of Palliative Care*, Vol.11, No.4, (2004), pp. 153-157, ISSN 1352-2779

Hudson P., Quinn K., O'Hanlon B. & Aranda S. (2008), Family meetings in palliative care: Multidisciplinary clinical practice guidelines, *BMC Palliative Care*, Vol.7, No.12, doi:10.1186/1472-684X-7-12, (August 2008), ISSN 1472-684X

Innes S. & Payne S. (2009), Advanced cancer patients' prognostic information preferences: a review, *Palliative Medicine*, Vol. 23, No.1, (January 2009), pp. 29-39, ISSN 0269-2163

Jack B., Hillier V., Williams A. & Oldham J. (2004), Hospital based palliative care teams improve the insight of cancer patients into their disease, *Palliative Medicine*, Vol.18, No.1, (January 2004), pp. 46-52, ISSN 0269-2163

Julian-Reynier C. (2007), Prédire sans médire: l'embarras médical face aux mauvaises nouvelles, *Sciences Sociales et Santé*, Vol.25, No.1, (March 2007), pp. 55-61, ISSN 0294-0337

Just J.M., Schulz C., Bongartz M. & Schnell M.W. (2010), Palliative care for the elderly--developing a curriculum for nursing and medical students, *BMC Geriatrics*, 20.09.2010, Available from http://www.biomedcentral. com/content/pdf/1471-2318-10-66.pdf, ISSN 1471-2318

Kallen M.A., Yang D. & Haas N. (2011), A technical solution to improving palliative and hospice care, *Supportive Care in Cancer*, (January 2011), doi: 10.1007/s00520-011-1086-z, ISSN 0941-4355

Kirk P., Kirk I. & Kristjanson L.J. (2004), What do patients receiving palliative care for cancer and their families want to be told? A Canadian and Australian qualitative study, *British Medical Journal*, Vol.328, No.7452:1343, 19.05.2004, Available from http://www.bmj.com/content/328/7452/1343.full, ISSN 0959-8138

Kurella Tamura M. & Cohen L.M. (2010), Should there be an expanded role for palliative care in end-stage renal disease?, *Current Opinion in Nephrology and Hypertension*, Vol.19, No.6, (November 2010), pp. 556-60, ISSN 1062-4821.

Lautrette A., Ciroldi M., Ksibi H. & Azoulay E. (2006), End-of-life family conferences: rooted in the evidence, *Critical Care Medicine*, Vol.34, No.11 Suppl, (November 2006), pp. S364-S372, ISSN 0090-3493

Madhavan S., Sanders A.E., Chou W.Y., Shuster A., Boone KW., Dente MA., Shad AT. & Hesse BW. (2011), Pediatric palliative care and eHealth opportunities for patient-centered care, *American Journal of Preventive Medicine*, Vol.40, No.5 Suppl 2, (May 2011), pp. S208-S216, ISSN 0749-3797

Mangan P.A., Taylor K.L., Yabroff K.R., Fleming D.A. & Ingham J.M. (2003), Caregiving near the end of life: unmet needs and potential solutions, *Palliative & Supportive Care*, Vol.1, No.3, (September 2003), pp. 247-259, ISSN 1478-9515.

McFarland K.F. & Rhoades D.R. (2006), End-of-life care: a retreat format for residents, *Journal of Palliative Medicine*, Vol.9, No.1, (February 2006), pp. 82-89, ISSN 1096-6218

McIlfatrick S. (2007), Assessing palliative care needs: views of patients, informal carers and healthcare professionals, *Journal of Advanced Nursing*, Vol.57, No.1, (January 2007), pp. 77-86, ISSN 0309-2402

Meyer E.C., Ritholz M.D., Burns J.P. & Truog R.D. (2006), Improving the quality of end-of-life care in the pediatric intensive care unit: parents' priorities and recommendations, *Pediatrics*, Vol.117, No.3, (March 2006), pp. 649-57, ISSN 0031-4005

Mills M.E., Murray L.J. & Johnston B.T. (2009), Cardwell C, Donnelly M, Does a patient-held quality-of-life diary benefit patients with inoperable lung cancer ?, *Journal of Clinical Oncology*, Vol. 27, No.1, (January 2009), pp. 70-77, ISSN 0732-183X

Miyashita M., Hirai K., Morita T., Sanjo M. & Uchitomi Y. (2008), Barriers to referral to inpatient palliative care units in Japan: a qualitative survey with content analysis, *Supportive Care in Cancer*, Vol.16, No.3, (March 2008), pp. 217-222, ISSN 0941-4355

Mystakidou K., Parpa E., Tsilika E., Kalaidopoulou O. & Vlahos L. (2002), The families evaluation on management, care and disclosure for terminal stage cancer patients,

BMC Palliative Care, Vol. 1,No.3 (April 2002), 10.04.2002, Available from http://www.biomedcentral.com/1472-684X/1/3, ISSN1472-684X

Nanton V., Docherty A., Meystre C. & Dale J (2009), Finding a pathway: information and uncertainty along the prostate cancer patient journey, *British Journal of Health Psychology,* Vol. 14, No.3, (September 2009), pp. 437-458, ISSN 1359-107X

National Agency for Accreditation and Evaluation in Health (ANAES) (2000), *Information des patients, Recommandations destinées aux médecins,* 59 p

National Agency for Accreditation and Evaluation in Health (ANAES) (2002), *Modalités de prise en charge de l'adulte nécessitant des soins palliatifs, texte des recommandations,* 33 p

National Assembly (2002), *Law n°2002-303 du 4 mars 2002, relative aux droits des malades et à la qualité du système de santé.*

National Assembly (2002), *Rapport d'information sur la loi n°2002-303 du 4 mars 2002 relative aux droits des malades et à la qualité du système de santé,* Enregistré à la Présidence de l'Assemblée nationale le 11 avril 2002 et déposé par MM. Claude Evin, Bernard Charles et Jean-Jacques Denis, Députés

National Council of the Order of Physicians (1995), *Decree n°95-1000 du 6 Septembre 1995, portant Code de déontologie médicale,* Article 35

National Hospice and Palliative Care Organization (2008), *International standards/guidelines of Practice,* 08.05.2008, Available from http://webcache.googleusercontent.com

Ngo-Metzger Q., August K.J., Srinivasan M., Liao S. & Meyskens F.L. (2008), End-of-Life care: guidelines for patient-centered communication, *American Family Physician,* Vol.77, No.2, (January 2008), pp. 167-174, ISSN 0002-838X

Norton S.A., Tilden V.P., Tolle S.W., Nelson C.A. & Eggman S.T. (2003), Life support withdrawal: communication and conflict, *American Journal of Critical Care,* Vol. 12, No.6, (November 2003), pp. 548-555, ISSN 1062-3264

Parker P.A., Aaron J. & Baile W.F. (2009), Breast cancer: unique communication challenges and strategies to address them, *The Breast Journal,* Vol.15, No.1, (January-February 2009), pp. 69-75, ISSN 1075-122X

Pautex S., Herrmann F.R. & Zulian G.B. (2008), Role of advance directives in palliative care units: a prospective study, *Palliative Medicine,* Vol.22, No.7, (October 2008), pp. 835-841, ISSN 0269-2163

Rainbird K., Perkins J. & Sanson-Fisher R. (2009), Rolfe I, Anseline P, The needs of patients with advanced, incurable cancer, *British Journal of Cancer,* Vol.101, No.5, (September 2009), pp. 759-764, ISSN 0007-0920

Ruszniewski M. (2004), Faut-il dire la vérité au malade ?, *Revue des Maladies Respiratoires,* Vol.21, No.1, (February 2004), pp. 19-22, ISSN 0761-8425

Schaefer KG. & Block SD. (2009), Physician communication with families in the ICU: evidence-based strategies for improvement, *Current Opinion in Critical Care,* Vol.15, No.6, (December 2009), pp. 569-577, ISSN 1070-5295

Serryn D. (2008), Quelle vérité pour quelle prise en charge?, Synthèses documentaires, Centre de ressources national soins palliatifs François-Xavier Bagnoud, 20.05.2008, Available from http://www.croix-saint-simon.org

Tibi-Lévy Y. (2007), *Les équipes hospitalières de soins palliatifs dans le processus de rationalisation des soins. Entre engagement idéologique et contraintes financières (Hospital palliative care teams in the process of rationalizing health care. Between ideological commitment and financial constraints*), Thèse de santé publique (spécialité: Economie de la santé), Université Paris XI, 459 p., tel-00351978, 12.01.2009, Available from http://halshs.archives-ouvertes.fr

Tibi-Lévy Y. & de Pouvourville G. (2007), *L'activité palliative hospitalière - Enquête qualitative sur l'adaptation de l'activité des Unités de Soins Palliatifs (USP) aux besoins et attentes des patients et de leurs proches*, Rapport Inserm-Cnrs, Haute Autorité de Santé (HAS) dans le cadre de son appel d'offre «Place et rôle de l'usager dans la démarche d'amélioration de la qualité des soins à l'hôpital», 81 p

Tibi-Lévy Y. & de Pouvourville G. (2009), Qu'est-ce qu'une unité de soins «performante» du point de vue des malades relevant de soins palliatifs et de leurs proches ? (*What is an «efficient» care unit, from the perspective of patients in palliative care and their families?*), *Médecine Palliative*, Vol.8, No.2, (April 2009), pp. 53-65, ISSN 1636-6522

Tuffrey-Wijne I. & McEnhill L. (2008), Communication difficulties and intellectual disability in end-of-life care, *International Journal of Palliative Nursing*, Vol.14, No.4, (April 2008), pp. 189-194, ISSN 1357-6321

Yennurajalingam S., Dev R., Lockey M., Pace E., Zhang T., Palmer J.L. & Bruera E. (2008), Characteristics of family conferences in a palliative care unit at a comprehensive cancer center, *Journal of Palliative Medicine*, Vol.11, No.9, (November 2008), pp. 1208-1211, ISSN 1096-6218

Yoshida S., Hirai K., Morita T., Shiozaki M., Miyashita M., Sato K., Tsuneto S. & Shima Y. (2011), Experience with prognostic disclosure of families of Japanese patients with cancer, *Journal of Pain and Symptom Management*, Vol.41, No.3, (March 2011), pp. 594-603, ISSN 0885-3924

14

Palliative Care in Children

Huda Abu-Saad Huijer
American University of Beirut, Lebanon

1. Introduction

In recent years the incidence of incurable disease and disability has been on the increase in developed and developing countries which in turn is increasing the need for pediatric palliative care all over the world (Gwyther & Cohen, 2009; Rogers et al., 2011). Medical and technological advances have certainly reduced infant and child mortality rates and, at the same time, have improved the survival rate of children with severe and potentially lethal pathologies, not always, however, offering the hope of a cure. This has produced an increase in the overall number of gravely ill children who continue to suffer from life-threatening problems.

For many years palliative care was not offered to pediatric patients and, even today, only a small percentage of children with incurable illness can actually benefit from palliative care services. Many of these children will die in inadequate conditions; without relief from distressing symptoms, usually in a hospital setting and rarely in their own home (Feudtner et al., 2011; Gwyther & Cohen, 2009).

Multiple cultural, organizational, educational and economical reasons have given rise to and have influenced the persistence in these shortcomings in patient care.

The purpose of this chapter is to examine the state of the art and need for palliative care in children. It sets out evidence for policy development, documents the importance of palliative care for children, describes the needs of children and their families, provides arguments for integrating palliative care across health services, summarizes evidence for effective care solutions, and formulates recommendations for health care policy.

2. Why palliative care for children?

The World Health Organization (WHO, 1998) defines Palliative care for children as:

"The active total care of the child's body, mind and spirit, and also involves giving support to the family. It begins when illness is diagnosed, and continues regardless of whether or not a child receives treatment directed at the disease. Health providers must evaluate and alleviate a child's physical, psychological, and social distress. Effective palliative care requires a broad multidisciplinary approach that includes the family and makes use of available community resources; it can be successfully implemented even if resources are limited. It can be provided in tertiary care facilities, in community health centers and even in children's homes".

Childhood diseases requiring palliative care differ from those of adults; they are usually rare and familial and are either life-limiting or life threatening.

Life-limiting illness *is defined as a condition where premature death is usual, for example Duchene muscular dystrophy.*

Life-threatening illness *is one where there is a high probability of premature death due to severe illness, but there is also a chance of long-term survival to adulthood, for example children receiving cancer treatment.*

It is important to draw a distinction between 'palliative' and 'terminal' care. 'Terminal care' refers to the care of the patient and family during the period when death is imminent (weeks, days, hours). Palliative Care is not terminal care but includes end-of-life care (EAPC Taskforce, 2007). This misunderstanding seriously conditions eligibility criteria, specific needs and the way services are offered, particularly in the pediatric sector.

2.1 Spectrum of illness

Four different categories of childhood diseases have been identified (Aldrich, 1995):

Group 1	Life-threatening conditions for which curative treatment may be feasible, but can fail (for example, cancer, organ failure of heart, liver or kidney, infections)
Group 2	Conditions requiring long periods of intensive treatment aimed at prolonging life, but where premature death is still possible (for example, cystic fibrosis, HIV/AIDS, cardiovascular anomalies, extreme prematurity)
Group 3	Progressive conditions without curative options, where treatment is palliative after diagnosis (for example, neuromuscular or neurodegenerative disorders, progressive metabolic disorders, chromosomal abnormalities, advanced metastatic cancer on first presentation)
Group 4	Irreversible, non-progressive conditions with severe disability causing extreme vulnerability to health complications (for example, severe cerebral palsy, genetic disorders, congenital malformations, prematurity, brain or spinal cord injury)

It is difficult to predict the duration of palliative care in children: in some cases (congenital disease), it may be limited to the first years of life; in others (neurological, cardiac and autoimmune pathologies) it can be long-term; while in others, it is concentrated in a brief period before death. In all these situations, there is no distinction between curative practices aimed at prolonging and enhancing the quality of life and treatment that is purely 'palliative'. Both approaches coexist, each prevailing depending on the phase of the disease and the circumstances (Fig. 1).

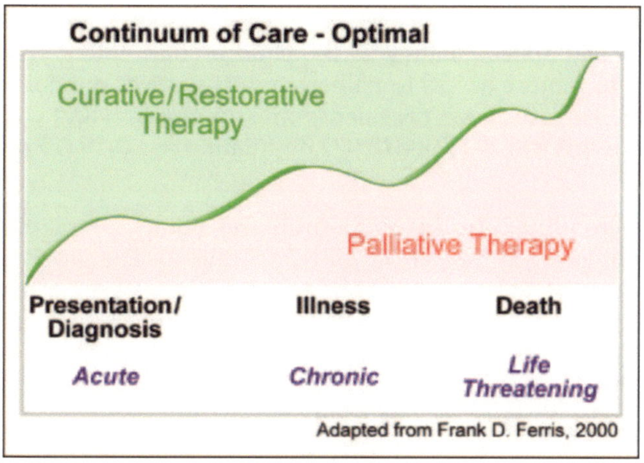

Fig. 1. New Model of Palliative Care (Korones, 2007)

Cognitive development and age along with child's experiences form the basis for a child's understanding of the concepts of illness and death which tend to change over time and vary between one child and another. Palliative care is as a result different in children in the following areas (Korones, 2007):

- Different spectrum and duration of illness
- Smaller, more varied patient population
- Specificity and complexity of services required.
- Parents are generally more involved as care-givers and decision-makers
- Developmental factors influence the child's understanding of illness and death, as well as their ability to communicate and participate in decision-making
- Sibling and extended family needs
- Grief in parents is more likely to be severe, prolonged and complicated

3. Epidemiological evidence

According to van de Wetering and Schouten-van Meeteren (2011), in developed countries the survival rate of children with cancer exceeds 75%. Children can tolerate more intense and combination therapies that have improved survival rates. 25% of children in developed countries will enter the palliative phase and ultimately die from their disease, while this rate exceeds 70% in developing countries.

Comprehensive epidemiological data is not available or is imprecise in many countries. In order to provide effective palliative care solutions, information relative to numbers, diagnostic category, age range and location of children with life-limiting or life-threatening conditions is essential. The available data regards mainly two statistics: mortality from life-threatening or life-limiting illness and the prevalence of life-threatening or life-limiting cases.

The published literature in the UK indicates that the prevalence of some conditions requiring palliative care is increasing, probably because of improvements in the survival rate of low birth weight babies and increased life expectancy (Department of Health, UK, 2007). It is estimated that approximately 20,100 children and young people in the UK aged 0-19 years are likely to require access to palliative care services annually (18,000 if neonatal deaths are excluded). The estimated prevalence rate for children and young people likely to require palliative care services is 16 per 10,000 population age 0-19 (15 per 10,000 if neonatal deaths are excluded).

In England, there were 42,400 deaths of children and young people from causes likely to have required palliative care in the period 2001-2005 (Fig. 2). The proportion of deaths likely to require palliative care is highest among children less than 1 year and lowest among older children (15-19 years) and young adults (20-24 years). There have been on average 2,109 neonatal deaths per year from causes likely to require palliative care in the period 2001-2005 (Department of Health, UK, 2007).

Three-quarters of non-neonatal deaths likely to require palliative care among children and young people aged 0-19 occurred in hospitals. The proportion of deaths in hospitals is lower for young adults aged 20-39 (61%) than it is for young children under one year (88%) or 1 - 4 years (74%). Almost all (98%) of neonatal deaths occurred in hospitals. In the years 2002-2005, the average proportion of deaths requiring palliative care at age 0-19 (excluding neonates) that occurred at home ranged from 14.5% to 25% in London (Department of Health, UK, 2007).

There are variations in mortality figures among countries. In the UK and Ireland the mortality from life-limiting and terminal illness is 1.2 in 10,000 in the UK (Department of Health, UK, 2007) and 3.6 in 10,000 in the Republic of Ireland (Department of Health and Children, the Irish Hospice Foundation, 2005).

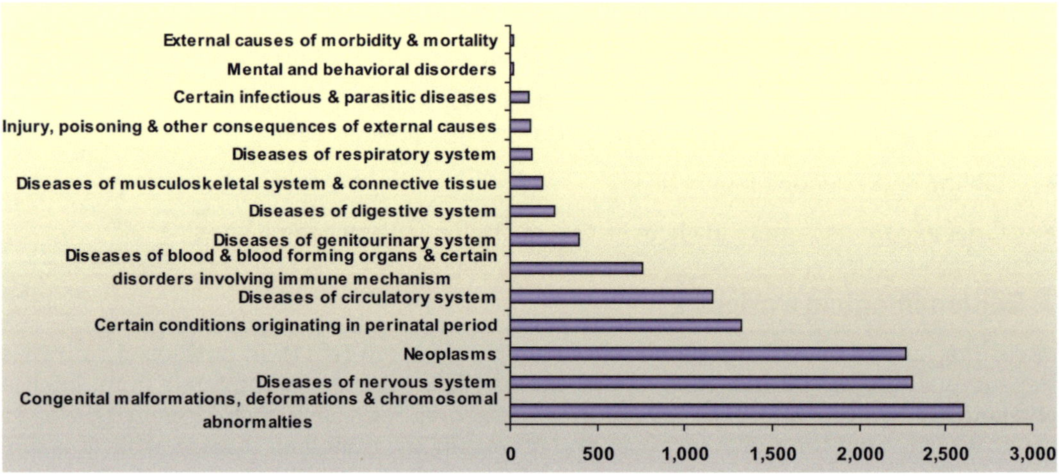

Fig. 2. Data from causes likely to require palliative care for ages 0-19, England 2001-05, excluding neonatal deaths (Department of Health, UK, 2007)

As for causes of death, in the UK 83% of the palliative care deaths in the neonatal period are from "conditions originating in the neonatal period". This group of conditions also accounts for 34% of the deaths in the 28 day to 1 year group. After the age of 1 year the most common causes of palliative care related death are congenital malformations, deformations and chromosomal abnormities, neoplasm, and diseases of the nervous system. During the year

2001-6, 68% of palliative care related deaths in the 1-19 year age group took place in a hospital setting, 8% occurred in hospices and 22% occurred at home (NHS, 2011).

In the United States, in 1900, children 5 years of age or younger accounted for 30% of all deaths; in 1999, that number dropped to 1.4%. Despite this change, more than 50,000 children die every year, and more than 500,000 children suffer from life-threatening conditions in the US (Korones, 2007).

According to the American Academy of Pediatrics, 50% of pediatric deaths in the USA are one year of age or younger; most of these infants die from complications of prematurity, perinatal complications, or congenital abnormalities. The death of older children (1 to 19 years) is from accidents, homicide, or suicide. However, a minority of infants and children (approximately 10,000 a year) die from complex chronic conditions that encompass a broad spectrum of disorders such as neuromuscular disease, cardiac abnormalities, renal failure, metabolic abnormalities, chromosomal anomalies, blood disorders, and malignancies. Children who have complex chronic conditions are the primary potential beneficiaries of palliative care services (Korones, 2007).

4. Needs of children

Pediatric palliative care is based on the same principles as adult palliative care but also recognizes the unique needs of the children, the adolescents, and the families faced with a child's illness and death (Liben & Goldman, 1998; Pritchard et al., 2011).

Physical needs: Pain and other symptoms are common and should be managed in a timely and skilled manner. This requires that healthcare providers be knowledgeable with pharmacologic and non-pharmacologic treatments for pain, dyspnea, nausea, and vomiting and other symptoms (Himelstein et al., 2004; Wolfe et al., 2000). Planning ahead can reduce pain and other symptoms; providing the child with the adequate pain killers and using distraction or other forms of non-pharmacologic therapies before an invasive procedure can assist in reducing the stress and anxiety associated with the procedures (Mercadante, 2004).

Psychological needs: The developmental stage of children affects their emotional and spiritual needs. The use of non-verbal and expressive communication methods such as drawing pictures, writing stories, and playing music can help children express their anger, fears, hopes and dreams (Himelstein et al., 2004). Honest and open communication with the terminally ill child is very important; children need to have hope and need to trust the healthcare provider (Abu-Saad Huijer, 2001; Hilden & Chrastek, 2000). Additionally, children need to feel safe in the environment they are in, and hence presence of a familiar person like a family member or a close friend, is of great assistance (Hynson & Sawyer, 2001).

Social needs: Children undergo a process of physical, emotional, cognitive and spiritual development. Religious and cultural beliefs, patterns of coping, disease experience, previous experience with loss and death, sadness, and other emotions associated with grief, all influence a child's understanding of death (Canadian Hospice Palliative Care Association, 2006). Additionally, children are members of many communities, including families, neighborhoods and schools. School is an integral part of their lives, and it is essential they have ongoing opportunities to pursue their education. Their continuing role in these communities should be incorporated into their dying journey.

Spiritual needs: Spiritual support should be available if and when requested taking into consideration the religious and cultural background of the family.

Special attention is given to the needs of adolescents and young adults who require palliative care (Pritchard et al., 2011). The emotional and social needs of this population are complex and vary significantly, depending on the level of maturity of the patients and the extent to which they have made the transition from complete dependence on parents and family to independence. Newly gained independence can be lost with severe illness and the patients again find themselves dependent on their parents for physical, financial, and emotional needs. In addition, peer involvement and support are vital in this period of life especially because adolescents feel isolated from their social surroundings and friends while on treatment and whenever they are being hospitalized. Social support is often provided by other adolescents and young adults of a similar age group being treated for cancer and receiving palliative care (Pritchard et al., 2011).

5. Needs of family

The unit of care is the family, defined as the persons who provide physical, psychological, spiritual and social comfort to the child, and who are close in knowledge, care and affection, regardless of genetic relationships. Family members may include biological, marital, adoptive, and custodial families (Canadian Hospice Palliative Care Association, 2006).

Parents of children with life threatening illnesses become healthcare provider, mental health counselor, spiritual counselor, home health aide, in addition to being parent, spouse and employee. They perform roles for which they receive little or no training and no payment, in order to avoid institutionalizing their child. They bear heavy responsibilities which may include making decisions in the best interest of the child at a time when they are highly stressed and grieving the loss of their child's health (Goldman, 1998; Hinds et al., 2005; Hynson et al., 2003; National Hospice and Palliative Care Organization, 2001).

The needs of the family can be categorized as follows (Texas Children's Cancer Center, 2000):

Educational needs: preparation and education that is specific to the unique needs and concerns of family members in various aspects of care provides a sense of competence and ease during a frightening transition.

Emotional needs: anticipatory grief and guilt can be addressed by social workers, support groups, and counselors. Relationships between couples and among families might weaken due to the increased stress and tension; encouraging individual family members to seek support outside the family circle can ease this burden.

Religious and spiritual needs: resources such as chaplain, other spiritual leaders, or social worker may be of help to the child and family who seek spiritual comfort. They can offer support by learning to be comfortable with death, listening to the family, and performing small acts of kindness.

Financial needs: changes in lifestyle can affect employment status and the financial security of the family. An examination of the economic resources available to the family, coupled with early planning, can help families manage finances.

In a study following up the needs of families of children who died from cancer (Monterosso, Kristjanson, & Phillips, 2009), parents reported the need for clear and honest information about their child's condition and prognosis throughout the trajectory of illness. Parents also requested access to, and advice from, multidisciplinary health professionals when caring for their child at home. Parents verbalized their preference to care for their child at home wherever possible and reported being well supported by immediate and extended family and friends.

6. Needs of siblings

Siblings of chronically ill, dying children are at risk of becoming forgotten. They feel isolated because the priorities of the parents shift to the care of the sick child, and their own needs are not considered as priority. They are at high risk for school problems, problems with parent-child relationships, and other psychological and social problems following their siblings' deaths.

Siblings have unique needs during and after a child's death (Lauer et al., 1985). Grief for a child is a process that might take time to resolve; it can last weeks to months. Grief can be manifested differently in children: shock and numbness, anger, guilt, disobedience, temporary regression, and believing deceased is still alive. One should be aware of this range of manifestations in order to intervene and help the grieving sibling accordingly (Table 1) (American Academy of Pediatrics, 2000; Texas Children's Cancer Center, 2000).

Siblings of children who die at home cope better with the loss than children whose siblings die in the hospital. At home, they are more likely to know what is going on, to take part in the care, and to be present at the time of death. In the months and years following the death, they are more comfortable with what happened and have better relationships with parents and friends (American Academy of Pediatrics, 2000; Texas Children's Cancer Center, 2000; Lauer et al., 1985).

• Siblings should be included in discussions of care from the time of diagnosis, through death of the child, and beyond.
• "Protecting" siblings by excluding them may cause long-term harm.
• Siblings should be included in discussions about end-of- life care.
• Siblings should be included in funeral planning.
• Certain resources should be made available to support siblings through their grief and bereavement.

Table 1. Guidelines for Assistance to Siblings of Children Who Have Cancer (Korones, 2007; Spinetta, 1999)

7. Effectiveness of pediatric palliative care

When comparing the availability of palliative care services for children with cancer in economically diverse regions of the world, low income countries were most likely to report self-payment for oncologists, palliative care services, and symptom management medications. Availability of specialized palliative care services, pain management, bereavement care, high-potency opioids and adjuvant drugs was significantly less likely in low income countries. Physicians in low income countries were significantly less likely than others to report high-quality symptom management, emotional support, bereavement support, interdisciplinary care, and parental participation in decisions (Delgado et al., 2010).

7.1 Symptom assessment and management

Children dying in the hospital suffer from many symptoms that are often distressing. In the last week of life, symptom prevalence increases and some symptoms like lack of energy, drowsiness, skin changes, irritability, pain, and edema of the extremities occur in 50% or more of children (Saad et al., 2011; Drake, 2003).

The most common symptoms reported are pain, lack of energy, fatigue, dyspnea, nausea, lack of appetite, drowsiness, cough, and other psychological symptoms like sadness, nervousness, worrying, and irritability (Collins et al., 2000; Hongo et al., 2003; Saad et al 2011; Wolfe et al., 2000). Overall, the majority of children (Fig. 3) experience a great deal of suffering from at least one symptom (Saad et al 2011).

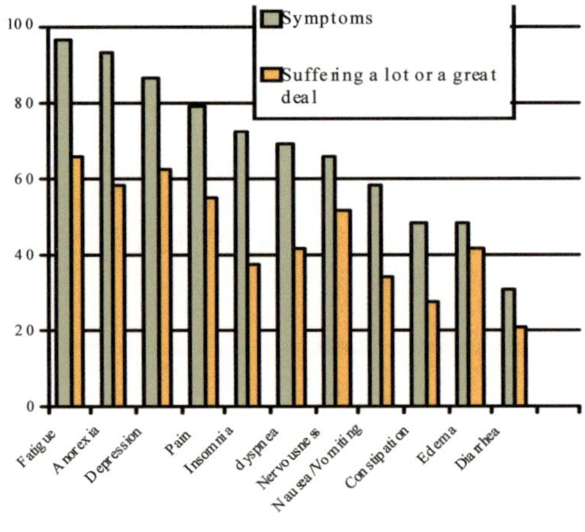

Fig. 3. Symptoms and their burden (Saad, Abu-Saad Huijer, Noureddine, Muwakkit, Saab, & Abboud, 2011)

Although pain is a major symptom in pediatric palliative care (Breau et al., 2003; Wolfe et al., 2000), pain assessment, pain management, and post-intervention reassessment are underreported in the medical charts by both physicians and nurses (Carter et al., 2004). Symptoms can be controlled if clinical guidelines including effective drug treatment combined with practical, cognitive, behavioural, physical and supportive therapies are followed (Canadian Hospice Palliative Care Association, 2006; Charlton, 2005; Korones, 2007; Selove et al., 2006; Texas Cancer Council, 1999).

7.2 Communication and information-giving

Informative, effective communication between health care providers, the child, and the family is critical when addressing end-of-life issues. In a study conducted by Saad et al. (2011), lack of communication was seen by parents as a barrier to effective and holistic care. The main concerns raised by the parents were: accessibility to healthcare services & empathy and acceptance of parents' situation and behaviors by the healthcare team. Providing parents with the information they desire in order to participate in informed decision-making should be a primary goal. Compassionate delivery of distressing news to the parents is an important step in facilitating adjustment. Parents can maintain a sense of hope for their child's survival even after being told that their child's death is certain (Hinds et al., 2005).

The child's right to be informed about his or her illness, available treatment options, clinical trials and their potential benefits, risks and burdens depends on the child's stage of development (Canadian Hospice Palliative Care Association, 2006). Parents determine how, when, and what information is shared with the child, with the guidance of professionals, taking into account the child's temperament, cognitive abilities, developmental level, and cultural beliefs and values (Canadian Hospice Palliative Care Association, 2006).

Parents have the right to know about the child's disease condition, available treatment options, and their potential benefits, risks and burdens, and palliative care. They have the right to make decisions about all treatments including the right to withhold treatment, and to determine goals for care (Canadian Hospice Palliative Care Association, 2006). In lower income countries, where poverty, limited resources, cultural norms and the absence of laws safeguarding self-determination are present, parents were seen to participate less in decisions regarding their child's care than in higher income countries (Delgado et al., 2010).

Language and cultural differences create barriers to information-sharing by healthcare providers to parents who are in need of pediatric palliative care. Inadequate information sharing contributes to frustration, anger, and sadness for parents long after their child's death. Therefore, healthcare providers are in a very critical position when providing information to parents from a diverse cultural background and need to be very sensitive to this issue (Davies et al., 2010).

8. Pediatric palliative care services

The needs of each family are unique and change over time; therefore a spectrum of services is needed in order to provide flexible care (ACT, Royal College of Pediatrics and Child Health, 2007):

- A locally based palliative care service led by a pediatrician or other appropriate senior professional and including a multidisciplinary network.
- Access to a children's hospice for short term respite, terminal and emergency care and bereavement support.
- Training, information, and psychological support for all carers (health carers, social workers, volunteers, family members).
- Specialists/tertiary hospital services (diagnosis, treatment, clinical management, and specialist palliative care services).
- District hospital services (inpatient and outpatient services for symptom management).

- Short term breaks or respite care services
- Medications, medical equipments, and supplies.
- Bereavement support services.
- Specialist palliative care support services

Providing care to children using community services is more cost effective than allowing children to spend inappropriate time in hospitals. Community services can manage for example children with cystic fibrosis who require intensive courses of antibiotics to be treated at home rather than in the hospital. Similarly, children who need long-term intravenous nutrition or tube feedings can be managed more effectively at home (York Health Economics Consortium/Department of Health Independent Review Team, 2007).

Bereavement services are provided for parents who have lost a child and for children who have lost a sibling (Rolls & Payne, 2003). Despite the growing evidence that families would prefer their children to die at home (Collins, 1998; Hannan & Gibson, 2005; Himelstein, 2006; Vickers & Carlisle, 2000), for the last decade, most children used to die in hospital. Recently, a new study published in the UK reported that similar proportions of children are dying at home (45%) and in hospital (47%), and the percentage dying in a hospice or care home has increased from 2% to 10% between 1996 and 2006 (Shah et al., 2011).

Deciding on the place of care and place of death for children is difficult and depends on several factors (Hearn & Higginson, 1998):

- Families value time left with children and therefore want their child to remain at home, in part to retain normality, but also because it is what the child often wants.
- Families want to feel safe and secure, having control but also wanting support. This leads some families to choose hospital in the absence of good community support.
- Families do not know what to expect, knowing how long a child will live is important. Having a child living longer than expected is emotionally and physically problematic, and conversely if the child dies sooner the family feels cheated of time spent with child.
- Specialist services are known to differ from conventional care (Department of Health and Children, the Irish Hospice Foundation, 2005). Specialist teams improve satisfaction by managing patient and family needs at home, improving symptom control, reducing hospitalization, and decreasing overall costs.

9. Ethical issues

Ethical issues about care for infants and children with life-limiting or life-threatening conditions have mainly focused on decisions (Institute of Medicine of the National Academics, 2003).

Decisions about who decides: Parents have the legal right to make decisions about medical care for the child but this does not mean that parents and physicians should exclude children from decisions about their care. Decisions may be constrained by culture, organizational or governmental policies, and environmental factors.

Decisions about treatment: Stopping versus not starting treatment: most physicians and ethicists consider these two options as the same. It is important for those deciding such interventions to be extremely knowledgeable about all clinical aspects that are in the best interest of the child.

Life-sustaining treatments: examples include cardiopulmonary resuscitation, mechanical ventilation, mechanical provision of nutrients or fluids, blood transfusions, antibiotics, and dialysis. It is now generally accepted by physicians, ethicists, policymakers, and the public that abstaining from life-sustaining treatment is appropriate when death is near.

Decisions about the criteria for decisions: a major goal of palliative care is to enhance the quality of life of the child, and not only to prolong it. When taking decisions in the course of care, parents and physicians should identify and weigh the potential benefits and burdens and their influence on the quality of life. As health care costs have increased in the past decades, disagreements often rise about the provision of services that are not beneficial. Consensus in the clinical field has been that resources should not enter the physicians' judgments about patient care unless supported by available scientific knowledge.

Not all conflicts can be avoided but it depends on the way they are handled can increase or decrease the potential for damage. Developing evidence-based and consensus based guidelines, improving communication skills and sensitivity to cultural differences, and developing organizational policies and procedures are possible strategies to deal with conflicts.

10. Pediatric palliative care solutions

10.1 Holistic and family-centered care

Palliative care for children is an active and total approach to care, embracing physical, emotional, social and spiritual elements. It focuses on enhancement of quality of life for the child and support for the family, and includes the management of distressing symptoms, provision of respite and care through death and bereavement. Pediatric palliative care is a holistic approach, and as such enhancing the quality of life needs to be family-directed and should serve as the guiding principle in determining the plan of care throughout the illness.

10.2 Place of care

"Children, during the trajectory of illness from diagnosis to end of life care and bereavement support for their families, require care from different services. Acute care may be provided by inpatient hospital services, whilst ongoing support may be provided by community teams. Respite care may be provided by hospices, whilst end of life care may be provided by hospices, hospitals or community teams in the families' own homes" (Hynson & Sawyer, 2001). Palliative care for children has a combined hospital, hospice and community focus for care delivery.

Home is the preferred place for care during the illness trajectory and more specifically during the end-of-life period and it has been verbalized by children and their families (Monterosso, Kristjanson, & Phillips, 2009; van de Wetering, & Schouten-van Meeteren, 2011). In the UK, the number of children provided with palliative care at home and eventually dying at home is increasing gradually (Shah et al., 2011).

10.3 Care coordination and management

Since no one person can provide all necessary support for the child and family, palliative care is best provided using an integrated interdisciplinary approach. The provision of palliative care for children involves coordination between the child, family, teachers, school staff, and health care professionals including nurses, primary care physicians, social workers, chaplains, bereavement counselors, and consultants (American Academy of Pediatrics, 2000).

The following has been recommended as a core standard concerning the care coordinator on the palliative care team (European Association of Palliative Care (EAPC) Taskforce, 2007): One professional from the palliative care team must be identified as the family's care coordinator or key worker. The care coordinator will help the family to build and maintain an appropriate support system of professionals so the family will be ensured access to social services, practical support (including appropriate aids and home adaptations), spiritual and respite care. The care coordinator will act as the main link, providing continuity, ensuring that the care provided is consistent with the needs of the child and family.

Since chronically ill children are often cared for by a number of healthcare providers and across a variety of settings, including clinics, inpatient units, home and school, the absence of clinical leadership and effective interdisciplinary communication across care settings may cause conflicting therapeutic goals among providers, placing unnecessary burdens on the children and their families (Department of Health and Children, the Irish Hospice Foundation, 2005; National Hospice and Palliative Care Organization, 2001; Wolfe et al., 2000).

10.4 Respite care

Respite is defined as "the provision of care, for the ill child by alternate care providers, rather than the parents, when a child is medically stable, enabling time off from the exhausting care these children require. Parents of children with life threatening conditions need time and energy to attend to their own basic physical and emotional needs and to be available to care for other members of their family. Respite care can be provided in the home by a trained professional, family member, volunteer, or paid sitter. Out-of-home respite can be provided by hospital units, residential facilities, licensed foster parent respite care or medical daycare programs" (National Hospice and Palliative Care Organization, 2001). Respite for family carers and the child is essential, whether for few hours or a few days; it should be possible to provide respite care in the family home and away from home (European Association of Palliative Care (EAPC) Taskforce, 2007).

10.5 Caregiver support

Health care professionals must be supported by the palliative care team, their colleagues, and institutions in dealing with the child's dying process and death. Institutional support may include paid funeral leave, routine counseling with a trained peer or psychologist, and regularly scheduled remembrance ceremonies or other interventions such as inviting bereaved families to return and celebrate with staff the deceased child's life (American Academy of Pediatrics, 2000).

The following are some guiding principles and norms of practice for caregivers support (Groot et al., 2005):

Formal and informal caregivers' physical, psychological, and spiritual well-being should be integral to the provision of pediatric palliative care. Ongoing programs should be in place to address employee issues and improve work life satisfaction. The institution should work to identify and minimize occupational risks and stresses. Formal caregivers should have access to ongoing support, including grief and bereavement support. Formal caregivers should have the opportunity to reflect on their own comfort and ability to enter into difficult conversations with children and families.

10.6 Education and training of health care professionals

Studies evaluating the knowledge and understanding of physicians and nurses regarding palliative care in several countries, whether developed or developing, depicted lack of knowledge and skills in that area and were considered as barriers to daily practice (Abu-Saad Huijer & Dimassi, 2007; Amery et al., 2010; Groot et al., 2005; Raudonis et al., 2002; Rogers et al., 2011; Walker & MacLeod, 2005). Lack of knowledge was mainly seen in pain and symptom management, referring patients to palliative care services, and talking to dying children and their families (Abu-Saad Huijer, 2006; Abu-Saad Huijer & Dimassi, 2007; Feudtner et al., 2007; Groot et al., 2005; Raudonis et al., 2002; Walker & MacLeod, 2005). This lack of knowledge is attributed to the absence of formal education and training in palliative care (Abu-Saad Huijer & Dimassi, 2007; Barclay et al., 2003; Rogers et al., 2011). Improvement in the knowledge and attitudes of nurses and physicians towards palliative care after educational interventions have been reported in several studies (Cramer et al., 2003; Duong & Zulian, 2006; Ersek et al., 2005; Fischer et al., 2003) and several others stressed the importance of integrating palliative care in undergraduate curricula (Ury et al., 2000). A study conducted recently in Lebanon recommended that pediatric palliative care would be improved with the implementation of structured educational programs for the staff, especially symptom management and communication, improvement of psychological, social and spiritual support for families with a seriously ill child (Saad, Abu-Saad Huijer, Noureddine, Muwakkit, Saab, & Abboud, 2011).

The following recommendations are made regarding the education and training of health care professionals including nurses (Wolfe et al., 2000): Appropriate faculty expertise, time and resources must be mandated to address pediatric palliative care issues. Pediatric residency and subspecialty fellowship programs must incorporate pediatric specific palliative care information. Continuing education programs and certification is needed to make pediatric palliative care more available and accessible. Training in pediatric palliative care for home care and hospice workers, parents, and volunteers must be provided to enable competent care for children living with life threatening conditions, particularly in the terminal phase. Finally, counselors, psychologists, school teachers and officials need training to effectively accommodate the needs of terminally ill children and their classmates.

10.7 Public education

A survey conducted in Scotland (Scottish Partnership for Palliative Care, 2003) on public awareness of palliative care in general showed the majority of respondents reporting some knowledge of palliative care, with 32% reporting no knowledge and 3% high levels of knowledge. Almost 90% felt palliative care should be offered to all those with terminal illnesses, with cancer ranking top on the list. Twenty percent preferred staying at home as long as possible, 10% had a preference for hospitals and the majority favored hospice care. The majority would like to see issues of death and dying more openly addressed and information about palliative care services more generally available.

Public education is one area in palliative care that has not received adequate attention. The public needs to be educated regarding the services provided, treatment modalities, and that pain and other symptoms can be adequately treated and relieved. These issues create challenges for palliative care that should be taken seriously (Abu-Saad Huijer, 2001).

11. Conclusion

In conclusion, the number of children needing palliative care is small and geographically spread over large areas. The duration of care can be prolonged and is difficult to predict. Children have complex palliative care needs that require the interventions of an expert multi-disciplinary team. Pediatric palliative care services must be an integral part of community health services. Home care improves the quality of life of the child and family provided skilled support and assistance are available. Hospital-based palliative care does not always offer the best solutions for the child and family. Education and training of health care professionals in pediatric palliative care is insufficient.

A considerable body of evidence shows that children, adolescents and young people suffer unnecessarily due to underassessment and undertreatment of their problems and due to lack of palliative care services to meet their needs. Children experience a multitude of unique problems and disabilities and as such require a family-centred approach to treatment and care. The predominant focus of the existing palliative care services in this age group is still on cancer; children with other life-threatening conditions are left out.

There is a misperception among healthcare professionals, legislators, administrators and the general public that palliative care is only of use when all curative efforts have been exhausted and that it is mutually exclusive with life-prolonging care. Very few practitioners are experienced in guiding decision-making or in caring for dying children and their families. Variation in the cognitive, emotional and social development of the child affects communication and decisional capacities. Determining the best interests of a child is as a result difficult for families and professionals.

Societies do not expect children to die. Families often believe medicine can currently or imminently cure all diseases. Death is inherently a social/community event, not a medical event. At the present time, it is placed in the hands of a medical community ill-prepared to meet these unique needs, particularly for children, who frequently die in the hospital. Poor communication, guilt, and societal expectations, often force children to endure therapies that adults, given the choice, reject for themselves. Families willing to forgo life-prolonging therapy are at risk of being accused of not caring about their child.

There is a huge disparity in Western countries in resource allocation for research, favoring "cure oriented" acute care interventions over palliative care. Adequate funding for research in pediatric palliative care must be allocated. Only then will children and families be assured that they are receiving proven therapies. Outcome measures relevant to the child and family must be developed. Research applied to children must be derived from children and their families. Research should build on evidence that already exists, be innovative, and fill existing gaps in knowledge and applied practice (National Hospice and Palliative Care Organization; 2001).

The conduct of research in palliative care or end-of-life care, and the recruitment of participants remain a major challenge (Tomlinson et al., 2007). The potential that the child is unaware that he/she is dying, and the possibility that parents have not yet come to terms with the inevitability of their child's death are some of the prevailing reasons. The ethical issues around pediatric palliative care and end-of-life research are significant; researchers must consider and address all the challenges in order to eliminate potentially preventable emotional burden on the child and the parents.

12. References

Abu-Saad Huijer, H. (2001). *Evidence-based palliative care, across the life span.* London: Blackwell Science.

Abu-Saad Huijer, H. (2006). Palliative care: Views of patients, home carers, and health professionals. *Supportive Palliative and Cancer Care,* Vol. 3, pp. 97-103.

Abu-Saad Huijer, H., & Dimassi, H. (2007). Palliative Care in Lebanon; knowledge, attitudes, and practices of physicians and nurses. *Lebanese Medical Journal,* Vol.55, pp. 121-128.

ACT, Royal College of Pediatrics and Child Health. Children palliative care services. A guide to the development of children's palliative care services, Second Edition. 2003.

Aldrich, L.M. (1995). Sudden death: crisis in the school. Thanatos Magazine; Fall.

American Academy of Pediatrics. Committee on Psychosocial Aspects of Child and Family Health (2000). The pediatrician and childhood bereavement. *Pediatrics,* Vol.105, No.2, pp. 445-447, ISSN 0031 4005.

American Academy of Pediatrics, Committee on Bioethics and Committee on Hospital Care (2000). Palliative Care for Children. *Pediatrics,* Vol.106, No.2, pp. 351-357.

Amery, M.J., Rose, C.J., Byarugaba, C., & Agupio, G. (2010). A Study into the Children's Palliative Care Educational Needs of Health Professionals in Uganda. *Journal of Palliative Medicine;* Vol.13, No.2, pp. 147-153.

Barclay, S., Wyatt, P., Shore, S., Finlay, L., Grande, G., & Todd, C. (2003). Caring for the dying: how well prepared are general practitioners? A questionnaire study in Wales. *Palliative Medicine,* Vol.17, pp. 27-39.

Breau, L.M., Camfield, C.S., McGrath, P.J., & Finley, G.A. (2003). The incidence of pain in children with severe cognitive impairments. *Archives of Pediatrics & Adolescent Medicine,* Vol.157, No.12, pp. 1219-1226.

Canadian Hospice Palliative Care Association, 2006. Pediatric Hospice Palliative Care, Guiding Principles and Norms of Practice. Retrieved October 10, 2007 from http://www.chpca.net/marketplace/pediatric_norms/Pediatric_Norms_of_PracticeMarch_31_2006_English.pdf

Carter, B.S, Howenstein, M., Gilmer, M.J., Throop, P., France, D., & Whitlock, J.A. (2004). Circumstances Surrounding the Deaths of Hospitalized Children: Opportunities for Pediatric Palliative Care. *Pediatrics.* Vol.114, No.3, pp. e361-e366, ISSN 0031 4005.

Charlton, J.E. (Ed). (2005) *Core Curriculum for Professional Education in Pain* (3rd edition), IASP Task Force on Professional Education, IASP Publications, Seattle.

Collins, J.J., Byrnes, M.E., Dunkel, I.J., Lapin, J., Nadel, T., Thaler, H.T., Emanuel, E.J., & Weeks, J.C. (2000). The measurement of symptoms in children with cancer. *Journal of Pain and Symptom Management,* Vol.19, No.5, pp. 363-377.

Collins, J.J., Stevens, M.M. and Cousens, P. (1998) Home care for the dying child, *Australian Family Physician,* Vol.27, No.7, pp. 610-614.

Cramer, L.D., McCorkle, R., Cherlin, E., Johnson-Hurzeler, R., & Bradley, E.H. (2003). Nurses' attitudes and practice related to hospice care. *Journal of Nursing Scholarship*, Vol.25, pp. 249-255.

Davies, B., Contro, N., Larson, J., & Widger, K. (2010). Culturally-sensitive information-sharing in pediatric palliative care. *Pediatrics*, Vol.125, No.4, pp. e859-e865, ISSN: 1098-4275

Delgado, E., Barfield R.C., Baker, J.N., Hinds, P.S., Yang, J., Nambayan, A., Quintana, Y., Kane, J.R. (2010). Availability of palliative care services for children with cancer in economically diverse regions of the world. *European Journal of Cancer*, Vol.46, pp. 2260-2266.

Department of Health (Editor): Palliative Care Statistics for Children and Young Adults. Health and Care Partnerships Analysis. Cochrane, H., Liyanage, S., Nantambi, R. 2007 (a). Retrieved October 22, 2007 from http://www.dh.gov.uk/prod_consum_dh/idcplg?IdcService=GET_FILE&dID=140063&Rendition=Web

Department of Health and Children, the Irish Hospice Foundation (Editor): A Palliative Care Needs Assessment for Children (2005). Retrieved October 22, 2007 from http://www.dohc.ie/publications/needs_assessment_palliative.html

Drake, R., Frost, J., & Collins, J.J. (2003). The symptoms of the dying children. *Journal of Pain and Symptom Management*, Vol.26, No.1, pp. 594-603.

Duong, P.H., & Zulian, G.B. (2006). Impact of a postgraduate six-month rotation in palliative care on knowledge and attitudes of junior residents. *Palliative Medicine*, Vol.20, pp. 551-556.

Ersek, M., Grant, M.M., & Kraybill, B.M. (2005). Enhancing end-of-life care in nursing homes: Palliative Care Educational Resource Team (PERT) program. *Journal of Palliative Medicine*, Vol.8, pp. 556-566.

European Association of Palliative Care (EAPC) Taskforce (2007). IMPaCCT: standards for paediatric palliative care in Europe. *European Journal of Palliative Care*, Vol.14, pp. 2-7.

Feudtner, C., Kang, T.I., Hexem, K.R., Friedrichsdorf, S.J., Osenga, K., Siden, H., Friebert, S.E., Hays, R.M., Dussel, V., Wolfe, J. (2011). Pediatric Palliative Care Patients: A Prospective Multicenter Cohort Study. *Pediatrics*, Vol.127, pp. 1094-1101

Feudtner, C., Santucci, G., Feinstein, J.A., Snyder, C.R., Rourke, M.T., & Kang, T.I. (2007). Hopeful thinking and level of comfort regarding providing pediatric palliative care: A survey of hospital nurses. *Pediatrics*, Vol.119, No.1, pp. e186-e192, ISSN: 1098-4275.

Fischer, S.M., Gozansky, W.S., Kutner, J.S., Chomiak, A., & Kramer, A. (2003). Palliative care education: An intervention to improve medical residents' knowledge and attitudes. *Journal of Palliative Medicine*, Vol.6, No.3, pp. 391-399.

Goldman, A. (1998). ABC of palliative care: Special problems of children. *British Medical Journal*, Vol.316, No.7124, pp. 49-52.

Groot, M.M., Vernooij-Dassen, M.J.F.J., Crul, B.J.P., & Grol, R.P.T.M. (2005). General practitioners (GPs) and palliative care: perceived tasks and barriers in daily practice. *Palliative Medicine*, Vol.19, pp. 111-118.

Gwyther, L., & Cohen, J. (2009). Introduction to Palliative Care, In: *Legal Aspects of Palliative Care*, Hospice palliative Care Association of South Africa, pp. 2-6. Retrieved from http://www.osf.org.za/File_Uploads/docs/Legal_Aspects_of_Palliative_Care-Entire_book.pdf

Hannan, J., & Gibson, F. (2005). Advanced cancer in children: how parents decide on final place of care for their dying child. *Health and Social Care in the Community,* Vol.13, No.5, pp. 441-450.

Hearn, J., & Higginson, I. (1998). Do specialist palliative care teams improve outcomes for cancer patients? A systematic literature review. *Palliative Medicine,* Vol.12, pp. 317-332.

Hilden, J.M., & Chrastek, J. (2000). Tell the children. *Journal of Clinical Oncology,* Vol.18, No.17, pp. 3193-3195.

Himelstein, B.P. (2006) Palliative Care for Infants, Children, Adolescents and their Families, *Journal of Palliative Medicine,* Vol.9, No.6, pp.163-181.

Himelstein, B.P., Hilden, J.M., Boldt, A.M., & Weissman, D. (2004). Pediatric palliative care. *New England Journal of Medicine,* Vol.350, No.17, pp. 1752-1762.

Hinds, P.S., Schum, L., Baker, J.N., & Wolfe, J. (2005). Key factors affecting dying children and their families. *Journal of Palliative Medicine,* Vol.8, S.1, pp. S70-S78.

Hongo, T., Watanabe, C., Okada, S., Inoue, N., Yajima, S., Fujii, Y., & Ohzeki, T. (2003). Analysis of the circumstances at the end of life in children with cancer: Symptoms, suffering, and acceptance. *Pediatrics International,* Vol.45, No.1, pp. 60-64.

Hynson, J.L., Gillis, J., Collins, J.J., Irving, H., & Trethewie, S.J. (2003). The dying child: how is care different? *Medical Journal of Australia,* Vol.179, pp. S20-S22.

Hynson, J.L., & Sawyer, S.M. (2001). Pediatric palliative care: Distinctive needs and emerging issues. *Journal of Pediatrics and Child Health,* Vol.37, pp. 323-325.

Institute of Medicine of the National Academics (2003). Ethical and legal issues. In When children die. Improving palliative and end-of-life care for children and their families (pp.293-327. The National Academy Press: Washington.

Korones, D.N. (2007). Pediatric palliative care. *Paediatrics Review,* Vol.28, pp. e46-e56, ISSN: 1526-3347.

Lauer, M.E., Mulhern, R.K., Bohne, J.B., & Camitta, B.M. (1985). Children's perceptions of their sibling's death at home or hospital: the precursors of differential adjustment. *Cancer Nursing,* Vol.8, No.1, pp. 21–27.

Liben, S., & Goldman, A. (1998). Home care for children with life-threatening illness. *Journal of Palliative Care,* Vol.14, No.3, pp. 33-8.

Mercadante, S. (2004). Cancer pain management in children. *Palliative Medicine,* Vol.18, pp. 654-662.

Monterosso, L., Kristjanson, L.J., & Phillips, M.B. (2009). The supportive and palliative care needs of Australian families of children who die from cancer. *Palliative Medicine,* Vol.23, pp. 526–536.

National Hospice and Palliative Care Organization; 2001. *A Call for Change: Recommendations to Improve the Care of Children Living with Life Threatening Conditions.* Alexandria, VA: Retrieved November 26, 2007 from www.nhpco.org/files/public/ChIPPSCallforChange.pdf

NHS East of England (March 2011). Better care, better lives: Achieving the vision for the palliative care of children & young people in the east of England. Retrieved June 03, 2011 from http://www.eoe.nhs.uk/page.php?page_id=2073

Pritchard, S., Cuvelier, G., Harlos, M., & Barr, B. (2011). Palliative care in adolescents and young adults with cancer. *Cancer,* Vol.117, No.10 suppl, pp. 2323–8.

Raudonis, B.M., Kyba, F.C.N., & Kinsey, T.A. (2002). Long-term care nurses' knowledge of end-of-life care. *Geriatric Nursing,* Vol.23, pp. 296-301.

Rogers, S.K., Gomez, C.F., Carpenter, P., Farley, J., Holson, D., Markowitz, M., Rood, B., Smith, K., & Nigra, P. (2011). Quality of life for children with life-limiting and life-threatening illnesses: Description and evaluation of a regional, collaborative model for pediatric palliative care. *American Journal of Hospice and Palliative Medicine,* Vol.28, No.3, pp. 161-170

Saad, R. Abu-Saad Huijer, H. Noureddine, S. Muwakkit, S. Saab, R. Abboud, MR. (2011). Bereaved Parents' Evaluation of the Quality of a Palliative Care Program in Lebanon. *Pediatric Blood & Cancer,* Vol.28, No.3, pp.161-170 Scottish Partnership for Palliative Care (2003). Public Awareness of Palliative Care. Retrieved November 28, 2007 from http://www.palliativecarescotland.org.uk/publications/aware.pdf

Selove, R., Cochran, D., & Todd Cohen, I. (2006). End-of-life pain management in children and adolescents. In The Hospice Foundation of America, *Pain management at end-of-life: Bridging the gap between knowledge and practice.* Retrieved July 3, 2008 from http://www.hospicefoundation.org/teleconference/books/lwg2006/selove.pdf

Shah, A., Diggens, N., Stiller, C., Murphy, D., Passmore, J., & Murphy, M.F.G. (2011). Place of death and hospital care for children who died of cancer in England, 1999–2006. *European Journal of Cancer,* in press.

Spinetta, J.J., Jankovic, M., Eden, T., et al. (1999). Guidelines for assistance to siblings of children with cancer: report of the SIOP working committee on psychosocial issues in pediatric oncology. *Medical and Pediatric Oncology,* Vol. 33, pp. 395–398

Texas Cancer Council (1999). Pain Management in Children with Cancer. Retrieved on November 10, 2007 from http://www.childcancerpain.org/

Texas Children's Cancer Center, Texas Children's Hospital. (2000). End-of-Life Care for Children. The Texas Cancer Council.

Tomlinson, D., Bartels, U., Hendershot, E., Constantin, J., Wrathall, G., & Sung, L. (2007). Challenges to participation in pediatric palliative care research: a review of the literature. *Palliative Medicine,* Vol.21, pp. 435-440.

Ury, W.A., Reznich, C.B., & Weber, C.M. (2000). A needs assessment for palliative care curriculum. *Journal of Pain and Symptom Management,* Vol.20, No.6, pp. 408-416.

van de Wetering, M.D., & Schouten-van Meeteren, N.Y.N. (2011). Supportive care for children with cancer. *Seminars in Oncology,* Vol.38, No.3, pp. 374-379.

Vickers, J.L. and Carlisle, C. (2000) Choices and control: parental experiences in pediatric terminal home care, *Journal of Pediatric Oncology Nursing,* Vol.17, No.1, 12-21.

Walker, S., & MacLeod, R. (2005). Palliative care knowledge of some South Island GPs. *New Zealand Family Physician,* Vol.32, No.2, pp. 88-93.

Wolfe, J., Grier, H.E., Klar, N., Levin, S.B., Ellenbogen, J.M., Salem-Schatz, S., Emanuel, E.J., & Weeks, J.C. (2000). Symptoms and suffering at the end of life in children with cancer. *New England Journal of Medicine,* Vol.342, No.5, pp. 326-333.

World Health Organization, (1998). Cancer Pain Relief and Palliative Care in Children. Geneva, WHO.

York Health Economics Consortium/Department of Health Independent Review Team: Independent Review of Palliative Care Services for Children and Young People: Economic Study. Final Report (2007). Retrieved November 15, 2007 from: http://www.york.ac.uk/inst/yhec/downloads/Final%20Report-may07v1.pdf

15

Palliative Care and Terminal Care of Children

Luis Pereda Torales
Instituto Mexicano del Seguro Social, México

1. Introduction

While modern palliative care movement began with the opening of St. Christopher's Hospice in London in 1960, it was not until 1990 that became widely used, when the World Health Organization adopted the definition of Palliative Care European Society for Care Palliative as "the active total care of patients whose disease does not respond to curative treatment", even if it is in advanced stage and progressive, yet pediatricians took longer to recognize the needs of some pediatric patients who require this type of attention, these patients still do not have access to specialists in palliative medicine than adults do have. As in all pediatric specialties, palliative medicine in children can not simply be imported, the more aspects are examined, children and adults look less and that is why palliative care should be developed from practice and experience pediatricians. [1]

While adults often terminally be referred to specialized equipment, in contrast, pediatricians continue to accompany the patient and family. The advantages of this approach include the combination of skills and knowledge, professional presence known and felt that the patient and his family are not neglected.

Palliative care in children should be considered as an integrated model of care to seriously ill patient or a medical condition that may threaten your life and your family. Begins at diagnosis and continue to be the result of survival or death of the child, or coexisting with healing therapies that prolong life. The model must meet the physical, psychological, social and spiritual needs of children and their families, in order to enhance their quality of life while supporting members of the family members. That is why palliative care can be integrated into care plans of children and their families, whether the goal is to get the cure, prolong life, or only palliate and provide comfort until death.

Terminal illness is defined when a medical condition expected to cause death in a short period of time (three to six months), no matter whether treated or not. There are diagnostic criteria for establishing the condition of terminal illness, such as the presence of a progressive and incurable disease, there is no reasonable likelihood of response to specific treatment, the presence of numerous problems or severe symptoms, multiple, multifactorial and changeable and a great emotional impact on the patient, family and treatment team, with the possibility of death.[2]

This diagnosis should be performed for at least two doctors, one of which is in charge of the patient or physician, and (the) other (s) unrelated to the patient. To make the diagnosis of terminal illness we can support the therapeutic proportionality principle, this principle holds that there is a moral obligation to implement all those measures which have a therapeutic relationship due proportion between the means employed and expected outcome and those measures that this relationship is not met ratio is found to be disproportionate and would not be morally obligatory. Importantly, the trial about the proportionality of a medical intervention should be determined by reference to the overall benefit of therapy, and not just in relation to possible physiological effects that she is able to induce.

As a child, when the family receives the news that one of his sons is in a position incurable and fatal disease in a relatively short time the entire structure is turned upside down: there will be uncertainty, fear, change roles, and changes family functioning and way of life of each of its members is for them that during the course of the disease the family will need psychosocial support of various kinds: information, facilitating the organization, access to social support structures, hold on stages of internal conflict and timely recognition of the moments of "exhaustion family."

This chapter points out the importance of integrating pediatric palliative care in the process of care of hospitalized children, and reviewing the needs of pediatric patients as family and medical staff who serve them. In addition, some recommendations that can help health personnel to serve these children and families.

2. Characteristics of palliative care in the pediatric patient

The terminal phase of disease is a destructive experience for the child and their family members, especially in long-term diseases, inexorable course, where curative options are no longer a reality. Therefore the focus of attention must change radically and move to help pediatric patients and their family, have a better quality of life possible time left to live, through a multidisciplinary effort and qualified. The short life of a child, spent her brief and limited future, deprived of opportunities to see him live and enjoy their existence can generate anxiety, sadness, despair, anger, helplessness in the people around him, including both their parents and close relatives and health personnel in charge of your care is why it is considered palliative medicine as active and total care of patients and their families by a multiprofessional team when the disease is no longer responds to curative treatment and life expectancy is relatively short. The word "palliative" comes from the Latin word pallium, meaning blanket or deck. Thus, when the cause can not be cured, the symptoms are "covered" or "covered" with specific treatments, such as analgesics, and so on.

The traditional view is that the main objectives that must be considered in palliative medicine are:

- Relieve pain and other distressing symptoms;
- Address psychological pediatric patients according to their chronological age;
- Offer a support system to help the child understand his illness to promote active communication between family members and health personnel;
- Provide a support system to help families cope with the patient's illness and cope with the mourning period.

Palliative care affirms life and recognizes that dying is a normal process, seeks neither to hasten nor postpone death, and this requires health professionals with high-level skills and expert care, individualized for each patient, attentive to details and sensitive, which is time consuming and palliative medicine is an attempt to restore the traditional role of doctors and nurses "to heal the sick, relieve when you can not cure, but always follow."

Whatever the type of care should be implemented the philosophy of palliative care in five specific categories, which provide evidence for discussions, evaluations and reflections and contribute to learning:

1. Initial assessment of the patient. Vital as it provides the physical, pathophysiological, social, environmental and spiritual illness.
2. Developing a work program. Options should include medical, ethical and humanitarian offers palliative medicine. Share concerns and perspectives of the patient's family, and medical equipment contributes to the pursuit of consensus and formulate a plan of care.
3. Review monitoring and updating treatment plan. Evaluates the information of the multidisciplinary team, patient and family, to judge the medical component of the treatment plan.
4. Assistance in the terminal phase and elaboration of grief. Allows to acquire knowledge about the symptoms of approaching death, fears, and beliefs of the family, preparing for the outcome, physical care of the dying, relief from suffering and elaboration of mourning for who is dying, with spiritual help needed.
5. Take an active role in her interdisciplinary group. It relates to supporting the work of other members, participation in the development and growth of the multidisciplinary team and training health staff and community about the philosophy, importance, needs and scope of palliative medicine. [3]

In general, states that a patient is terminally ill with a disease that acute, subacute or chronic, the most common, of course subject to inexorable and palliative care, but also could be considered as a patient whose condition is classified as irreversible , treated or not and probably will die in a period of three to six months. Many ailments can lead to children prematurely to the terminal phase, mostly cancer, neurological damage, kidney disease, the immunopathy, congenital malformations, acquired immunodeficiency syndrome and liver disease, each with specific characteristics that share similarities end.

Cancer is largely responsible for the terminal phase in the pediatric age and is considered a serious public health problem and a major cause of morbidity and mortality worldwide. The mere mention of the word cancer mortified generates distress and immediate relationship with an incurable disease, although at present the cancer in children is no longer lethal, and many will have a chance to heal, but other have an unrelenting course and reach the terminal phase, though it is used all available treatments, testing new strategies and even experimental, but without the possibility of cure. In these particular cases life expectancy is very short, perhaps a few months and most patients die shortly after diagnosis. An estimated 2 to 10% of patients attending a highly specialized hospital are terminally ill, so accept that a child is at this stage involves a great responsibility, so the diagnosis must be made by a group of experts and staff in a trial.

It is difficult to establish a precise definition of palliative care to include all children in need and to provide international standards for their implementation, as each country has different health resource models, models of care, philosophy, culture, politics, legal rules, and so on. However, there are children dying from cancer or other diseases that fail to be addressed in all their needs, and there are many reasons why this happens, among others, that childhood is not the age of death (kills more adults) seems easier to care for the children by their parents, but not the pain and other symptoms that society, medicine, have taken less severe disease and death in children, which allegedly curative treatments are rarely abandoned, and yet, even in intensive care units raises increasingly limited therapeutic child care from the palliative approach is increasing in importance.

Death has always been something that people tend to ignore out of fear. When death occurs in children is more striking because the parents expect to see healthy growth and development, represents the continuation and perpetuation of individuals, families, cultures, nations, even said that people who do not treat their children have no future also be considered "the hope of humanity." In addition to the immeasurable suffering in those parents happen all kind of feeling guilt, helplessness, failure, anger and punishment. For medical and paramedical staff, the meaning of the death of a child usually involves feelings of failure, helplessness and guilt, just as a great sense of grief for parents who suffer from this devastating loss. That is why parents are an essential part of palliative care of children, contributing to the care of affected are receiving care and instructions by the medical staff and paramedics should be encouraged so assertive communication, and and offer all possible facilities for this purpose.

2.1 Care for the relief of physical suffering of the child

Children have needs in end-organic, psychological, familial, social and spiritual order to fulfill specific and if possible, requires the participation of a multidisciplinary team of health professionals. Palliative care is divided into specific and nonspecific. First used in surgery, radiotherapy, chemotherapy, blood transfusions, and so on. (Large tumors, hydrocephalus in children with Chiari syndrome Ardnold, among others) in non-specific changes are analgesia, nutrition, hydration, constipation, management of pressure sores, vomiting, hygiene, insomnia, anxiety, depression treatment, counseling , social and spiritual management of other organic symptoms and signs.

Respecting the former management types (specific and nonspecific), we must also consider what you are like kittens maneuvers needed to integrate them into the following four aspects:

- The power, which can be provided in natural form or by nasogastric tube, instead of parenteral nutrition is not part of palliative treatment only if patients with short bowel and intestinal absorption problems.
- Maintaining the hydration status of patients, through a baseline fluid intake, contributing to the welfare of children, as well as the best removal of bronchial secretions and oropharyngeal. This type of hydration is preferably orally.
- Good oxygen through their various modes of application, but preferably without mechanical ventilatory support. Otherwise when the patient is under the support of a ventilator, when establishing its terminal state, extubation is part of the palliative management, but must be considered the minimum respiratory parameters assists.
- It is necessary to consider the child's comfort, this can be done by placing it in a bed with adequate support for the patient with appropriate clothing. The comfort should be extended to visiting relatives, seeking a physical area of privacy in which to have a child living in an environment as comfortable as possible. In any case the room should be adequately ventilated. Try to avoid many people stay in the room and the presence of noise. It is important to maintain physical contact with the patient, touch is the last sense to the patient loses.
- The child's hygiene is also critical, which is needed for both the nursing staff that treats you like family doing their daily bathroom cleaning personal clothing and bedding. To hydrate the skin can be massaged with moisturizing cream soft, provided it does not bother the child or cause pain.
- Frequent changes of position, which must be common to modify support points that reduce circulation which may predispose to the appearance of scars and / or pressure ulcers.

- Finally, consider the use of blood transfusions for severe anemia, when the child is likely to live for several days or weeks. The wet mouth and lips there for that commercial preparations that may be useful as parenteral hydration is not improving xerostomia. [4]

It is also necessary to establish what are the purposes of a hospice program in pediatrics which should consider the following points:

- The income of a pediatric patient to a hospice program should be considered only if it is highly unlikely that the child reaches adulthood.
- It is not intended to shorten life, but to control the physical and emotional symptoms in dignity for the patient and his family.
- Do not hasten or postpone death.
- Start from the beginning supported the diagnosis.
- Seek to improve the quality of life of children and their families.
- Provide comfort and pain relief is a fundamental right of the sick child and their management to be an essential part of treatment.
- Provide comprehensive care, individual and continuing, accepting the values, desires and beliefs of the child as part of a whole.
- Promote values and humanism.
- There should be promotion of the truth.
- Management should be made by a multidisciplinary team, 24 hours a day, 365 days a year, with the proviso that any of the team members are trained to provide support in the child's needs or their families.
- Provide tools to parents, guardians and other family members for communication and interaction with the child about his illness, condition, expectations, etc.
- Provide ongoing emotional and spiritual support.
- Complement the curative treatment when applicable.
- Reaffirm life and see death as a natural process.
- Palliative care does not end with the death of the patient, support the duel should take place as long as necessary to all those affected by the death of the child.
- Set goals and limits for therapy in a child with chronic illness.
- Make appropriate decisions at the end of life. [5]

The management of symptoms is a vital part of palliative care. Pain is the most prominent symptom, its frequency and impact on patient and family, but should not be left aside other symptoms such as dyspnea, nausea, vomiting, salivation and convulsions. Pain is a prominent symptom, not only in cancer patients, but also in other diseases such as cystic fibrosis, acquired immunodeficiency syndrome (AIDS) and neurodegenerative diseases. It is essential for the management of pain, knowing the cause of it, since the treatment will depend on having a correct diagnosis. Opioids are of great value for moderate to severe pain. Neuropathic pain is caused by direct irritation of nerves and drugs such as amitriptyline, nortriptyline and gabapentin have demonstrated efficacy in controlling this type of pain. Another type of pain is somatic, which affects the bone and soft tissue treatment for this is given with nonsteroidal antiinflammatory drugs. Visceral pain, which can be caused by distention or obstruction, requiring treatment with glucocorticoids or octreotide.

The relief of pain and other distressing symptoms of is considered, rightly, the primary goal of palliative care in this way is considered palliative medicine as an expert in the management of end-stage patients to keep them virtually free of pain. You can also expect a high degree of relief from many symptoms. However, not being distracted and exhausted by unrelieved pain, patients may experience greater emotional and spiritual anguish when contemplating the nearness of death. Few do it with balance, most are psychologically defend themselves in various ways, and some are overwhelmed by anxiety, anger or fear of what is happening as the relatives and it is necessary to offer a personalized attention. The health team should seek to assist the patient has given his best, according to their personality, their family, their culture, beliefs, age, disease, its symptoms, anxieties and fears. It is necessary flexibility you need to know to find the patients where they are socially, culturally, psychologically, spiritually and physically.

Sometimes the patient's symptoms in the dying phase can not be controlled with standard treatments and have to use palliative sedation which is defined as the deliberate administration of sedative drugs specifically to reduce intolerable suffering, derived from refractory symptoms, by decreased level of consciousness of the patient. The intolerable suffering should be determined by the patient as a symptom or condition which can not continue to endure. When the patient can not communicate is the opinion of caregivers and / or family members who must determine the nature intolerable suffering. Refractory symptoms are those for whom all possible treatment has failed or, at least, the use of other measures is not appropriate given the margin benefit / risk from the patient's situation. Because palliative sedation is done with refractory symptoms always mean a situation of great anxiety for the health care team. In the days that passed from the onset of sedation until the end of treatment, usually marked by the death of the patient, many decisions are taken to try to achieve the ultimate goal of a good death. Physicians should be aware of the anxiety from this situation and the importance that their anxiety has no effect on the decisions taken with the patient. The consensus in the health team for each of the decisions is essential to prevent an emotional overload at the time

2.2 Psychological needs, emotional and spiritual

In addition to pain management specialists in this symptom, there are alternative therapies such as biofeedback (which corresponds to behavioral therapy for the relief of human suffering, with empirical and theoretical foundations, solidly scientific, which is an essential feature in your application), hypnosis, massage and acupuncture, all play a vital role, more always go hand in hand with other therapies. Agitation can be treated with benzodiazepines; itching with a variety of oral antihistamines, nausea and vomiting with prochlorperazine or ondansetron. Seizures with diazepam and secretions with hyoscyamine.

There are countless situations that generate conflict related to the treatment of children in its terminal phase, with serious birth defects, with severe or irreversible neurological damage and the complexity of this situation presents a series of feelings and conflict of values between the medical staff and paramedics so that you can not give absolute criteria but a series of recommendations to parents of these children, including:

1. Parents or guardians are solely responsible for the decisions about treating your child in appropriate interaction with the treating physician who knows the child's illness. In these cases it is recommended the participation of the Ethics Committee of the institution for advice relevant to each particular case.
2. All children in the terminal phase have inherent dignity, values and rights as human beings and must receive all medical care considered reasonable to take them to the best possible existence.

3. The moral obligation of health workers towards the child is always sick, so the decision to withdraw or not to apply intensive management can be justified when it serves the best interests of the child, that is, when your near future is grim, full suffering or when new interventions only cause greater risks.
4. You should always consider the application acceptable minimum of palliative care in the following cases: those involving greater agony of the child or prolong the life of the unnecessary if, when suffering severe pain and intolerable only if the child is in state persistent vegetative or in the agonal phase of the disease. [6]

In these cases it is also important ethical review but with certain peculiarities of the characteristics of his being in development and maturation. First and foremost, remember that life and human health have intrinsic value derived from the same human dignity. For the sanctity of life, every person, regardless of age and psychophysical characteristics, has-without exception-the same basic right to life and deserves respect and protection of society and all professionals dedicated to your care. This is helpful to the implementation of a set of ethical standards including casuistry, virtue ethics (aretológico), utilitarianism, the ethics or medical duties, however we must consider the bioethical model and of paramount are beneficence, autonomy, justice and nonmaleficence that might work well at the time of decision making by physicians and can be summarized in the fact that all the therapeutic actions tend to benefit patients, avoid damage with an appropriate and relevant information to parents or legal guardians choose the best decisions for their children that children receive the best treatments available to date and supported by quality scientific research proven methodology, but not excessive when is in final stage, always consider the good, proper and fair to them, thinking only in their best interests and to avoid unnecessary suffering.

The contribution of psychology in this context includes aspects of care both for children with terminal illness and their families as different members of the multidisciplinary team. Psychological intervention can be carried out in at least four periods with both patients and relatives, before the impact caused by the onset of the disease after diagnosis of the disease and the start of the intervention during the disease progression and the process of death and finally after the death of the child.

In relation to the patient, the task from the psychological point of view, focuses on the welfare assessment, pain and suffering as a result of the situation which is in addition to psychopathological symptoms such as anxiety, fear of death, depression or loss of control of the situation, this can be directed to the alleviation of the emotional impact while facilitating the process of adaptation to the disease. This assessment should be carried out continuously and flexible, as there are rapid changes in disease evolution, adapting to the characteristics and needs of each individual child.

In relation to family assessment and intervention focus on work overload and emotional impact that occurs as a result of the proximity of the disease and its possible consequences. Do not forget that many times family members are the only ones who know the patient's diagnosis, hidden so that it does not suffer. Therefore, psychological intervention will aim to reduce psychosocial problems that this causes in family functioning and to assist the family in anticipation of mourning.

As it relates to health workers providing palliative care, the action aims to facilitate both the management of emotions to the terminal as the communication situation between the different members of the health team towards further professional effectiveness . The latter at the organizational level is a powerful resource that can help prevent or reduce the risk of discouragement and decreased quality and quantity of efficiency. In this sense, communication skills with patients, families and among health professionals is essential from the first contact established to give the diagnosis to the patient's death. It is therefore necessary to raise the team development through techniques such as counseling, both to encourage training in assertive communication that allows people to show what they feel, what they think and what they need. [7]

Finally the doctors and parents, with proper informed consent, must make decisions taking into account the benefits and burdens then they mean, also assessing alternative treatments. But as we have seen, with due respect for the thoughts, feelings or wishes of the child when their age and maturity you gain experience and judgment. Therefore desirable to add palliative care units in all hospitals and pediatric primary care teams working so that, with the terminal disease, lengthen or shorten not intended life but provide comfort while the child left to live while helping his family.

2.3 Legal aspects of palliative care in children

Once the provider accepts medical services patient care, it also establishes a legal relationship (doctor-patient relationship) and is required to provide appropriate service and quality, conforms to the rules of law applicable in each country. It must be emphasized the need to recognize and protect the right to palliative care, likewise, is a responsibility of governments to ensure that palliative care accessible to all who need them. These recommendations emphasize the need to develop a coherent national policy framework and comprehensive palliative care that includes the following sections: principles and guidelines on palliative care services and structures that should tell the health care system, welfare policy and organization of the plan of palliative care, quality improvement and research on relevant issues in health care programs, education and training of specialist staff for the care of terminally ill patients, family support, communication, teamwork and mourning.

Palliative care should be an integral part of the Health Committee of the countries and as such should be an element of general health plans, and on specific programs, such as cancer, AIDS, or any patient in a terminal. The implementation of government programs should meet the need of any health system where there are patients in advanced stages and terminals of any kind, in all care settings and where it is considered a fundamental right and a priority in health programs public.[8]

3. Role of paediatrician in the provision of palliative care

The role of pediatricians at the death of a child in the hospital is not easy to define, and the lack of guidelines leads to question if it works correctly. Supporting families after a sudden and unexpected death is particularly difficult. No time to prepare families and health personnel for the event, and it is likely that any further contact with the family involving the staff who do not know well. Offering a bereavement follow-up meeting to the families is an accepted part of clinical practice and is perceived as useful to help them. Unfortunately, there is little guidance on the objectives of these meetings or training to carry them out.

The pediatric specialists we bring in our own references to death, which are formed along personal and professional experiences. Starts walking toward death when born, talk about it so widespread and yet death is a preventable and ignored issue. For many it is difficult to talk about death in a society that denies and trying desperately to forget their finitude and that is why death is just means suffering. Always without medical training to defend life against the death of patients. In the last hundred years there was an important step to reduce mortality at all levels, purpose made significant steps in terms of public health as well as major advances in diagnostic and therapeutic resources so the emphasis in medical education but the scientific and biomedical research as the basis of scientific knowledge applicable to the medical activity in contrast to the hitherto prevailing empirical knowledge in courses at the beginning of last century, this new model of medical education introduced significant advances in the effectiveness and efficiency of treatments, as well as contributing to the improvement of health indicators in the world.

However as a result of technological development in medicine was a fragmentation of knowledge within the medical training that led to multi-specialty discipline, which today produce serious difficulties in communicating with each other, along came the disintegration of the individual as a patient, an approach that little organ systems interact with each other, and that has led to the dehumanization of medical education. Pain, anxiety, suffering and death are concepts that are not included in the process of care and therefore has no place in the curricula of medical schools. Only sometimes the emphasis is on techniques and medical management to save lives and little or nothing to the development of clinical skills to deal with the pain and suffering, the death of patients and support for families facing the loss of a loved one.

Pediatricians in their education in schools and hospitals where they perform their clinical fields learn to engage with life, all their training is geared towards healing and save the patient, not letting die, so the healing is the meaning of learning or reward the effort. That is why when death occurs, it brings frustration, feelings of inadequacy and limitation, may perceive the child's death as a particularly stressful event. There may also be feelings of helplessness, stress, moral and spiritual suffering, and the emergence of depressive symptoms and burnout syndrome. These aspects must be recognized and addressed proactively to prevent the loss of highly skilled medical personnel. The lack of respect between doctors of different environments, poor interdisciplinary communication, a hierarchical structure of authority, and feelings of helplessness in morally problematic situations contribute to stress and burnout of medical staff, rather than the death of children per se, It is therefore necessary supporting staff work better health while learning to develop adaptive responses to the demands of their work. In environments where demands are particularly intense a reasonable starting point would be to acknowledge this point and go beyond crisis intervention. So the challenge that is the pediatrician is to encourage interdisciplinary and collaborative nature of clinical practice and training to improve pediatric palliative care and child-centered family.

Can you give some examples of ways to improve the quality of the workplace for medical staff that handles children in their terminal phase, including clear orders recorded as well as the following:

- Establish a systematic interdisciplinary meetings.
- Create and actively maintain an atmosphere of open communication and respect.
- Conduct regular ethical discussions between the medical and paramedical personnel.
- Assign experienced clinicians with whom it is safe to discuss concerns and emotional responses on the patient or care plan.
- Have team meetings relief after difficult cases, providing access to crisis intervention teams and psychologists when desired.
- Carrying out acts of commemoration after the death of some patients.

- Encourage follow up with the grieving families.
- Recognize the grief associated with personal and professional losses.
- Recognize the value of the provision of palliative care. [10]

Health staff and particularly the pediatrician also goes through a grieving process, you may feel overwhelmed by having to help the bereaved parents as they have to develop their own grief, so it is necessary to the development of programs aiming at monitoring the mourning families and the healthcare professional. It takes scientific research to learn the process of learning to cope with multiple losses and accumulated health professionals and also consider interventions designed to improve the kind of education and support needed in the experience of dueling doctors in particular pediatricians who have daily contact with children in its terminal stage, such as oncologists, nephrologists, intensivists, and so on.

Medical schools, including the chairs of Pediatrics, the importance of what has been the subject of this dissertation, should be included as part of medical training, content related to child rights and family informed consent of parents and patients less capable of understanding the duty to maintain the privacy of children, protect their identity and knowledge of the behaviors for the care of critically ill children or risk death.

4. The role of family in palliative care of the child

We know that living the illness of a loved one, suffering and death is one of the most difficult life events faced by humans. When a boy joins innocence, helplessness and think he has not had time to live. The death of a child is the loss more traumatic for a parent as it also faces the experience of destruction of a part of himself, the most linked to projects and future hopes. The father's feelings are mixed feelings towards himself, towards the child and toward the couple. The death of a child can affect physical health and psychological well-being of members of the family for the rest of their lives.

When a family is informed that the child will die, a process of confusion and anguish in which decisions about the care and treatment of disease of a child and in desperate need of hope mixed.

Their children do not suffer pain or disability. Parents can express feelings of worthlessness and guilt for having subjected her son to treatments that have not had the expected outcome. It is essential that before the change of therapeutic approach for parents to have confidence that has done everything possible to cure disease and save the life of her son and that he will provide comfort and symptom control. They may also feel conflicting emotions: protection / decoupling; hopelessness / guilt for surviving, disbelief and denial by the change in prognosis, fear of pain and suffering, the capacity to provide care, the emotional loss of control.

Studies of grief in parents suggests that pain control, care during the time of death, and conducting follow-up after the death of the child are factors that may reduce long-term distress in the grief of parents . In other words, improving the care of the sick child, symptom control and care in the dying can also be beneficial for long-term parents. In addition to caring for a child at the end of life at home facilitates the development of mourning. The family perspective is critical to advancing healthcare quality of pediatric palliative care.

There is a cultural trend, especially in urban areas, to set aside the brothers of these situations and sometimes they are not even explain what is happening. But children are highly sensitive to the mood of your family and know that something is happening, then replace the lack of information on their fantasies and draw their own conclusions, for example, that your loved one have been abandoned or their misbehavior is the cause of the disease. Siblings may fear for the life of his ailing brother, to be able to get sick and die. Also face a loss of parental attention they can get angry, less time at home when the child is hospitalized, fewer gifts to his ailing brother, difficulty in understanding the gravity if no physical changes in the patient, shame about being a different family because his brother is disfigured. Sometimes they feel guilt for having escaped the disease, or have wished for the death of his brother. You will need to adapt to being provided with information tailored to their level of development, to be included in care, and that their care is delegated to trusted people and stable.

The child can be cared for at home at the end of his life will facilitate the involvement of the brother in the situation, strengthen the bond between brothers and share games and joint activities, and farewell. Reactions to the death of a brother are varied: from no apparent response to the presence of somatic problems, nightmares, aggression, manipulation, learning difficulties, resentment toward parents for failing to be closer or more time with his brother. The clear and open communication, attention to the needs of the brothers for the rest of the family and maintaining a more normal life as possible, integrated into the serious situation of the sick sibling, will facilitate the adaptation process of dying, fired and the elaboration of grief.

Other significant family for the child and grandparents also suffer at the news of the evolution of the disease and its end of life, and will also be essential support for parents and siblings. The health team must identify the family dynamics and to address the emotional needs of siblings and other relatives integrating them into care when treating the sick child.[11]

4.1 Communication with the family physician's

The final stage of the disease is the stage when the family needs more support as they go through the same stages as the patient but in different ways, trying to deny even imminent death, it is here to provide privacy, access to patient, show kindness, give comfort as with the patient. The doctor and the multidisciplinary team should get the patient to die decently in explaining a positive way to face death, treating patients in their dignity, not dependence. It is often the physician in charge of announcing the death and should provide the best conditions to face this task, this way the family will be satisfied with the care they provide.

The contribution of psychology in this context includes aspects of attention both to terminally ill patients and their families as different members of the multidisciplinary team. In relation to family assessment and intervention focus on work overload and emotional impact that occurs as a result of the proximity of the disease and its possible consequences. Do not forget that many times family members are the only ones who know the patient's diagnosis, hidden so that it does not suffer. Therefore, psychological intervention will aim to reduce psychosocial problems that this causes in family functioning and to assist the family in anticipation of mourning.

Many families are unfamiliar with medical information, and are facing their own shock and anxiety during this critical hospital. Being aware that these circumstances may contribute to the confusion of families, many physicians state that all personnel involved and their different styles of communication, contribute to these difficulties. Very often, parents are lost with the new concepts, detailed explanations and unfamiliar terms when they need time and clear communication to assimilate and process information, so that improvements in communication increase the sense of parental control.

Parents whose child is in the terminal stage of their disease may develop PTSD, and emotional disorders (anxiety and depression). Admission to a hospital medical establishment also negatively affects the family unit. The severity at admission and length of stay in services or departments of a hospital may have negative consequences for the family.

Several studies have documented the psychological benefits for parents and children, medical and economic needs emotional parents whose children are admitted to a hospital in terminal stage, so the medical and paramedical staff should be more sensitive to the needs of aid psychological family members to seek the help of the most qualified professionals in this work and also to provide, within its capabilities, continuous emotional support.

In recent years, has developed an awareness on the emotional and spiritual needs all patients, their families and support staff. Terminal in each patient, these issues must become an indispensable part of treatment. That is why the doctor needs the support of parents, guardians and other staff responsible for patient care because it is important to keep routines before detection of the disease. The first step in treating depression and anxiety is the recognition thereof through communication with the child, which requires knowledge of normal development and spiritual development. To work with these patients is necessary to evaluate based on drawings, games, stuffed animals, stories, music and creating rituals, allowing children to express their fears and anxieties, and thus manage their emotional distress.

The attitude of medical and health personnel to the severely ill or dying in a hospital, and to his family, and the type of information that these professionals provide can have a direct effect on the family's ability to adapt the loss of a loved one and spending a proper grieving process. Parents perceived slights or emotional distance from the health staff usually show a duel inadequate short and long term. Also, a caring emotional attitude has beneficial effects in the short and long term.

4.2 Recommendations to support the child's family in terminal stage

Despite the lack of specific guidelines that help medical personnel how to act in the last moments of a child's life so that they can support the family, some authors have proposed some recommendations:

- Try to predict questions that may have parents but are afraid or unable to verbalize.
- It is helpful for any family to know the expected course of death, even the unpleasant physical circumstances.
- Leave plenty of time for goodbyes, visits and rituals. Privacy and familiar presence, if they want the child and family is another important aspect to provide comfort to both parties.
- It is important to tell the family that may or may not happen during and after the withdrawal of life support. Moreover, even if parents do not accept the possibility of abandoning the medical interventions that extend life, the evidence suggests that some families do not only want, but can also benefit from the opportunity to be present during resuscitation efforts.
- Do not forget to ask family members if they want to hold your baby with you or be with them in bed.

- Should be told that the child will not feel pain and the medical staff will provide all necessary medication to ensure patient comfort.
- The answer to the question of how long the child will survive after the limitation of life support is very important information, since families may develop unrealistic expectations about the time of death. It is very important to prepare for the fact that the child might not die, or death can occur within minutes or weeks, depending on many conditions associated with the disease and the patient's general condition.
- Some children do not die in the highly complex services such as intensive care units so they must communicate this to parents and the medical team to properly ascertain both the transfer of the patient and the services they receive child .
- Children need to know that they are not going to forget and parents shared experiences to remember. (Ensuring the importance, the continuing legacy and love are important aspects of parenting the child who will die). When death can be anticipated, measures to create memories during times of relative health or ongoing claims that they are loved and that they are not going to forget, are important.
- For a child who dies suddenly, for example victims of trauma, some innovative approaches may be to create molds the child's hand, save a lock of hair, or take pictures or videos at moments when the family visit the child. Those involved in caring for the child will die, should seek to provide opportunities to create legacies or inheritances.
- When the child was deeply sedated, parents may have the opportunity to see your child smile and see with open eyes before his death, an experience that sometimes has a great value.
- Parents, siblings, other family members and friends may have to spend the final moments of the dying child, so that policies restricting visits to the different services of a hospital need a thorough discussion and review. [12]

5. Conclusion

For the management of end-stage patients is necessary to integrate a multidisciplinary and interdisciplinary team who can take charge of the complex needs of these children, and the problems they face inside and outside the health institutions, especially in view of relieving their suffering and achieve an improvement in quality of life standards. It is essential for teamwork (which would include pediatricians or neonatologists, nurses, pain specialists, psychologists, thanatologists, social workers, physiotherapists, occupational therapists and a spiritual leader within the team), which must prevail in a spirit binding, collaboration among its members, and a shared competence, ie a single goal, and a great patience and high tolerance for frustration.

Undoubtedly optimal care to patients and families in the service environment that serve patients in terminal stage, would also imply an institutional sensitivity to allow or permit the reflection of the team, including structural and organizational changes and the provision minimum financial resources that would enable the adequacy of care according to need.

Finally, the necessarily humanistic medicine, palliative care and a multidisciplinary unit that should work with the patient and his family twenty-four hours a day, 365 days a year, it is desirable that all members involved in the process to be the same philosophy and specific goals for the welfare and tranquility of the children and their families.

6. References

[1] Salas M, Gabaldón O, Mayoral ML, Pérez YG Amayra I. (2005) El pediatra ante la muerte del niño: integración de los cuidados paliativos en la unidad de cuidados intensivos pediátricos. *An Pediatr (Barc),* Vol. 62 Nº 5, (mayo de 2005) pp 450-457

[2] Korones N. (2007) Pediatric palliative care. *Pediatr Rev*, Vol. 28 pp 46-56.

[3] David E. Weissman , Diane E. Meier . (2011) Identifying Patients in Need of a Palliative Care Assessment in the Hospital SettingA Consensus Report from the Center to Advance Palliative CareIdentifying Patients in Need of a Palliative Care Assessment in the Hospital SettingA Consensus Report from the Center to Advance Palliative Care. *Journal of Palliative Medicine,* Vol.14 Nº 1, (enero 211) pp 17-23.

[4] Postovsky S, Ben Arush W. (2004) Care of a child dying of cancer: The role of the palliative care team in pediatric oncology. *Pediatr Hematol Oncol* Vol. 21 pp 67–76

[5] Hinds PS, Drew D, Oakes LS, Fouladi M, Spunt S, Church C, Furman W. (2005) End-of-life preferences of children and adolescents with advanced cancer. *J Clin Oncol* Vol.23 Nº 36, pp 9146–9154

[6] American Academy of Pediatrics. Committee on Bioethics and Committee on Hospital Care. (2000) Palliative care for children. *Pediatrics* Vol. 106 pp 351-357

[7] Studdert M, BurnsJP, Mello M, Puopolo L, Truog D, Brennan A. (2003) Nature of conflict in the care of pediatric intensive care patients with prolonged stay. *Pediatrics* Vol. 112 pp 553-558

[8] Aulisio M, Chaitin E, Arnold R. (2004) Ethics and palliative care consultation intensive care unit. *Crit Care Clin* Vol. 20 pp 505-523

[9] Bruera E, Palmer JL, Bosnjak S, Rico MA, Moyano J, Sweeney C, Strasser F, Willey J, Bertolino M, Mathias C, Spruyt O, Fisch M. (2004) Methadone versus morphine as a firstline strong opioid for cancer pain: A randomized, doubleblind study. *J Clin Oncol* Vol. 22 pp 185–192.

[10] Sepúlveda C, Marlin A, Yoshida T, Ullrich A. (2002) Palliative Care: The World Health Organization's Global Perspective. *J Pain Symptom Manage* Vol. 24 pp 91–96

[11] Goldberg L. (2004) Psychologic issues in palliative care: depression, anxiety, agitation, and delirum. *Clin Fam Pract Vol.* 6 pp 441-70

[12] Billings A, Dahlin C, Dungan S, Greenberg D Krakauer L, Lawles N, Montgomery P, Reid C. (2003) Psychological training in a palliative care fellowship.*International Journal of Palliative Nursing* Vo. 6 pp 355-363.

16

Meeting the End of Life Needs of Older Adults with Intellectual Disabilities

Philip McCallion[1], Mary McCarron[2], Elizabeth Fahey-McCarthy[3] and Kevin Connaire[4]
[1]*University at Albany,*
[2,3]*Trinity College Dublin,*
[4]*St Francis Hospice, Raheny,*
[1]*USA*
[2,3,4]*Ireland*

1. Introduction

Palliative care for adults with intellectual disabilities has come to the fore as an issue only in recent years. This was and to some extent continues to be a largely hidden population in general health care, services were largely provided within their own intellectual disabilities services system, aging was the exception rather than an expectation and there were beliefs that people with intellectual disabilities themselves were not able or ready to made decisions about their end of life care. Some of these assumptions were never true but increases in longevity, onset of chronic diseases such as Alzheimer's disease and the development of palliative delivery in multiple countries are changing this picture (Fahey-McCarthy et al., 2009; McCallion & McCarron, 2004; & Tuffrey-Wijne, et al., 2007).

2. The demography of aging and chronic illness in people with an intellectual disability

Estimates suggest that life expectancy for people with an intellectual disability have increased from an average 18 years in 1930 to 59 years in 1970 to 66 years in 1993 (Braddock, 1999), with projected continued growth to match life expectancy of the general population (Janicki, Dalton, Henderson, & Davidson, 1999). By 2020 the number of persons with intellectual disability aged over 65 is projected to double from 1990 estimates (Janicki & Dalton, 2000). Many of the same socioeconomic and environmental factors in longevity improvement for the general population (clean water, decline in infectious diseases, improved living and nutritional standards, and disease and risk factor management - see Friedman, 2010) have been a feature for people with intellectual disability, but other contributors have been advances in and extension of medical care, advocacy and self-advocacy, and the development by providers of quality living environments and their support of enriching lives (McCallion & McCarron, 2007). Living in the community and improved economic status are likely to be the socioeconomic and environmental factors to drive continued increases in longevity for people with intellectual disability, but attention to disease and risk factor management are increasingly a feature for this population too, as an augmented life expectancy also exposes a growing number of persons with intellectual disability to age-related diseases and challenges the health care they receive.

- Individuals with intellectual disability (ID) have a greater variety of health care needs compared to those of the same age and gender in the general population (US Department of Health and Human Services, 2002; Haveman, *et al.*, 2010)
- People with intellectual disability have 2.5 times the health problems of those without ID (Van Schrojenstein Lantaman-De Valk *et al.*, 2000)
- Rates of psychopathology are considerably higher in individuals with an intellectual disability compared to the general population (Fletcher *et al.*, 2007)
- People with intellectual disability are more likely to lead unhealthy lifestyles which contribute to the development of physical ailments in later life (Evenhuis *et al.*, 2001; WHO, 2001).
- Health problems of persons with intellectual disability are not being recognised (Merrick, *et al.*, 2002; Cooper *et al.*, 2004).
- The experience of poor health and early mortality among people with ID may be related to the location and types of health care services people with ID have received over a life time as well as in their older years (see for example Strauss et al., 1998).
- There is a lack of specialist knowledge and training amongst multidisciplinary and health team members (McCarron & Lawlor, 2003).
- People with intellectual disability do not access health promotion and health screening services to the same extent as peers without disability (Iacono & Sutherland, 2006).

3. The challenge of Alzheimer's disease

Another feature of older age is exposure to risk of Alzheimer's disease and other dementias. This is particularly true for older people with Down syndrome who are uniquely at risk of developing Alzheimer's dementia at earlier ages. Current estimates are that 15-40% of persons with DS over the age of 35 years, present with symptoms of dementia and consequently, their related declines are precipitous (Prasher, 1995; Prasher et al., 1998). Onset is also earlier with the mean age of dementia in persons with Down syndrome being estimated at 51.3 years.

Despite the pressing concerns, responses to Alzheimer's disease issues for people with intellectual disability have tended to be reactive rather than proactive. Providers are faced with unanswered questions regarding how their resources and skills may best be pooled, as well as what service models/developments need to be undertaken, and by whom (Bigby, 2002). A question remains as to what care setting is most useful in addressing and responding to dementia care needs in terms of both cost effectiveness and quality of life outcomes. Differences in philosophies, terminologies, fiscal arrangements and priorities complicate these issues (McCallion & Kolomer, 2003; Wilkinson & Janicki, 2002).The impact on family carers is at an even earlier stage of response (McCallion, Nickle & McCarron, 2005).

In fairness to providers, staff and families, these are new care situations and there is a need for evidence-based models for care if resolution is to be realized, institutionalization and re-institutionalization avoided, quality of life maintained and costs contained. Research is still responding to this challenge.

Very different issues present when individuals have symptoms of dementia and they challenge traditional staffing approaches and philosophies. Staffing numbers and patterns, and the training of staff has more usually been focused upon client groups who are young and middle adult, and on supporting and promoting the independence of persons with intellectual disability who are in jobs and interested and ready for community participation. The inevitable decline associated with dementia challenges this programming philosophy and there has been a danger within intellectual disability services that when dementia presents, providers will seek transfer to other, often more expensive and restrictive alternatives. Instead, there are opportunities in supporting aging in place and in understanding the role of specialized units for people with intellectual disability and dementia (Janicki, et al.2002). Finally, the traditional intellectual disability services funding assumption of fixed needs is challenged by new needs, e.g., 24-hour staffing where overnight staff were not previously needed, more frequent hospitalizations and emergency room use as symptoms of both dementia and co-morbidities increase and environmental management challenges such as falls, wandering and safety concerns occur. Responses to these new challenges are too rarely planned and are often unprepared for the end stage of disease even when maintaining a person in place is intended (Janicki, et al., 2002; McCallion et al., 2005). Data gathered to date suggests that service redesign for dementia is needed at individual, staff, residential/programming unit and organizational levels (McCallion & McCarron, 2004). Equally, approaches and assumptions may need to be re-examined at end stage disease (McCarron et al., 2010). It is also important to recognize that the living situations and social networks of people with intellectual disability may be different from those of other patients with whom palliative care comes in contact.

3.1 Living situations

The majority of people with an intellectual disability live with family or independently but a considerable number have lived most of their adult lives in staffed out of home situations, and rather than being employed have attended workshops and day programs specifically for people with intellectual disability (Haveman et al., 2011). There is a strong likelihood that as adults with intellectual disability get older that they will have small social networks and that paid staff will have significant roles in those networks often occupying personal and friendship roles equivalent to those usually seen in family members (McCarron et al., 2011). It is important that palliative care staff recognize and include in their planning and service delivery this unique aspect of lives of people with intellectual disability.

3.2 Responding to end of life issues

The core philosophy that has shaped current intellectual disability services has emphasized a citizenship model of care, i.e., that a person with an intellectual disability be recognized by other people as an individual who is a full member of society (Duffy 2003). As a citizen, the person with intellectual disability should have choice about where to be cared for and where to die and staff are challenged by how then to respond to the additional care needs of the person who is on a journey with a terminal illness (Blackman & Todd, 2005). Many intellectual disability services are poorly prepared to meet and respond to end-stage dementia in terms of the suitability of the service environments and the skill mix and knowledge base of staff (McCallion & McCarron, 2004).

The need to consider palliative care for persons with an intellectual disability is now receiving attention (Blackman & Todd, 2005; Ryan & Mc Quillan, 2005) as it is for the care of persons with dementia (Kitwood, 1997). However, a University of Sydney review (DADHC, 2004) reports difficulty still exists in the initiation of palliative care for persons with intellectual disability particularly since staff in intellectual disability services do not normally hold palliative care skills. Ng and Li (2003) go further, specifically citing a lack of knowledge of effective communication with the dying person and a lack of knowledge about bereavement support for carers of persons with intellectual disability.

Similarly, palliative care services have traditionally been provided predominantly to persons with malignant disease. There are challenges such as the lack of recognition and acceptance that dementia is a terminal illness and the difficulty in defining of the terminal stage of dementia (Lynn & Adamson, 2003; Lloyd-Williams & Payne, 2002). This is often further confounded in persons with intellectual disability by the level of pre-existing intellectual impairment and sometimes pre-existing high dependency levels (McCarron et al., 2010). Palliative care specialists often lack the knowledge and skills necessary to communicate effectively with persons with intellectual disability and may have limited experience in working with persons with dementia (Ryan and McQuillan, 2005). Although generally accepted that palliative care principles should be extended to other groups with terminal illnesses such as dementia, much work remains from a policy, resource and educational perspective to operationalize this intent (Luddington et al., 2001; Lloyd-Williams & Payne, 2002).

3.3 Merging palliative care, dementia and intellectual disability care principles

Lynn and Adamson (2003) suggest that models of hospice care do not apply well to persons with chronic illness such as dementia because palliative care is seen as turning away from conventional (active/acute) care when persons with dementia instead require a mix of both kinds of care, particularly in the early stages of the disease. Others (Sachs et al., 2004) cite barriers such as the unpredictable nature of dementia and issues with assessment and symptom management. In addition, professionals and family have difficulty in viewing dementia as a terminal condition. Yet the person centered approaches in dementia care concerned with maintaining a quality of life for the person, supporting the persons in living until they die and ensuring that family/carers or persons close to him/her are included in their care (Downs et al., 2006) marry well with the palliative philosophy.

Indeed, opportunities lie within person-centered care to address both dementia and intellectual disability concerns. But in the application of palliative care, there is also a need to consider knowledge and skill issues in 1) relationship-centered care, 2) caring for a person with an intellectual disability, 3) caring for a person with dementia, 4) facilitating grief and loss, and 5) disenfranchised grief.

3.4 Person-centered care

The person-centered challenge for palliative care lies in finding agreement amongst the individual, the physician(s), the primary caregiver, and the hospice team on expected outcomes in relief from distressing symptoms, the easing of pain and/or the enhancement of quality of life. Such ideas are not new to intellectual disability services or to dementia care. In intellectual disability services, there are well established systematic processes for the discovery of an individual's gifts, capacities, experiences, core beliefs and dreams. The collaborative development of plans by service providers to realize those dreams is enhanced by the commitment to the individual by valued persons who help to realize the plan (Abery & McBride, 1998). In dementia care, Kitwood (1997) argued that as well as meeting physical needs, the enabling of the exercise of choice for the person, the use of the person's abilities, the fostering of the expression of his/his feelings and enabling him/her to live in the context of relationship, were also critical to his/her care. Being included means being part of a group and if this need is not met the person can go into decline or retreat.

3.5 Relationship-centered care

Critiques of person-centered care are beginning to emerge (Adams & Grieder, 2005). Nolan, et al., (2001) acknowledge that person-centered care has had a far reaching impact on care in dementia but it is not enough to consider the individual without considering his/her relationships. Relationship-centered care is proposed for situations where relationships have developed over long periods of time such as in care homes (Nolan et al. 2006) and intellectual disability care settings. Dementia care triad, models of relationship-centered care recognize that there are at least three people, the person being cared for, the carer and one or more health and social care professionals (Adams & Grieder 2005), and may further include other people involved in the care of the person. The approach to care sees health care as a human activity given meaning by people within relationships (Tresoloni & Pew-Fetzer 1994). This view also resonates for people with intellectual disability (McCarron et al., 2010)

3.5.1 Knowledge and skills of caring for a person with an intellectual disability

A lack of knowledge of the needs of persons with intellectual disability by staff in general acute medical settings has been identified as leading to diagnostic overshadowing and unexpected and unexplained deaths (MENCAP 2007). Tuffrey-Wijne (1998) and Lindop and Read (2000) have identified (1) a need to be able to interpret non-verbal and alternative communication strategies and (2) the assessment and management of pain as two major educational needs for nurses in general practice to care efficiently for this population. For staff in intellectual disability settings there is an additional need for training and education about the ageing of persons with intellectual disability and the implications of care for a person presenting with symptoms of dementia (McCarron & Lawlor 2003). As persons with intellectual disability experience terminal illness and approach their end of life, this poses further challenges for the staff in intellectual disability settings. Hospice and other palliative care staff must also be equipped to understand the care of persons with intellectual disability (McCallion & McCarron, 2004).

3.5.2 Knowledge and skills of caring for a person with dementia

Regarding care for the general population with dementia, McCallion, (1999) reported that care assistants in nursing homes identified a need for education on communicating with the person with dementia and on managing behavioral issues. Despite such requests, there has been minimal training for staff or carers. Kitwood (1997) argues that this may result from society's fear of ageing, illness, mental illness and death as well as the lack of understanding of dementia. He argues that good quality and sensitive interactions between carers and individuals with dementia are essential for good care (Kitwood 1997). Similar needs have been identified for staff in intellectual disability settings including their need to know how to recognize and manage dementia-associated changes in the person (McCarron & Lawlor, 2003). Sachs et al., (2004) go further, observing that staff should understand the need for early planning of care for the person with dementia, and ensuring continuity of care throughout the trajectory of the illness at early, mid and late stages. The diagnosis of dementia in persons with intellectual disability is complex and the up-skilling of staff in intellectual disability services in the assessment and support of the person with dementia has become crucial, as has on-going education of staff and family on the needs and care issues for the person (McCarron & Lawlor, 2003). Nutrition and hydration also cause concern for family and staff because often "the act of providing sustenance symbolizes love and caring" (Solomon & Jennings, 1998:138). A new culture of care emerges that does not pathologize dementia. Instead it focuses on the uniqueness of each person and respects what s/he has accomplished and allows what s/he has endured to be understood compassionately.

3.5.3 Knowledge and skills of culturally competent caring

There is a need to deliver culturally competent care (Tuffrey-Wijne,1998). Culture affects every aspect of a person's being (Tracey & Ling, 2005). Broad culture-specific issues have previously been identified in relation to terminal illness disclosure, breaking bad news, advance planning and locus of decision-making (Searight & Gafford, 2005). Some cultures advocate explicit disclosure of diagnosis and frank planning for end-of-life care (Candib, 2002). Other cultural groups place higher value on family connectedness than on individual autonomy and may value life at all costs over an easy death. In intellectual disability services there are long established trends of differences in culture between the person, the staff carer and the organization providing care (McCallion & Grant-Griffin, 2000). In intellectual disability settings, more concretely, in many aspects of care McConkey (2004) identified that new staff members tend to rely heavily on verbal communication; yet asking too many questions of the person and the family may actually make situations more complex and impede decision-making. Looking specifically at issues in aging and health, McCallion et al., (1997) identified that professional staff in intellectual disability services may also not be sufficiently sensitive to cultural differences and influences among family and among care staff and may fail to recognize the strengths in other cultures. Culturally appropriate care respects and recognizes the contributions of everyone involved including care staff.

3.5.4 Knowledge and skills of palliative care

Staff in intellectual disability services are not generally prepared in palliative care skills (DADHC 2004). This is compounded by a clear lack of literature about the palliative care needs of persons with intellectual disability (Tuffrey-Wijne, 1997). Tuffrey-Wijne (1997) reported that while staff supported offering death and dying care in principle, they did not feel they had the expertise in practice. Furthermore, staff may be unprepared for the family dynamics around caring for someone with a terminal illness and the emotions involved. In later work, Tuffrey-Wijne (2002) suggests that a more collaborative working relationship between intellectual disability staff and palliative care staff may improve care. Collaboration with specialist palliative care would also encourage greater exchange of expertise. Todd (2004) agrees that carers in intellectual disability services would benefit from education on what to report to the palliative care team and from information on what to expect in the progression of the disease/illness and how to interpret important changes which could indicate pain.

Findings elsewhere suggest that nursing staff who acquired knowledge about the use of drugs commonly used in the symptomatic and palliative management of patients, developed new confidence and found ways to make their assessments of the end-of life care needs of the patients more explicit to other practitioners, thus improving care (Watson et al., 2006). Whittaker et al., (2007) argue that frontline staff and their skills determine the quality of care delivered to people and there is a need for more training in psycho-social care, spiritual care and meeting cultural needs. Solomon and Jennings (1998) also report that medical and nursing staff would benefit from training in the pharmacological and non-pharmacological management of pain and other symptoms to improve palliation. These findings for care of the general population have been confirmed as needs too for care staff, nursing staff and medical staff within intellectual disability services (Fahey-McCarthy et al., 2010).

3.5.5 Knowledge and skills of addressing nutrition, hydration and pain concerns

Feeding difficulties and challenges experienced as part of end-stage dementia care by persons with intellectual disability mirror those difficulties described in the generic care literature in persons with Alzheimer's dementia (Norberg et al., 1994; Biernacki & Barratt 2001; McCarron & McCallion, 2007). Lack of ability to self-feed, the difficulty of holding food in one's own mouth, chewing and swallowing concerns, agitation and distress, spitting, and food inhalation/aspiration all culminate in stress for the person, the family and staff (McCarron et al., 2003). For example, staff report that watching someone they know and care for who is now unable to eat/drink is difficult and they describe feelings of guilt and remorse when faced with this concern (Service, 2002). Staff carers and family are often attracted to what they perceive as the benefits of artificial nutrition and hydration (ANH), including the use of feeding tubes. End stage dementia and related end of life decision making is an emotional and value laden time. Given influences of cultural and religious values of the person, the family and at times care staff, emotions and relationship bonds and conflicts, limited ability to know and understand the wishes of the person, and a lack of undisputed outcome data to support or discourage use of feeding tubes (or alternative approaches) and other life sustaining treatments, making decisions regarding sustaining treatments such as feeding tubes for persons with intellectual disability and dementia present formidable clinical and care challenges. Work is needed on understanding the utility of tube feeding for persons with intellectual disability, where it fits within the continuum of palliative care, and how best to present and discuss these issues with persons with intellectual disability and dementia, their family members and staff carers.

Within the generic care literature there is little evidence to support the use of tube feeding in persons with advanced dementia (Mitchell et al., 1998; Finucane et al., 1999, Volicer, 2005). Perceived benefits of tube feeding in persons with advanced dementia such as preventing malnutrition and reducing risk of pressure sores, preventing pneumonia, promoting comfort and improving functional status have not been upheld in the reported research (see Finucane & Bynum, 1996; Finucane et al., 1999; Volicer, 2005). However, there is a history of successful use of tube feeding among children and adults with intellectual disability that confounds the discussion of its implementation in end stage disease meaning that it is important that there be education around its implication at end of life (McCarron & McCallion, 2007).

Similarly, the assessment of pain in persons with cognitive impairment or intellectual disability has also always been identified as problematic (Regnard et al., 2003; 2006). Assessing pain in patients with Alzheimer's dementia appears to be even more complex again (Regnard et al., 2006). Specialist palliative care services must also recognize that the assessment instruments used for the general population for both pain and nutrition needs are rarely helpful for people with intellectual disability (McCallion & McCarron, 2004; McCarron & McCallion, 2007). Staff in intellectual disability services therefore would benefit from additional guidance from generic palliative care services on such issues as pain management.

3.5.6 Knowledge and skills of facilitating grief and loss

Loss is broadly divided into the two categories of physical loss and psycho-social loss. When someone experiences the death of any loved one, there will be the potential for the loss to manifest in grief (Rando, 1993), the process of experiencing the psychological, behavioral, and social reactions to the experience of the loss. Mourning is then the cultural and/or public display of grief, often described in terms of uncomplicated grief versus complicated or unresolved grief.

Grief issues are often reported to be different in dementia compared to other terminal conditions (Sachs et al., 2004). Despite the findings of Moss and Moss (2002:202) that staff in hospitals and nursing homes are "not kin" and have "no lifelong ties with the resident" others argue that staff form relationships with the person with dementia and have their own grief issues (Whittaker et al., 2007). A services framework that emphasizes physical and medical care and sees psycho-social needs in relation to death as secondary (Moss & Moss 2002) fosters staff ideologies such as 'professional distance' that are linked to "disenfranchised" grief. In intellectual disability services many staff have lifelong ties with the person with dementia.

Staff caring for persons with an intellectual disability have also been found to be heavily involved in the rituals around the death of a person in their care (Dodd et al., 2005). Yet palliative care staff and some intellectual disability services administrators may still respond to staff in intellectual disability services as if the Moss and Moss 'distance" model applies, making this group particularly prone to disenfranchised grief.

Disenfranchised grief as a concept was first put forward by Doka (1989:4) as "the grief that persons experience when they incur a loss that is not or cannot be openly acknowledged, publicly mourned or socially supported". This concept validates grief which had not previously been acknowledged (Corr, 2002). Health care professionals "rarely grieve the death of patients", and "usually do not participate in funerals or mourning rituals for deceased patients" according to Lamers (2002:183). "Disenfranchised grief occurs when staff members perceive that their loss is not legitimized and that their relationship with the deceased does not entitle them to feel or express grief" (Moss & Moss, 2002:205).

Care-giving staff may also experience vicarious grief (Kastenbaum, 1989) where they identify with a surviving resident who was a long-term friend or room-mate. In intellectual disability services such grief challenges staff in their supporting of surviving peers. Many staff in intellectual disability services want the people they care for to die in their own home and actively attempt to keep other services at a distance in the belief that they are more knowledgeable and sympathetic to this group (Todd, 2004).

Staff are often unprepared educationally to care for the dying and they struggle to give end-of-life care to the best of their abilities, providing lots of love and personal care (Todd, 2004). Institutional policies and procedures compound disenfranchised grief of staff when they do not support an overt grieving process (Lamers, 2002).

There is also disenfranchised grief for the other persons with intellectual disability in the home and for the family. There is both a long-standing belief that persons with intellectual disability do not experience the range of emotions of others including feelings of grief at the loss of family members and close friends/neighbors and, conversely, that they will not be able to "manage" the associated feelings (Yanok & Beifus, 1993). These beliefs and concerns are often used by family members to justify not informing persons with an intellectual disability of the death of parents and for not involving them in funerals and other death and mourning rituals.

It is not just a "family" problem. Todd (2002) points out that staff too have difficulties with the issue of death; family desires to "protect" the person become a convenient explanation for a lack of advocacy for death experiences and education for persons with intellectual disability. Yet persons with intellectual disability, as they age, are likely to experience losses through death often with major implications such as with the death of a parent that may mean they will have to move to a sibling's home or to an out-of-home placement (McHale & Carey, 2002). Not having experienced death and mourning also means that many persons with intellectual disability will poorly understand death and not be prepared for their own deaths (Clegg & Lansdall-Welfare, 2003).

While death and bereavement in this population remains a poorly researched area (Todd, 2004), there is evidence that persons with intellectual disability do indeed understand the finality of death and have often formed bonds with family members and others and feel personal loss and grief. However, being shielded from funerals, even the announcement of death may mean that people with intellectual disability do not know how to or have the opportunity to express their grief (Yanok & Beifus, 1993).

Grief does surface. Symptoms of normal grief as defined by ICD-10 occur within one month of the bereavement and do not exceed 6 months duration. For persons with intellectual disability, later onset and longer duration of grief symptoms are more likely. Also, as well as with increased levels of depression, anxiety and distress, grief reactions in persons with intellectual disability are often manifested in behavioral difficulties. These behaviors are more likely to be viewed by family members and professionals as psychosocial concerns rather than as the expression of grief (Hollins & Esterhuyzen, 1997; McHale & Carey, 2002). Reflecting these findings, Dodd et al., (2005) identified a need for staff training to support the grieving process for people with intellectual disability.

4. Best practices

A recent study of collaboration and training needs among intellectual disability services and a specialist palliative care provider (Fahey-McCarthy et al, 2010) highlighted a number of critical steps in successful delivery of palliative care for people with intellectual disability:

- Raising awareness among staff in both systems of the philosophies underpinning care and the expertise inherent in both intellectual disability and specialist palliative care services.
- Recognizing staff in intellectual disability services as highly dedicated and committed to providing optimal care but sometimes lacking knowledge and specific skills, particularly in managing symptoms such as pain, constipation, dyspnoea and fevers and the skills needed in the siting sub-cutaneous lines, managing nutrition and hydration, and assessing pain/distress.
- Recognizing that staff in specialist palliative care offer skills around symptom management and an external source of support that may be vital to navigating final days.
- Equipping specialist palliative care staff to address their communication difficulties with persons with ID, and need for understanding of dementia, care needs of people with ID, current services structures in ID and where specialist palliative care fits and bests addresses the gaps in current service provision.
- Given that many staff working in community group homes in intellectual disability services do not have nursing expertise/training, recognizing a need to re-evaluate the skill mix among staff in some of these care settings as more persons present with advanced dementia.

Tuffrey-Wijne (2002) and Todd (2004) have highlighted that when staff working in intellectual disability care are equipped to report important changes to palliative care staff, this has proven critical to good symptom management in terminal care.

A lack of understanding, experience, and skills in the management of pain and distress is reported to frequently result in the person with an intellectual disability being transferred from their usual home/care setting to a generic care setting/hospital and "bad deaths" are also described when staff have been unable to keep the person comfortable or at home to die (Fahey-McCarthy et al., 2009). Such reports support practices of collaboration, cross training, multi-disciplinary teams empowered to promote collaboration and the development of an understanding of when and how to involve specialist palliative care input into end of life care. Such involvement of specialist palliative care appears particularly needed for symptom management, i.e., the control of pain and dyspnoea and in the management of nutrition and hydration (Fahey-McCarthy et al., 2009). Due respect by palliative care for the competency and services offered by the intellectual disability services system should not preclude the development of supportive and consultative relationships between the two service systems and indeed comfort, caring and support of persons with intellectual disability in the advanced stages of dementia requires it.

Additional education and palliative care intervention guidelines are also needed. As Tuffrey-Wijne et al (2007) point out, available curricula are not usually targeted at staff responsible for day to day care. This gap in training needs to be addressed and policy and service provision should also ensure that there is specialist palliative support available to assist staff to operationalize guidelines and approaches (Fahey-McCarthy et al., 2009). Operationalization should include coordinating care with multidisciplinary care teams, increasing collaboration, communication and building of bridges with acute care settings and community based physicians working in intellectual disabilities, dementia and palliative care settings, and working with intellectual disability services staff to develop the ability to care for dying persons on site (Fahey-McCarthy et al., 2009; Solomon & Jennings 1998).

Approaches that draw upon the perspectives of staff within intellectual disability services and specialist palliative care encourage and support greater understanding of the core philosophies, common strengths and contributions to care offered by each service system. Such approaches offer insights that will potentially encourage greater creativity in determining the roles and timing of palliative care for persons with intellectual disabilities and advanced dementia (McCarron et al., 2010).

4.1 Sources for best practice materials

Among the resources available, five deserve particular attention:

1. *Supporting Persons with Intellectual Disability and Advanced Dementia: Fusing the Horizons of Intellectual Disability, Dementia and Palliative Care: A training Curriculum.* The curriculum emerged from an effort to understand staff experiences in supporting persons with intellectual disability and advanced dementia. A cross section of intellectual disability service providers and a specialist palliative care provider in the Republic of Ireland were involved in the study. Their experiences were interpreted to gain an understanding of their education and training needs and this information was then the basis for an educational intervention which was designed, delivered and evaluated as a pilot effort with these services. A partnership approach which involved the Trinity College School of Nursing and Midwifery research team, intellectual disability service providers and a specialist palliative care service was crucial to success.
2. End of Life Care: A guide for supporting older person with intellectual disabilities and their families (Botsford & Force, 2004; McCallion, 2006).
   http://www.nysarc.org/files/3213/0995/7606/Advocacy_Monograph_No._3_2.22.11.pdf
   A collaborative report involving both intellectual disability and hospice/palliative professionals providing guidance for staff and families on the policy context and day to day management strategies when persons with intellectual disability approach the end of life. The guide is supported with a cd-rom supplement also available through NYSARC, Inc.
3. http://ddhospiceandpalliativecare.org/
   An online forum was developed in response to a series of training workshops organized across New York State to bring together Developmental Disabilities, Hospice and Palliative Care providers and advocates who have an interest in improving end-of-life and supportive care for persons with developmental disabilities, as well as their families and their staff caregivers
   Goal: to improve end-of-life care for persons with developmental disabilities through greater utilization of hospice and palliative care services.
   The forum was developed to provide a safe and accessible platform that would encourage a learning dialog and features a professionally facilitated discussion board where registered members are able to post questions and concerns and then receive answers from experts and/or their peers. Forum members also receive monthly E-Newsletters that provide up to date news, policy information, advocacy opportunities, education resources, practical materials and a current events calendar centering on Hospice, Palliative care and Developmental Disabilities.
4. *Let's Talk about Death.* A booklet about death and funerals for people who have an intellectual disability available from Down syndrome Scotland. This booklet may be

used both to prepare individuals with an intellectual disability to participate in decisions about their end of life care and to support peers of individuals who are dying. http://www.dsscotland.org.uk/resources/shop/talkaboutdeath

5. *The Palliative Care and End of Life Training Project* (Hahn et al., 2011). A handbook, specialized curriculum and short, intensive "Train-the-Trainer" training program for staff to address the unique palliative and end of life care needs of individuals with developmental disabilities who live in developmental centers. When training is developed in partnership with the staff who will use these training resources, it has the potential to sustain its use and to alter the care practices to address the palliative care needs of persons with intellectual disabilities. Joan.Hahn@unh.edu

5. Conclusion

Both United Nations and European documents on the rights of people with disabilities (Council of Europe, 2006; United Nations, 2006) emphasize that health and social care should be most influenced by the needs of the individual with a disability and call for equal enjoyment of rights and freedoms and respect for the inherent dignity of people with disabilities. Such a view is consistent with person-centered planning philosophies and World Health Organization (http://www.who.int/cancer/palliative/definition/en/) encouragement for "impeccable" assessment, prevention and relief of physical, psychosocial and spiritual suffering. There is much within the intellectual disability services system that will support such approaches for people with intellectual disability. However, Alzheimer's disease and other dementias are fundamentally challenging this service system and there is a need for assistance, particularly with complex symptom management, assistance available through palliative care. Palliative care services are also being challenged; they have not traditionally served people with an intellectual disability, are not skilled in some of the unique communication and assessment challenges and also may not have extensive experience in dementia care. As noted in the best practice resource section, there are models for collaborative and supportive practice among intellectual disability and palliative care service providers but more work and related research is clearly needed if people with intellectual disability are to experience the same choice and comfort at end of life that is hoped for by everyone in society.

6. References

Abery, B. and McBride, M. (1998). Look - and understand – before you leap. Feature issue on person-centered planning with youth and adults who have developmental disabilities. *Impact 11* (2): 2-3, 26.

Abu-Saad, H. (2001) *Evidence Based Palliative Care across the Lifespan*, Blackwell Publishing, 9780632058181, Oxford.

Adams, N & Grieder, D.M. (2005). *Treatment Planning for Person-centered Care: The Road to Mental Health and Addiction Recovery*, Elsevier Academic Press, 0120441551, San Diego, CA.

Biernacki, C. & Barratt, J. (2001). Improving the Nutritional Status of People with Dementia. *Journal of Nursing 10*, 1104–1114.

Bigby, C. (2002). Ageing people with a lifelong disability: Challenges for the aged care and disability sectors. *Journal of Intellectual and Developmental Disability, 27*(4), 231–41.

Blackman, N. & Todd, S. (2005) *Caring for People with Learning Disabilities who are Dying.* Worth Publishing Ltd, 1903269172, London.

Botsford, A., & Force, L. (2004). *End of Life Care: A guide for supporting older person with intellectual disabilities and their families.* Albany, NY: NYSARC & NYSDDPC.

Candib, L.M. (2002). Truth telling and advance planning at the end of life: Problems with autonomy in a multicultural world. *Families, Systems and Health, 20*(3): 213-228.

Clegg, J. & Lansdall-Welfare, R. (2003). *Death, disability and Dogma. 10*(1), 67-79.

Cooper, S.A. (1997) High prevalence of dementia among people with learning disabilities not attributable to Down's syndrome. *Psychological Medicine. 27*, 609-616.

Cooper S.A., Melville C., Morrison J. (2004). People with intellectual disabilities. Their health needs differ and need to be recognized and met. *British Medical Journal , 329*, 414-415.

Corr, A. (2002). Revisiting the Concept of Disenfranchised Grief. In K. Doka, (Ed.)., *Disenfranchised Grief: New Directions, Challenges and Strategies for Practice.* Research Press, 9780878224272, Illinois.

Council of Europe Council (2006). *Council of Europe Disability Action Plan 2006-2015. A plan about how to make things better for people with disabilities in Europe;* retrieved from http://www.coe.int/t/e/social_cohesion/soc-sp/Action%20Plan%20CoE%20 - %20Easy%20to%20Read%20%2013.11.08%20_EN_.pdf on 12 August 2011.

Department of Ageing, Disability and Homecare (DADHC) (2004). *Palliative care in people with congenital or acquired intellectual disability and high nursing support needs Report to the Department of Ageing, Disability and Home Care.* University of Sydney: Centre for Developmental Disabilities studies.

Dodd, P. et al (2005). Attitudes to bereavement and intellectual disabilities in an Irish context. *Journal of Applied Research in Intellectual Disabilities, 18*, 237-243.

Doka, K.J. (1989). *Disenfranchised Grief: Recognising Hidden Sorrow.* Lexington, 066917081X, Lexington, MA.

Downs, M., Small, N. and Froggatt, K. (2006). "Explanatory models of dementia: links to end-of-life care." *International Journal of Palliative Nursing, 12* (5): 209-213.

Duffy, S. (2003). *Keys to Citizenship: A Guide to Getting Good Support Services for People with Learning Difficulties.* Paradigm, 0954306821, Birkenhead, UK

Fahey-McCarthy, E., McCallion, P., Connaire, K., McCarron, M. (2008). *Supporting Persons with Intellectual Disability and Advanced Dementia: Fusing the Horizons of Care. An Introductory Education and Training programme.* Trainer's Manual. Dublin: Trinity College Dublin.

Finucane, T. E., Christmas, C., and Travis, K. (1999).Tube feeding in patients with advanced dementia: A review of the evidence. *Journal of the American Medical Association, 282*, 1365–1370.

Fletcher R., Loschen E., Stavrakaki C. and First M. (2007). *Diagnostic Manual – Intellectual Disability.* NADD and APA, 1572561017, Kingston, New York.

Haveman M., Perry J., Salvadoe-Carulla L., Noonan Walsh P., Kerr M., Van Schorojenstein lantman-DeValk H., Van Hove G., Berger DM., Azema B., Buono S., Cara AC., Germanavicius A., Linehan C. Maatta T., Tossebro J. & Weber G. (2011). Ageing and health status in adults with intellectual disabilities: Results of the European POMONA II study. *Journal of Intellectual and Developmental Disability, 36*(1) 49–60.

Haveman M., Heller, T., Lee L., Maaskant, M., Shooshtari S. and Strydom A. (2010). Major health risks in aging persons with intellectual disabilities: An overview of recent studies. *Journal of Policy and Practice in Intellectual Disabilities, 7*(1), 59-69.

Haveman M., Heller T., Maaskant M., Lee L., Shooshtari S. and Strydom A. (2009). Health risks in older adults with intellectual disabilities: A review of studies (IASSID report). Retrieved from http://www.IASSID.org on 1 August 2011.

Iacono T. & Sutherland G. (2006). Health screening and developmental disability. *Journal of Policy and Practice in Intellectual Disability, 3*(3), 155-163.

Janicki, M.P., & Dalton, A.J. (2000). Prevalence of dementia and impact on intellectual disability services. *Mental Retardation, 38*, 276-288.

Janicki MP., Dalton AJ., Henderson CM., and Davidson PW. (1999). Mortality and morbidity among older adults with intellectual disability: Health services considerations. *Disability Rehabilitation, 21*(5-6), 284-294.

Janicki MP., Henderson CM., Davidson PW., McCallion P., Taets JD., Force L.T., Sulkes SB., Frangenberg E., and Ladrigan PM. (2002). Health characteristics and health services utilization in older adults with intellectual disability living in community residences. *Journal of Intellectual Disability Research, 46*(4), 287-298.

Janicki, M.P., McCallion, P. and Dalton, A.J. (2002). Dementia related care decision making in group homes for persons with intellectual disabilities. *Journal of Gerontological Social Work , 38*(1/2): 179-195.

Kastenbaum, R. (1989). Vicarious Grief. In R. Kastenbaum, & B. Kastenbaum (Eds.). *The Encyclopaedia of Death.* The Oryx Press, 0205610536, Phoenix, AZ.

Kitwood, T. (1997). *Dementia Reconsidered: The Person Comes First.* Open University Press, 0335198554, Buckingham, UK

Klass, D., Silverman, P. and Nickman, S. (1996). *Continuing Bonds, New Understandings of Grief.* Taylor and Francis, 1560323361, Washington, DC.

Lamers, W.M. (2002). Disenfranchised Grief in Caregvers. In K. Doka (Ed.). *Disenfranchised Grief: New Directions, Challenges and Strategies for Practice.* Research Press, 9780878224272, Illinois.

Lindop, E. & Read, S. (2000). District nurses' needs: Palliative care for people with learning disabilities. *International Journal of Palliative Nursing, 6*(3), 117- 122.

Lloyd-Williams, M. & Payne, S. (2002). Can multi-disciplinary guidelines improve the palliation of symptoms in the terminal phase of dementia? *International Journal of Palliative Nursing, 8*(8), 370-375.

Luddington, L., et al (2001). The need for palliative care for patients with non-cancer diseases: a review of the evidence. *International Journal of Palliative Nursing, 7* (5), 221-226.

Lynn, J., & Adamson, D. (2003) *Living well at the end of life.* Rand Health http://www.rand.org/publications/WP/WP137/index.html (accessed 09th December 2005)

McCallion, P. (2006). *End of Life Care: Supporting older people with intellectual disabilities and their families.* A cd-rom curriculum supplement. Albany, NY: NYSARC & NYSDDPC

McCallion, P., Nickle, T., & McCarron, M. (2005). A Comparison of reports of caregiver burden between foster family care providers and staff caregivers in other settings. *Dementia, The International Journal of Social Research and Practice,* 4(3), 401-412.

McCallion P., & McCarron M. (2004) Aging and intellectual disabilities: A review of recent literature. *Current Opinion in Psychiatry ,17*(5), 349-352.

McCarron M., & McCallion P. (2007) *An Intellectual Disability Supplement to the Irish Longitudinal Study of Ageing: A proposal submitted to the Health Research Board*. Trinity College Dublin: Dublin.

McCarron, M. & Lawlor, B. (2003) Responding to the challenges of ageing and dementia in intellectual disability in Ireland. *Aging and Mental Health* 7(6), 413-417.

McCarron, M., McCallion, P. & Begley, C. (2005). Health co-morbidities in ageing persons with Down syndrome and Alzheimer's. *Dementia Journal of Intellectual Disability Research, 49*(7), 560-566.

McCarron, M., & McCallion, P. (2007). End-of-life care challenges for persons with intellectual disability and dementia: Making decisions about tube feeding. *Intellectual and Developmental Disabilities, 45*(2), 128-131.

McCarron, M., Swinburne, J., Burke, E., McGlinchey, E., Mulryan, N., Andrews, V., Foran S. and McCallion, P. (2011) *Growing Older with an Intellectual Disability in Ireland 2011: First Results from The Intellectual Disability Supplement of The Irish Longitudinal Study on Ageing*. Dublin: School of Nursing & Midwifery, Trinity College Dublin.

McConkey, R. (2004). The staffing of services for people with intellectual disabilities. P. Noonan-Walsh, & H. Gash (Eds.). *Lives and Times: Practice, Policy and people with disabilities*. Rathdown Press, 1903806755, Bray, Ireland.

Mitchell, S.L., et al (2003). Clinical and Organizational Factors Associated With Feeding Tube Use Among Nursing Home Residents With Advanced Cognitive Impairment. *JAMA:- Journal-of-the-American-Medical-Association, 290*(1), 73-80.

Moss, S.Z. & Moss, M.S. (2002). Nursing Home Staff Reactions to Resident Deaths. In K. Doka (Ed.). *Disenfranchised Grief: New Directions, Challenges and Strategies for Practice*. Research Press, 9780878224272, Illinois

Ng, J. and Li, S. (2003). A survey exploring the educational needs of care practitioners in learning disability settings in relation to death, dying and people with learning disabilities. *European Journal of Cancer Care, 12*, 12-19.

Nolan, M., Keady, J., & Aveyard, B (2001). Relationship-centred is the next logical step. *British Journal of Nursing ,10*(12), 757.

Nolan, M., Davies, S. & Brown, J (2006). Transitions in care homes: towards relationship-centred care using the 'Senses Framework'. *Quality in Ageing – Policy, Practice and Research, 7*(3), 5-14.

Norberg, A., et al (1994). Ethical reasoning concerning the feeding of severely demented patients: An international perspective. *Nursing Ethics, 1*(1), 3–13.

Prasher, V.P. & Krishnan, V.H.R. (1993). Age of onset and duration of dementia in people with Down's syndrome. *International Journal of Geriatric Psychiatry, 8*, 915-922.

Prasher, V.P. (1995). End stage dementia in adults with Down Syndrome. *International Journal of Geriatric Psychiatry, 10*, 1067-1069.

Rando, T.A.(1993). *Treatment of Complicated Mourning*. Research Press, 0878223290, Illinois.

Regnard, C. et al (2003). Difficulties in identifying distress and its causes in people with severe communication problems. *International Journal of Palliative Nursing, 9*(3), 173-176.

Regnard, C. et al (2006). Understanding Distress in people with severe communication difficulties: developing and assessing the Disability Distress Assessment Tool (DISDAT). *Journal of Intellectual Disability Research, 51*(4), 277-292.

Ryan, K., & McQuillan, R. (2005). Palliative care for disadvantaged groups: People with intellectual disabilities. *Progress in Palliative Care, 13*(2), 70-74.

Sachs, G.A., Shega, J.W., & Cox-Haley, D. (2004). Barriers to excellent end-of-life care for patients with dementia. *Journal of General Internal Medicine, 19*, 1057-1063.

Ryan, K. & McQuillan, R. (2005). Palliative care for disadvantaged groups: People with intellectual disabilities. *Progress in Palliative Care, 13*(2), 70-74.

Sachs, G.A., Shega, J.W., & Cox-Haley, D. (2004). Barriers to excellent end-of-life care for patients with dementia. *Journal of General Internal Medicine, 19*, 1057-1063.

Todd, S. (2004). Death counts: the challenge of death and dying in learning disability services. *Learning Disability Practice, 7*(10), 12-15.

Todd, S. (2007). Silenced grief: living with the death of a child with intellectual disabilities. *Journal of Intellectual Disability Research, 51*(8), 637-648.

Tuffrey-Wijne, I. (1997). Palliative care and learning disabilities. *Nursing Times, 93*(31), 50-51.

Tuffrey-Wijne, I. (1998). Care of the terminally ill. *Learning Disability Practice, 1* (1): 8-11.

Tuffrey-Wijne, I. (2002). The palliative care needs of people with intellectual disabilities: A case study. *International Journal of Palliative Nursing, 8*(5), 222-231.

Tuffrey-Wijne I., Hogg J. S. & Curfs L. (2007). End-of-life and palliative care for people with intellectual disabilities who have cancer or other life-limiting illness: a review of the literature and available resources. *Journal of Applied Research in Intellectual Disabilities, 20*, 331–344.

Watson, J. Hockley, J and Dewar, B (2006). Barriers to implementing an integrated care pathway for the last days of life in nursing homes. *International Journal of Palliative Nursing, 12*(5), 234-240.

Whittaker, E. et al (2007). Palliative care in nursing homes; exploring care assistant's knowledge. *International Journal of Older People Nursing, 2*, 36-44.

Wilkinson, H. and Janicki, M.P. (2005). Dementia - where crosscutting issues and technologies can become universal - sharing ideas from the intellectual disability field. *Dementia: the International Journal of Social Research and Practice*, 4(3): 323-325.

UN (2006) *United Nations Convention on the Rights of Persons with Disabilities.* UN Headquarters, New York.

vanSchrojenstein Lantman-De Valk HM., Metsemakers JF., Haveman MJ. and Crebolder HF. (2000) Health problems in people with intellectual disability in general practice: A comparative study. *Family Practice* 17(5), 405-407.

Yanok, J. & Beifus, J.A. (1993). Communicating about loss and mourning: Death education for individuals with mental retardation. *Mental Retardation, 31*(3), 144-147.

17

Palliative Care for the Elderly: A Japanese Perspective

Yoshihisa Hirakawa
Nagoya University Hospital, Japan

1. Introduction

Japan currently has the fast growing aging society among industrialized countries. In 1970, the Japanese population aged 65 years or older accounted for 7% and by 1990, this rate had climbed to 12%. However, by 2006, 20.8% of the Japanese population was aged 65 or older - the highest rate in the world **(National Institute of Population and Social Security Research, 2011)**. This trend is expected to continue for the next few decades and dealing with the country's aging population has become a serious concern for Japan.

Furthermore, in recent years, the number of elderly deaths has climbed very rapidly in Japan. The number of overall Japanese deaths is expected to continue rising from 1.1 million in 2007 to 1.7 million in 2040, a surge associated with the steady growth in elderly deaths **(Figure 1)(National Institute of Population and Social Security Research, 2011)**.

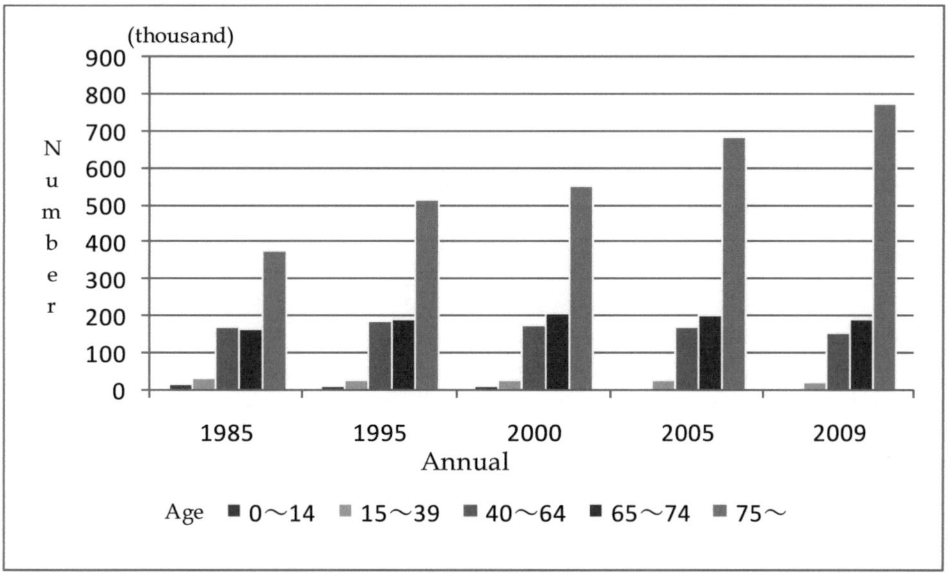

Fig. 1. Annual changes of mortality rates in the number of deaths by age class (**National Institute of Population and Social Security Research, Available from** http://www.ipss.go.jp/syoushika/tohkei/Popular/Popular2011.asp?chap=0

This sudden escalation in the number of elderly and elderly deaths is contributing to an explosion of need for long-term and palliative care. In other industrialized countries, where a more gradual shift to an aging society has occurred, innovative elderly care services are being explored and reforms are ongoing. Even after 1990, nursing home and home care were not widely available in Japan (although the government implemented the "Gold Plan" to expand long-term care services including institutional care in 1989, and the "New Gold Plan" in 1994 to further enhance the service infrastructure) **(Masuda, 2000)**. However, the elderly who required long-term care (LTC) often needed to stay in hospitals for months or even years, partly owing to the lack of long-term institutional or home care service. This situation has contributed to an increase in hospital deaths to the point where most Japanese elderly now die at the hospital. The proportion of elderly who die at long-term care facilities in Japan is still very low (1.7% in 1995, and 4.3% in 2009) **(Figure 2)**, and the use of hospitals to care for elderly patients until their death and the lack of LTC resources constitute urgent social problems for the country.

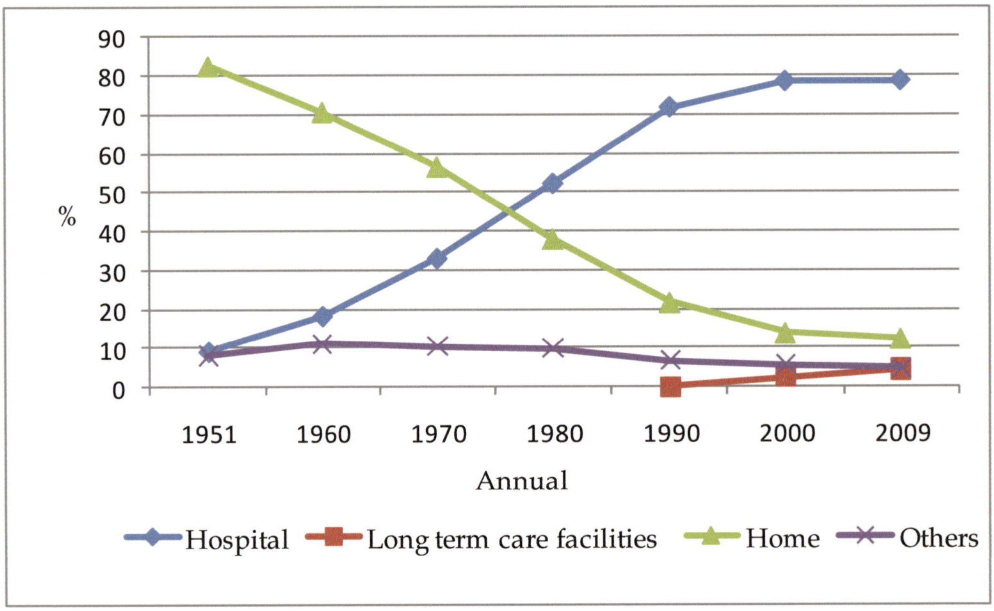

Fig. 2. Annual changes of the proportions seen in the number of deaths by place of death (**Ministry of Health, Labour and Welfare, Available from** http://www.mhlw.go.jp/toukei/saikin/hw/jinkou/suii03/deth5.html)

Given these circumstances, Japan has introduced a number of care systems modeled after schemes employed in Western countries. For example, following Germany and Holland's introduction of public long-term care insurance (LTCI) systems, Japan followed suit and launched its LTCI system to improve the quality of long-term and palliative care **(Tsutsui & Muramatsu, 2007)**. This system was part of a social security policy reform designed to address a prolonged economic slump and soaring medical and LTC expenditures for older people. Also, a key aspect of Japan's LTCI system, the Care Management System, was based on the experience of the United Kingdom **(Jacobs & Challis, 2007)**.

However, there are notable cultural differences between Japan and these countries **(Japan Geriatric Society, 2001; Shimizu, 2009)**. For example, in Japan, family members or physicians play a more critical role in making decisions when the patient lacks decision-making capacity. Also, the Japanese have developed a unique concept of life and death, represented by the patients' submissive attitudes to medical professionals or the acceptance of their own circumstances as fate. In addition, the Japanese hesitate to complain of pain because patience is a virtue in Japanese culture and Japanese elderly patients do not want to bother their physician. These values may differ from those in Western cultures, where patient autonomy is highly appreciated.

The purpose of this review is to offer a comprehensive view of the current palliative care situation for the elderly in Japan, including care system, education, symptom management, and ethical issues. The review also briefly examines the Position Statement of the Japan Geriatric Society Ethics Committee on the Terminal Care of the Elderly **(Japan Geriatric Society, 2001)**.

2. Medical and long-term care systems affecting palliative care for the elderly

In Japan, enrollment in the National Health Insurance Plan is compulsory for all residents, including the elderly. Japan's Health Insurance System allows people to choose their doctor or hospital freely, as long as they pay the fixed medical charges.

Moreover, for residents ≥ 40 years of age, enrollment in the Long-term Care Insurance Plan is mandatory; individuals aged ≥ 65 years who require long-term care can reap the benefits of this plan, as can individuals aged 40-65 years who require long-term care for diseases related to aging. The dramatic rise in the aging population in Japan has created serious economic problems as the social cost of medical care for the elderly has soared. More Japanese adults are surviving into old age, and older adults are facing physical or mental health problems that require LTC. To handle the anticipated explosion of need for long-term care for the elderly, Japan introduced the Public Long-term Care Insurance (LTCI) system in 2000 **(Matsuda & Yamamoto, 2001; Tsutsui & Muramatsu, 2007)**. This system provides professionals with official recognition as Care Managers whose primary responsibility is to oversee the co-ordination of care services and draw up care plans for elderly people. Licensed professionals such as nurses, physicians, social workers, and physical therapists, can be certified as 'Care managers' after undergoing a special training. Under this system, anyone aged 65 or older can benefit from institutional or community-based care services on the basis of need for long-term care and under the care service coordination of care managers.

3. Position statement from the Japan Geriatrics Society

In 2001, the Japan Geriatric Society released its Position Statement regarding palliative care for the elderly **(Japan Geriatric Society, 2001) (Table 1)**. The position statement was drafted in September of 2000 and reviewed and edited by the Ethics Committee, which was established in 1998 **(Uemura, 2000)**. The need for this position statement was founded on a questionnaire survey to the Japan Geriatric Society Council **(Iguchi, 2001; Iijima, 2009)**. A total of 95.5% of the respondents answered that a position statement was needed, and several members of the Japan Geriatric Society agreed with this stance.

Position statement from the Japan Geriatrics Society,13 June 2001
Position 1 : Elderly patients should not be deprived of opportunities to receive relevant care because of their limited independence or other age-related disabilities.
Position 2 : Care of dying patients should be carried out with full respect for each value, thought and faith.
Position 3 : Care of dying patients should be directed toward the maintenance or improvement of quality of life
Position 4 : The care of a dying patient includes support for the patient's family.
Position 5 : Terminal care of dying patients is multidisciplinary care that encompasses a broad realm of disciplines that involve medicine, nursing and socio-psychology.
Position 6 : Medical practice implemented in terminal care should warrant its profit to the patient.
Position 7 : In consideration of the patient's dignity and to show respect for the patient's autonomy,individual cultural background should be taken into account.
Position 8 : Medical professionals should receive special education in order to secure patients' right to receive optimal treatment and care.
Position 9 : Broad understanding about how the terminal care of dying patients can improve the quality of life of the patients should be promoted nationwide. Terminal care and death education should be made available to the general public in Japan.
Position 10 : Health care reform is necessary to improve the terminal care of dying patients.
Position 11 : Research on the optimal care of dying patients should be promoted by providing sufficient sources of funding.
Position 12 : It is strongly advised that each institution establish its ethical committee with a third party in attendance and discuss the propriety of its medical practices and care for dying patients. To achieve wide consensus, the general public should be allowed free access to the discussion through the disclosure of information.
Position 13 : This position statement is transitional, and its appropriateness should be examined in light of further experience and investigations using scientific methods.

Table 1. Position statement from the Japan Geriatrics Society

The intent of the position statement was to provide the elderly and their families the support they needed to benefit from optimal care in the last stage of their lives, in full respect of their values, philosophy and faith. The questionnaire survey revealed a strong opposition to ageism: "Elderly patients should not be deprived of opportunities to receive proper care because of their limited independence or other age-related disabilities" (Position 1), and "Care of dying patients should be carried out in full respect for their values, philosophy and faith" (Position 2). The statement also emphasizes the pressing need for the creation of ethical committees and for professional education.

However, the results of the questionnaire survey also suggested a need for guidelines concerning a number of ethical issues including artificial nutrition and decision-making **(Iijima, 2009)**. Some members of the society criticized the statement for being too abstract regarding the provision o palliative care. To improve the position statement, additional investigation, practice and education are needed.

4. Technical terms and definitions of palliative care for the elderly

In Japan, care for end-stage patients is generally called terminal care, hospice care, end-of-life care, or "palliative care". The terms "End-of-life care", "Hospice Care", and "Terminal Care" are considered synonyms for palliative care among Japanese professionals **(Higuchi, 2010)**. According to empirically obtained information, Japanese medical professionals generally use the term "terminal care" to refer to care for patients who face imminent death, and "palliative care" to describe care for end-stage patients **(Hirakawa, 2011)**. Incidentally, in the position statement from the Japan Geriatrics Society **(Japan Geriatric Society, 2001)**, dated 13 June 2001, the society uses "terminal care" as a synonym for palliative care.

In this position statement, "Final Stage Patients" refer to people who are considered to be at the terminal stage of life when their illness is progressive and irreversible, when no available treatment can improve their condition or halt its deterioration, and death is considered to be unavoidable in the near future. In defining 'terminal stage', the length of time until death is not considered due to a lack of clinical evidence for accurately predicting when the patient will die. The reason of this may include difficulty of prognostic prediction on a terminal care stage. As Lunney JR et al. **(2003)** show, dying process of elderly people has 4 different trajectories or its combinations as follows; each of which suggests that prognostic prediction is so difficult that dying process is unpredictable. First pattern is sudden death, which refers to a case where those who seem to be in a good shape leading a normal life die suddenly. Heart disease is among the most common cause and cerebrovascular disease follows. As older people get and more care people need, a much higher risk they would face to. Second pattern is a terminal illness such as cancer. This pattern is related to a functional decline which results in death after progressive debilitation with a variety of pain. In this case, it might be possible to make predictions of a clinical course and a prognosis to some extent from observing appearance of time and frequency of physical symptoms such as general malaise, pain, anorexia and wheezing or from monitoring degree of decline in limited independence. Third pattern is a case of organ failure. The clinic course of this organ failure such as chronic heart failure, chronic liver failure, liver failure and respiratory insufficiency is characterized by repetitive and combinational progressive decline of physical function and acute exacerbation. When an individual suffers from organ failure, metabolic function works with functional decline in organs. And more limited metabolic function could lead to acute exacerbation. Even if acute treatment works effective, the function doesn't recover completely in most cases. After repeating these processes, function becomes uncompensated and death will follow in the end. Fourth pattern is frailty observed in apoplexy, dementia and being bedridden. Those who suffer from this trajectory have a prolong course with pneumonia and result in death. Therefore, the question of when to start terminal care for the elderly is a very controversial question in Japan.

The World Health Organization has suggested, in its definition, that "palliative care is an approach that improves the quality of life of patients and their families facing the problems associated with life-threatening illness, through the prevention and relief of suffering by means of early identification and impeccable assessment and treatment of pain and other problems, physical, psychosocial and spiritual"**(Sepúlveda et al., 2002)**. Applying the definition to palliative care for the elderly, we can interpret that it is applicable early in the course of their increasing long-term care need, in conjunction with other usual therapies that are intended to prolong life and manage distressing clinical complications. In Japan, where access to a hospice program is at present only available to patients with cancer or AIDS, but not to other dying elderly patients, the concept that long-term care and palliative care are inseparable in elderly care settings is spreading through the literature and educational programs.

5. Educational issues

5.1 Medical profession

In its Position Statement, the Japan Geriatric Society suggests that education is one of the most important aspects concerning palliative care for the elderly, and that "the majority of health care professionals receive insufficient specialized training in the care of terminally-ill patients. Concrete and practical instruction in the care of dying patients, including the management of symptoms and communication skills, should be given"**(Japan Geriatric Society, 2001)**.

We performed a number of studies concerning palliative care education. In 2005, we conducted a national survey on the status of programs to teach end-of-life care to undergraduates of medical and nursing schools in Japan **(Hirakawa et al., 2005b)**. Most of the medical and nursing schools offered palliative care education programs, but the mean number of teaching hours was too low (7.6 hours in medical schools vs. 35.5 hours in nursing schools) to allow for the acquisition of proper experience with palliative care in medical schools. Because palliative care education programs include palliative care for cancer patients in general, we can say that the lack of education on palliative care for the elderly is actually a more serious problem than we had anticipated from our results.

Although information technology advances have enabled medical students and professionals to access a wider array of medical information, medical textbooks still play an important role in medical education. Quality textbooks contribute to higher standards in medical education. A number of studies on end-of-life content in foreign medical textbooks have revealed that coverage was indeed lacking in Japan **(Carron et al., 1999; Rabow et al., 2000)**. A preliminary study on this issue reveals that most top-selling Japanese end-of-life care or geriatric textbooks lack proper coverage on end-of-life care, and efforts need to be made to improve this **(Hirakawa et al., 2008a)**.

In 2009, we conducted an investigation concerning the syllabi of palliative care education or training course for undergraduates of medical and nursing schools in Japan to design a comprehensive undergraduate educational program model of palliative care for the elderly. We reviewed the syllabi in Japanese medical and nursing schools, and classified the content according to the items specified by the Japan Geriatric Society's position statement. Our findings, which were published elsewhere **(Hirakawa et al., 2009a)**, highlighted the need for education on quality of life of elderly who require palliative care and comprehensive geriatric assessment (CGA). Postgraduate clinical retraining on the palliative care of the elderly is important for long-term care facility physicians. Due to a lack of authorized and standardized palliative care or geriatric care education program for long-term care facility physicians in Japan, professionals in this field are not sufficiently educated on palliative care for the elderly. To get the information needed to develop a comprehensive palliative care education program for facility physicians, we conducted a questionnaire survey on educational needs concerning end-of-life care for the elderly at long-term care facilities in Nagoya City in 2008 **(Hirakawa et al., 2008b)**. Our results suggested that most directors wanted to receive additional training about their clients' decision-making process, communication skills, and legal issues related to palliative care.

In conclusion, medical care provider education on palliative care for the elderly is still lacking in Japan. There is a need to develop educational programs for medical professionals based on further research.

5.2 Care profession

Care staff education is one of the most important aspects of palliative care for the elderly. Also, as a result of new policies promoting home care as well as the recent changes in preferences of elderly patients and their families, greater numbers of frail elderly are now opting to spend their last years of life at home or at a long-term care facilities rather than a hospital. Therefore, staff involvement in delivering palliative care has increased **(Henderson et al., 2000)**. Improving the quality and quantity of palliative care provision at home or at long-term care facilities has become an urgent priority in Japan **(Hirakawa et al., 2009b)**.

The quality of palliative care at long-term care facilities, including group homes for demented elderly, greatly depends on the preparedness of care staff to deliver quality services. However, young care staff usually has little experience with death either on or off the job, and we therefore need to emphasize palliative care clinical training for care staff.

Palliative care educational programs or guides for care staff have been developed in several countries. In the United States, Henderson ML et al developed and published a palliative care training manual for long-term care staff **(Henderson et al., 2000)**. In Canada, the National Advisory Committee developed the "Guide to end-of-life care for seniors", which is a useful and informative document for care staff working at long-term care facilities and community care settings **(National Advisory Committee., 2000)**. Again in Canada, Kortes-Miller K et al developed a 15-hour interprofessional curriculum tailored to meet the needs of care staff **(Kortes-Miller K et al., 2007)**.

In Japan, a project to develop an educational program for long-term care staff delivering palliative care for the elderly was launched in 2011 under the scheme of a research project funded by the Ministry of Education, Culture, Sports, Science and Technology. However, as shown in the position statement of the Japan Geriatric Society, there has been insufficient support for research or education contributing to the improvement of palliative care for elderly **(Japan Geriatric Society., 2001)**.

In 2007, through a nationwide survey of chief nurses in geriatric health services facilities, we outlined the educational items which were frequently taught at long-term care facilities **(Hirakawa et al., 2007b)**. With these results a a guide, we also conducted action research concerning care staff education. Finally, we developed a 9-hour workshop program to educate care staff who provide palliative care, and reported the effects elsewhere **(Hirakawa et al., 2011b)**.

The attitudes of nurses and care workers toward death and caring for dying older adults are positively associated with the quality of palliative care at long-term care facilities. Matsui and Braun **(2010)** suggested, in their research, that better attitudes toward caring for the dying were positively associated with seminar attendance and negatively associated with fear of death. We introduced a number of tools we believe can be helpful in modeling positive attitudes toward death, such as group discussions on death and dying among care staff, reading picture books on the topic of dying, and others.

5.3 Community

Family education is an essential component of long-term care for Japanese elderly patients. Effective communication based on reliable and comprehensive health information between health professionals and elderly patients and their family is an important part of home elderly care **(Hirakawa et al., 2011a)**.

While television and newspapers have traditionally been common sources of health information for the general public, many people are now turning to the internet to gather information **(Hirakawa et al, 2011a)**. However, elderly patients vary widely in terms of health condition and daily living activities, and the issues surrounding their care are often complex. It is thus crucial that the elderly and their family caregivers not rely solely on general information through the mass media, but that they be provided with accurate, timely and tailored information about their condition and needs.

Family caregivers are often at a loss as to how to proceed to look after their loved ones. In 2009, we conducted a broad survey to find out about the kind of information family caregivers of home elderly patients seek and the way in which they generally obtain this information **(Hirakawa et al., 2011a)**. A total of 475 family caregivers of home elderly patients residing in Nagoya city took part in the survey. Our results indicated that the 3 items they perceived as of most concern were dementia (especially dementia care), first aid, and public long-term care insurance services. Also, nearly half of the caregivers were interested in food and nutrition. The respondents either received health information from their physician or from a care manager, despite the fact that care manager is not a medical profession. Our results suggested that care managers are an important source of health information in Japan, and that they should be trained on how to deliver appropriate and tailored information to family caregivers.

Comprehensive palliative care for the elderly places emphasis on elderly patients' values and preferences; it is therefore essential that health care providers discuss the prognosis or clinical course of advanced illness in detail with the elderly and their family. Therefore, palliative care education in community settings should include a unit on decision-making with an emphasis on advance directives. Matsui recently evaluated the effectiveness of an educational intervention in the form of a discussion on end-of-life directed at older Japanese adults and their attitude toward and acceptance of this intervention **(Matsui, 2010)**. The study revealed that, following the intervention, participants tended to view advance directives more favorably, while they began to view life-sustaining treatments by means of artificial nutrition more negatively.

It should be noted that there are some differences in attitudes toward palliative care education between Japan and other countries. The Institute for Health Economics and Policy of Japan conducted a study to assess the attitude of long-term care staff and residents' families toward a Canadian publication entitled: "Comfort Care at the End-of-Life for Persons with Alzheimer's Disease or Other Degenerative Disease of the Brain" **(Institute for Health Economics and Policy of Japan, 2010)**. The study showed that decision-making on palliative care is likely to be performed by discussing options among health care providers and families in Japan. The study also revealed a general dislike for guideline-based education by the Japanese people. It also stresses the fact that educating families concerning palliative care somehow tends to heighten their anxiety regarding the death of their loved ones or makes them uncomfortable as they view the approach as too aggressive.

6. Caregiver burden of family

Family caregivers play a critical role in caring for dying elderly relatives. At the request of family caregivers, health care providers should disclose available information on the elderly patient and provide support for the family in coping with the sorrow of losing an elderly patient. Because the quality of life of family caregivers has a direct influence on that of their elderly, providing the family the necessary support to cope will eventually help them better meet the needs of the patient. Within the framework of Japan's public long-term care insurance system, care managers play an important role in reducing the burden of family caregivers who care for elderly relatives at home.

Despite this support, Japanese family caregivers often suffer from stress caused by physical, psychological, social, and spiritual factors. Japanese elderly may also be reluctant to make decisions, and their family caregivers feel pressured into making decisions for their elderly relative **(Japan Geriatric Society, 2001)**.

The burden of caring for an elderly relative is especially heavy for female caregivers. According to a comprehensive survey of living conditions conducted by the Ministry of Health, Labor and Welfare, women represent about 70% of all caregivers in Japan **(Ministry of Health, Labor and Welfare, 2010)**. Many women caregivers find it extremely challenging to care for an elderly relative while also handling other responsibilities such as family, work and household duties, a feeling also shared by women rural areas of Canada **(Crosato & Leipert, 2006)**.

Due to women's increased life expectancy, a greater number of women now care for an elderly relative. In Japan, women live approximately 6 years longer than men, and are thus in a position to care for their spouse by default **(WHO, 2011)**.

In addition, Japanese women may feel that it is their duty to care for a spouse because Japanese cultural values place an expectation on women to provide care for an ill or ageing husband. Cultural values also influence the decision-making process regarding placement of an elder in a long-term care facility. Japanese female caregivers may also hold a negative view about placing their elderly relatives at long-term care facilities, even when such care is readily available. These beliefs and values place additional burdens on Japanese women, especially on those who cannot or do not wish to provide elder care. In rural Japan, there is a strong belief that women should assume the traditional caring role, and that being a caregiver is natural part of being a woman. Furthermore, the general belief is that caring for elderly parents is way for women to repay them for caring for them as children **(Okuyama, 2005)**.

7. Nutrition care

As Endevelt et al suggested, providing disabled elderly people with nutritional care has become important in community settings **(Endevelt et al., 2006)**. Elderly people who require care are likely to present with appetite loss, lower chewing ability, or protein energy malnutrition (PEM). PEM in elderly people is associated with loss of muscle tissue, impaired cognitive function, high risk of infection and increased morbidity and mortality. Thus, health care providers should offer their elderly clients tailor-made care services based on their detailed assessment of their nutritional and life conditions.

Dietitians working in the community are the main professionals responsible for counseling the elderly on nutritional issues. In Japan, under the medical and the long-term care insurance system, elderly patients and their family can benefit from home visits by dietitians **(Hirakawa et al., 2003)**. Typical visits include cooking lessons, advice on energy intake, sharing new recipes, and anthropometric examinations. They also include education on ways to cope with an inability to swallow and on artificial nutrition therapy.

8. Multidisciplinary care

As stated in the position statement of the Japan Geriatric Society, a multidisciplinary approach to the care of dying patients is preferable. Physicians are expected to develop a broad knowledge and experience in comprehensive care in order to function as key members of the team. In Japan, the public long-term care insurance system has promoted the use of multidisciplinary care conferences **(Hara, 2011)**. Unfortunately, few physicians ever attend these conferences because attendance is not compulsory.

The CGA is a multidimensional, interdisciplinary diagnostic process to determine the medical, psychological and functional capabilities of a frail elderly person that enables the development of a coordinated and integrated plan for treatment and long-term follow up **(Ellis et al., 2011)**. In Japan, CGA is a useful tool for health care providers who offer long-term and palliative care for elderly. The assessment tool is widely used in geriatric care settings including hospitals, long-term care facilities, and the community. Under the scheme of a comprehensive research project for longevity sciences funded by the Ministry of Health, Labor and Welfare, a research team developed a CGA-based tool for discharge support **(Hirakawa et al., 2010b)**.

9. Ethical issues

9.1 Tube feeding

Percutaneous endoscopic gastrostomy (PEG) tubes have become widely used among elderly patients. PEG tubes are now frequently used in elderly who have diseases or conditions that make it difficult to swallow or eat voluntarily. Though the procedure is fairly routine medically, there are many complex issues surrounding PEG use, particularly for elderly patients near the end of life. Clinical evidence supporting the use of PEG tube feedings in patients with advanced dementia is clearly lacking, yet PEG procedures continue to be performed in a large number of these cases. In Japan, artificial nutrition and hydration (ANH) for severely cognitively impaired elderly is considered standard care. Bito S and Asai A revealed, through an internet survey, that many physicians would initiate tube feeding for an 84-year-old bedridden man with dementia **(Bito & Asai, 2007)**. Aita et al **(2007)** identified five factors related to the decision to provide ANH through PEG to older Japanese adults with severe cognitive impairment: (1) the national health insurance system that allows elderly patients to become long-term hospital in-patients; (2) legal barriers with regard to limiting treatment, including the risk of prosecution; (3) emotional barriers, especially abhorrence of death by 'starvation'; (4) cultural values that promote family-oriented end-of-life decision making; and (5) reimbursement-related factors involved in the choice of PEG. There are also a few more factors including the caregiver burden of feeding orally, and the request for early discharge from hospital management.

In conclusion, the framework of Japan's medical-legal system unintentionally provides physicians with incentives to routinely offer ANH for this patient group through PEG tubes. End-of-life education should be imparted to medical providers in Japan to help change the automatic assumption that ANH must systematically be provided.

9.2 Decision making

Physicians and family members usually play a critical role in making decisions when the patient lacks decision-making capacity. Japan has developed a unique concept of life and death **(Japan Geriatric Society, 2001; Uemura, 2000)**, represented by patients' submissive attitude toward medical professionals and the acceptance of their own circumstances as fate (which probably originates from Buddhist philosophy). Moreover, for fear of losing hope, some elderly patients with severe conditions prefer not to be informed of the deteriorating state of their health. As a result, Japanese physicians and family members therefore need to make decisions on their behalf and are required to develop the ability and insight to judge the will of an elderly who is unable to express his or her own will explicitly. If the wishes of an elderly patient are unclear, both the physician and family are in a very difficult position.

Discussing palliative care options with the elderly and their family in advance may reduce the mental stress of making decisions for the physician and family. A growing number of Japanese people now chose to outline advance directives, especially living wills, although there is no legislation recognizing such legal documents **(Masuda et al., 2003)**. However, there are several problems associated with the use of advance directives in Japan. First, as stated in item 2 of the position statement, the will of the elderly patients may change, or the patients may be reluctant to make a decision. Hattori et al also stated in their paper that the will of elderly patients may easily change considering the feelings of others **(Hattori et al., 2005)**. Second, Japanese people traditionally dislike discussing death and related issues, which is perceived as taboo **(Okuno et al, 1999)**. The Japanese's hesitation to talk about death is exemplified in their avoidance of numbers 4 and 9 which are considered unlucky as they are pronounced the same as the words death and suffering. Also, the Japan Association of Geriatric Care Services Facilities **(2007)** as well as Tsuruwaka and Semba **(2010)** reported that discussing palliative care or life-sustaining treatment options on admission is psychologically difficult for care staff.

Third, the physician's explanations of advance directives have a strong influence on the decision-making of elderly patients and their families. We recently conducted a study to explore the factors affecting decision-making regarding cardiopulmonary resuscitate (CPR) and hospitalize orders at a long-term care hospital **(Hirakawa et al., 2007a)**. We observed a wide variation in the likelihood of opting for CPR and hospitalize orders in families who had been given information on advance directives. There is a need for standardized methods for eliciting the end-of-life preferences of residents and families upon their admission to long-term care facilities.

Fourth, although living wills and advance directives are gaining popularity, few people actually want to draw an official document. According to national data **(Ministry of Health, Labour and Welfare., 2004)**, less than half of the Japanese population wants to enact a living will or draw advance directives. Other studies suggest that Japanese people do not want to make a concrete plan of treatment but general instructions concerning end-of-life **(Akabayashi et al., 1997; Hirakawa et al., 2006b)**.

9.3 Dementia care

As a byproduct of the aging of the population, Japan has witnessed a dramatic rise in patients with dementia, and it is now important to ascertain how cognitive impairment is associated with acute or palliative care received. Several studies have suggested that patients with dementia often receive poor end-of-life care, with inadequate pain or other symptom control in the other industrialized countries **(Morrison et al., 2000; Sampson et al., 2005)**.

On the other hand, we have observed that Japanese physicians tend to ignore dementia in their patients. For example, we assessed the cases of 123 people aged 65 and older who died at two long-term care hospitals in order to clarify the use of aggressive and palliative treatments, artificial nutrition and sedation **(Hirakawa et al., 2004)**. Also, we observed that dementia itself was not a significant independent predictor of uncontrolled pain or use of end-of-life care in a home setting **(Hirakawa et al., 2006a)**. Our findings indicated that regardless of whether patients suffered from dementia, they received similar acute or palliative treatments in the end-stage.

A greater understanding of the course of dementia is needed to further discussions on the terminal care of people with dementia. A national consensus on how to treat end-stage demented patients is also needed.

9.4 Ethical committee and guidelines

In Japan, the need to set up ethical committees has been the focus of public attention at conferences discussing ethical issues **(Uemura, 2000)**. Recently, the realization of the impact of such issues as patient's rights, population aging and development of advanced medical techniques has intensified the relationship between health care providers and elderly patients and their families. In the position statement, it is strongly advised that each institution establish its ethical committee with a third party in attendance and discuss the propriety of its medical practices and care for dying patients (Position 12). Health care providers are now more likely to face important ethical issues surrounding death and palliative care.

However, institutional ethical committees are still not widespread in Japan. Nakao et al **(2003)** suggested that many nurses would rather discuss ethical issues with the persons directly involved or with complete outsiders to the situation than to consult an ethical committee. A national survey also suggested that there are currently few ethical committees at Japanese hospitals **(Hirakawa et al., 2007c)**.

In long-term care settings, death conferences are becoming an important tool. Reflecting on palliative care for the elderly after their death is important from an educational point of view. Death conferences also trigger a peer support effect among health care providers who have experienced the death of a patient. However, the death conference is not widely and frequently adopted at long-term care facilities. Hayasaka **(2010)** reported in a small study covering 10 long-term care facilities and 3 hospitals with a palliative care unit, that only 11% of the 200 care staff had participated in a death conference, while 100% of the 40 nurses had.

Palliative care discussions as part of ethical committee consultations or death conferences should be encouraged at hospitals and long-term care facilities.

There are a number of tools for the discussion of ethical issues, such as a contingency table reported in "A practical Approach to Ethical Decisions in Clinical Medicine"**(Jonsen et al., 2002)**. In addition, Higuchi et al **(2010)** developed a death conference sheet package which was published elsewhere. The conference package includes sheets on the will of elderly patients and families, care support, medical care, and care management, which are considered key factors of high quality palliative care.

Standardization through authorized palliative care guidelines for the elderly can help reduce the stress of facing ethical complications. The Ministry of Health, Labor and Welfare's "Guidelines for decision-making process for end-of-life care" outlines the following key components: 1) Team approach, 2) Discussion with and confirmation of the will of patients, 3) Discussion between family and health care team (if the will of the patient is unclear) **(Shimizu, 2009)**. Referring to the Ministry guidelines, we developed a decision-making process model for application at long-term care facilities **(Hirakawa & Uemura, 2009)**. With this model **(Figure 3)**, if an elderly resident get suddenly worse and possibly requires hospitalization, facility staff will convene a meeting to confirm the desire to transfer to a hospital. If there is a do-not-hospitalize order, facility staff will reach a decision after discussing the ethical implications of the case. If the resident needs to be provided palliative care at the facility, a palliative care team will be set up and will draw a palliative care plan based on the will of the resident and family. Care staff may also need to reexamine the care plan and make change1s if necessary.

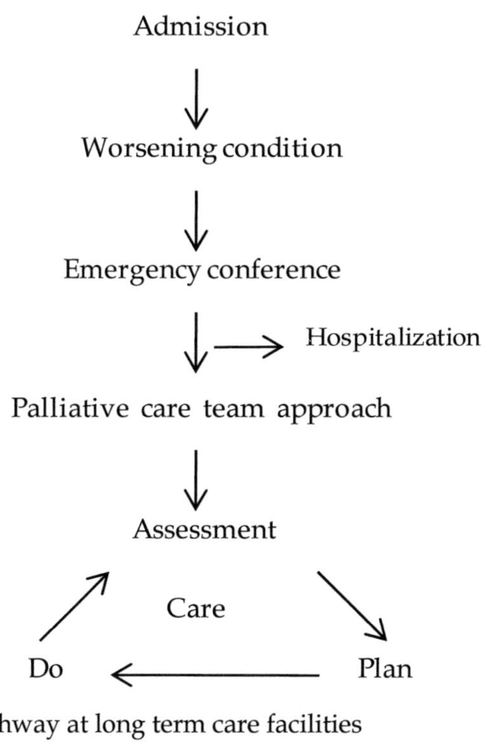

Fig. 3. Palliative care pathway at long term care facilities

10. Pain and distress symptom control

Pain and distress symptom management is one of the most important issues in palliative care. For elderly patients with advanced cancer or dementia, there are reliable and authorized guidelines for pharmacological approaches to the relief of pain.

Under-treatment and estimation are two critical issues of palliative care for the elderly. A few studies have suggested that many elderly residents at long-term care facilities feel uncontrolled pain **(Krulewitch et al, 2000; Morrison et al, 2000)**. Elderly people are likely to have difficulty communicating their symptoms due to poor hearing or dementia. In addition, Japanese elderly generally do not want to complain about pain or distress symptoms because they think that patience is a virtue.

To improve the situation, the author recently launched a project to develop a communication and symptom assessment tool called the "Nagoya Graphical Symptom Scale for the Elderly" (NGSSE) **(Hirakawa & Uemura., 2010)**. This project was geared toward elderly patients requiring palliative care under the scheme of a research project funded by the Ministry of Health, Labour and Welfare in Japan. The rating scale, which featured symptoms frequently observed among the elderly who require care, was drawn using "manga (cartoons) rather than text or illustrations. Manga is a good communication tool that can be used to convey important information in a humorous and pleasurable fashion across the generations.

11. Complementary therapies

Complementary medicine is another approach to palliative care for the elderly. The aged are vulnerable to various chronic medical problems that are difficult to alleviate by relying solely on Western medicine; attention has thus recently increasingly focused on ways to enhance the quality of life of the elderly through complementary and alternative medicine. The Japan Geriatrics Society's position statement emphasizes that geriatric medicine, a discipline that deals with aging and death, should be regarded as holistic medicine that stands on the achievements of the life sciences with particular emphasis on bioethics **(Japan Geriatric Society, 2001)**. Holistic medicine emphasizes the need to look at the whole person, from the combine perspective of physical, nutritional, environmental, emotional, social state as well as spiritual and lifestyle values. Thus, complementary therapies are considered non-pharmacological interventions used to enhance and support the patient's palliative plan of care, that should be integrated to palliative care for the elderly. For example, bathing in a hot spring ("onsen" in Japanese) or taking a bath is often recommended to elderly patients in Japan; as a matter of fact, the benefits balneotherapy have been widely examined in Japan. Also widely available in Japan are music therapy, aroma therapy, electroacupuncture, and thermotherapy.

Other very popular complementary therapies in Japan are acupuncture/moxibustion and massage which have been used since ancient times. These therapies are offered by trained professionals and are partially covered by public medical insurance as an alternative medical service. Home massage rehabilitation therapy by trained professionals is widely available to the bed-ridden elderly as an alternative home rehabilitation service in Japan **(Hirakawa et al., 2005a)**. Although relatively few studies have been conducted on the effect of acupuncture/moxibustion and massage on the frail elderly, a number of papers have highlighted their positive influence on their well-being, including pain and distress symptom relief **(Ferrell-Torry & Click, 1993; Meek SS, 1993; Weinrich & Winrich, 1990)**.

In Japan, tea is also widely available and popular as a complementary therapy. Scientific research has shown that drinking green tea promotes a healthy metabolism. Because of the health benefits of green tea, it is widely used in elderly care settings. Fujii et al **(2004)** used green tea as a foot care tool for elderly who require care. Their investigation highlighted the positive effect of green-tea based foot care for patients with BPSD. Fukuoka et al **(2009)** used green tea as a component for a finger grip bag to reduce the smell of the contracted hand grip of bedridden patients. Hirakawa et al **(2010a)** used "Persimmon Leaf Tea," which is also widely popular in Japan, as air freshener at a long-term care facility.

Post obitum treatment "Angel Care" and the embalmer' art "Angel Make" are also popular as a complementary therapy. At the terminal stage of life or even after death, paying attention to the appearance of the elderly could contribute to improving the quality of their life and that of their family members. Japanese health care providers often refer to post obitum treatment as "Angel Care", and to the art of the embalming as "Angel Make", which are generally practiced by nurses. The nurses who perform Angel Care or Angel Make have a certain level of formal training and they also benefit from informal training from senior staff.

12. Conclusion

This paper aims to examine characteristics observed in palliative care service in Japan. One of them is an ambiguity that Japanese elderly people often show when they express their intensions or demands based on their self-decision. And we show that providing elderly people with tube feeding such as PEG is very much common in care service and also show that elderly people hesitate to complain of pain because they don't want bother others. Though Japan have developed medical care by introducing a number of systems modeled after schemes employed in Western countries, we can not discuss palliative care without considering cultural backgrounds that differ between different countries. Therefore, in this paper we propose that it is important for us to take into account Japanese cultural characteristics to build an original care system for Japanese while reviewing and examining western schemes we have employed.

13. Acknowledgment

This review was supported by the Ministry of Education, Culture, Sports, Science and Technology of Japan and the Sasakawa Health Science Foundation.

14. References

Aita, K.; Takahashi, M.; Miyata, H.; Kai, I.& Finucane, TE.(2007) Physicians' attitudes about artificial feeding in older patients with severe cognitive impairment in Japan: a qualitative study. *BMC Geriatrics*, Vol.7, (August 2007), p.22, ISSN 1471-2318

Akabayashi, A.; Kai, I.; Ito, K.& Tsukui, K. (1997) [The acceptability of advance directives in Japanese society: a questionnaire study for health people in the physical check-up settings]. *Journal of the Japan Association for Bioethics*,Vol.7,No.1,(September 1997), pp.31-40.(in Japanese) ISSN 1343-4063

Bito, S.& Asai, A. (2007) Attitudes and behaviors of Japanese physicians concerning withholding and withdrawal of life-sustaining treatment for end-of-life patients: results from an internet survey. *BMC Medical Ethics* ,Vol.8, (June 2007), p. 7, ISSN 1472-6939

Carron, AT.; Lynn, J.& Keaney, P. (1999) End-of-life care in medical textbooks. *Annals of Internernal Medicine*, Vol.5, No.130(1), (January 1999), pp.82-86, ISSN 0003-4819

Crosato, KE.& Leipert, B. (2006). Rural women caregivers in Canada. *Rural Remote Health* Vol.6,(April-June 2006), p.520, ISSN 1445-6354

Ellis, G.; Whitehead, MA.; O'Neill, D.; Langhorne, P.& Robinson, D. (2011) Comprehensive geriatric assessment for older adults admitted to hospital. *Cochrane Database of Systematic Reviews*, (July 2011) 6;7:CD006211, ISSN 1469-493X

Endevelt, R.; Werner, P.& Stone, O. (2006) Dietitians' attitudes regarding elderly nutritional factors. *Journal of nutrition for the elderly*, Vol.26, No.1-2, (2006), pp.45-58, ISSN 0163-9366

Ferrell-Torry, AT. & Click OJ. (1993) The use of therapeutic massage as a nursing intervention to modify anxiety and the perception of cancer pain. *Cancer Nursing*, Vol.16, No.2, (April 1993), pp.93-101, ISSN 0162-220X

Fujii, M.; Sato, T. & Sasaki, H. (2004). Green tea for tinea manuum inbedridden patients, *Geriatrics and Gerontology International*, Vol.4, No.1, (March 2004), pp.64-65, ISSN 1444-1586

Fukuoka, Y.; Kudo, H.; Hatakeyama, A.; Takahashi, N.; Satoh, K.; Ohsawa, N.; Mutoh, M.; Fujii, M. & Sasaki H. (2009) Four fingergrip bags with tea to prevent smell of contractured hand andaxilla in bedridden patients. *Geriatrics and Gerontology International*,Vol.9, No.1, (March 2009), pp.97–99, ISSN 1444-1586

Hara, K. (2011) [Multidisciplinary approaches for the elderly at the end-of-life stage]. *Nippon Ronen Igakkai Zasshi*, Vol.48, No.3, (May 2011), pp. 257-259, (in Japanese) ISSN 0300-9173

Hattori, A. ; Masuda, Y. ; Fetters, MD. ; Uemura, K. ; Mogi, N. ; Kuzuya, M. & Iguchi, A. (2005) A qualitative exploration of elderly patients' preferences for end-of-life care. *Japan Medical Association Journal*,Vol48, No.8,(August 2005), pp.388-397, ISSN 1346-8650

Hayasaka, H. (2010) [Nursing staff's outlook on the necrobiosis, and it takes care and the following grief psychology: From the comparison with the nurse]. *Hokkaido Bukyo Daigaku Kenkyu Kiyo*, Vol.34, (March 2010), pp.25-32, (in Japanese) ISSN1349-3841

Henderson, ML. ; Hanson, LC. & Reynolds KS. Improving nursing home care of the dying: a training manual for nursing home staff. *NY: Springer Publishing Company*, (2003), ISBN0-8261-1925-5

Higuchi, K. [End-of-life care for elderly]. In : *[End-of-life care for elderly- four conditions for high quality care and care management tools]*, Higuchi, K et al.(Ed). *Chuohoki Publishing* (April 2010), pp.21-31, (in Japanese), Tokyo, ISBN978-4-8058-3275-2

Higuchi, K. ; Shinoda, M. ; Sugimoto, H. & Kondo, K. [End-of-life care for elderly- four conditions for high quality care and care management tools]. *Chuohoki Publishing* (April 2010) (in Japanese), Tokyo, ISBN978-4-8058-3275-2

Hirakawa, Y.; Masuda, Y.; Uemura, K.; Nait,o M.; Kuzuya, M.& Iguchi, A. (2003) [Dietitians' understanding of personalized nutritional guidance--proposals to increase home visits by dietitians]. *Nippon Ronen Igakkai Zasshi*, Vol.40, No.5, (September 2003), pp. 509-14, (In Japanese) ISSN 0300-9173

Hirakawa, Y. ; Masuda, Y. ; Kimata, T. ; Uemura, K. ; Kuzuya, M.& Iguchi, A. (2004) [Terminal care for elderly with dementia in two long-term care hospitals.] *Nippon Ronen Igakkai Zasshi,* Vol.41,No.1, (January 2004), pp.99–104 (In Japanese), ISSN 0300-9173, Japan

Hirakawa, Y. ; Masuda, Y. ; Kimata, T. ; Uemura, K. ; Kuzuya, M. & Iguchi, A. (2005a) Effects of home massage rehabilitation therapy for the bed-ridden elderly: a pilot trial with a three-month follow-up. *Clinical Rehabilitation,* Vol.19, No.1, (January 2005), pp.20-27, ISSN 0269-2155

Hirakawa, Y.; Masuda, Y.; Uemura, K.; Kuzuya, M.; Noguchi, M.; Kimiata, T.& Iguchi A. (2005b) [National survey on the current status of programs to teach end-of-life care to undergraduates of medical and nursing schools in Japan]. *Nippon Ronen Igakkai Zasshi*, Vol.42, No.5, (September 2005), pp.540-545, (In Japanese) ISSN 0300-9173

Hirakawa, Y. ; Masuda, Y. ; Kuzuya, M. ; Kimata, T. ; Iguchi, A.& Uemura, K. (2006a) End-of-life experience of demented elderly patients at home: Findings from DEATH project. *Psychogeriatrics,* Vol.6, (June 2006) pp.60-67, ISSN 1346-3500

Hirakawa, Y.; Masuda,Y.; Kuzuya, M.; Iguchi,A.& Uemura, K. (2006b) [Attitude of middle-aged healthy elderly toward location of end-of-life care and living will]. *Hospice and Home Care,* Vol.14, No.3, (December 2006), pp.201-205, (In Japanese) ISSN 1341-8688

Hirakawa, Y.; Masuda, Y.; Kuzuya, M.; Iguchi, A.& Uemura, K. (2007a) [Decision-making factors regarding resuscitate and hospitalize orders by families of elderly persons on admission to a Japanese long-term care hospital]. *Nippon Ronen Igakkai Zasshi,* Vol.44, No.4, (July 2007) pp.497-502, (In Japanese) ISSN 0300-9173

Hirakawa, Y.; Masuda, Y.; Kuzuya, M.; Iguchi, A.& Uemura, K. (2007b) Non-medical palliative care and education to improve end-of-life care at geriatric health services facilities: a nationwide questionnaire survey of chief nurses. *Geriatrics and Gerontology International,* Vol7,(September 2007), pp.266-270, ISSN 1444-1586

Hirakawa, Y.; Kuzuya, M.& Uemura, K. (2007c) [Current situation of hospital ethics committees in Japan].*Nippon Ronen Igakkai Zasshi*, Vol.44, No.6, (November 2007), pp.767-769, (In Japanese) ISSN 0300-9173

Hirakawa, Y.; Kuzuya, M.& Uemura, K. (2008a) [An analysis of content on end-of-life care for elderly in Japanese-language end-of-life care or geriatric textbooks]. *Hospice and Home Care* Vol.16, No.3 (December 2008), pp.213-217, (In Japanese) ISSN 1341-8688

Hirakawa, Y.; Uemura, K.& Kuzuya, M. (2008b) [Survey of directors of long-term care facilities on opinions about end-of-life care and director education] . *Medical Education Japan* ,Vol.39, No.4, (August 2008) pp.245-250, (In Japanese) ISSN 0386-9644

Hirakawa, Y.; Kuzuya, M.& Uemura, K. (2009a) [Topics of medical education concerning end-of-life care for the elderly] . *Medical Education Japan*,Vol. 40, No1, (February 2009) pp.61-64, (In Japanese) ISSN 0386-9644

Hirakawa, Y.; Kuzuya, M.& Uemura, K. (2009b) Opinion survey of nursing or caring staff at long-term care facilities about end-of-life care provision and staff education.

Archives of Gerontology and Geriatrics, Vol.49, No.1, (July-August 2009) pp.43-48, ISSN 0167-4943

Hirakawa, Y. & Uemura, K. (2009) [Clinical pathway for end-of-life care at long-term care facilities]. *Nippon Ronen Igakkai Zasshi*, Vol.46, No.4, (July 2009) p.366 (In Japanese) ISSN 0300-9173

Hirakawa, Y.; Suzuki, S. & Uemura, K. (2010a) [Trial to use persimmon leaf tea as air freshener at a long-term care facility]. *Hospice and Home Care*, Vol.18, No.1, (April 2010), pp.53-55, (In Japanese) ISSN 1341-8688

Hirakawa, Y.; Uemura, K. & Kuzuya, M. (2010b) [Comprehensive geriatric assessment (CGA)-based tool for discharge support]. *Nippon Ronen Igakkai Zasshi*, Vol.47, No.2, (March 2010) pp.162, (In Japanese)ISSN 0300-9173

Hirakawa, Y. & Uemura, K. (2010c) [Development of the Nagoya Graphical Symptom Scale for Elderly (NGSSE)]. *Nippon Ronen Igakkai Zasshi*, Vol.47, No.3 (May 2010), p.264, (In Japanese), ISSN 0300-9173

Hirakawa, Y. [Palliative care for elderly patients]. *Nippon Ronen Igakkai Zasshi*, Vol. 48, No.3, (May 2011), pp.216-220, (In Japanese) ISSN 0300-9173

Hirakawa, Y.; Kuzuya, M.; Enoki, H.& Uemura, K. (2011a) Information needs and sources of family caregivers of home elderly patients. *Archives of Gerontology and Geriatrics*, Vol.52, No.2, (March-April 2011), pp.202–205, ISSN 0167-4943

Hirakawa, Y.; Yasui, H. ; Aomatsu M. & Uemura, K. (2011b). [Effect of a end-of-life care workshop program for upper-class care staff]. *Hospice and Home Care*, (October 2011 in press), (In Japanese) ISSN 1341-8688

Iguchi, A. (2001) [How the terminal care in the elderly: a position statement from the Japan Geriatric Society started]. *Nippon Ronen Igakkai Zasshi*, Vol.38, No.4, (July 2001) pp.584-586, (In Japanese) ISSN 0300-9173

Iijima, S.(2009). [The terminal care in the elderly: a position statement from the Japan Geriatric Society and how it will develop]. *Geriatric Medicine*, Vol.47, No.4, (April 2009), pp.443-447, ISBN978-4-89801-316-8 C3047

Institute for Health Economics and Policy of Japan (March 2010). [International comparative study of end-of-life care for elderly patients with dementia]. Institute for Health Economics and Policy Study Report 2009. (in Japanese) Tokyo

Japan Geriatric Society (June 2001). [Announcement from The Japan Geriatrics Society Ethics Committee: The Terminal Care of the Elderly- position statement from the Japan Geriatrics Society], 01.08.2011, (in Japanese) Available from http://www.jpn-geriat-soc.or.jp.

Japan Association of Geriatric Care Services Facilities (March 2007). [Report of the study on development of guidelines on end-of-life care at geriatric care services facilities]. (in Japanese) Tokyo.

Jonsen, AR.; Siegler, M.& Winslade, WJ. (May 2002) Clinical ethics: A practical approach to ethical decisions in clinical medicine (5 edition). ISBN 0071387633. McGraw-Hill/Appleton & Lange; NY

Kortes-Miller, K. ;Habjan, S. ;Kelley, ML.& Fortier, M. (2007) Development of a palliative care education program in rural long-term care facilities. *Journal of palliative care*. Vol.23, (Autumn 2007), pp.154-162, ISSN 0825-8597

Krulewitch, H. ; London MR. ; Skakel VJ. ; Lundstedt GJ. ; Thomason H. & Brummel-Smith K. (2000) Assessment of pain in cognitively impaired older adults: a comparison of pain assessment tools and their use by non-professional caregivers. *Journal of the American Geriatrics Society,* Vol.48, (December 2000), pp.1607-1611, ISSN 0002-8614

Lunney, JR. ; Lynn, J. ;Foley, DJ. ;Lipson,S. &Guralnik, JM. (2003) Patterns of functional decline at the end of life. *JAMA,* Vol.289, No18, (May 2003), pp.2387-2392, ISSN 0098-7484

Masuda, Y. (May 2000). [Long-term care, medical care and welfare], In: *Korekarano Ronengaku,* Iguchi A(Ed), pp.239-242, (in Japanese) The University of Nagoya Press, ISBN4-8158-0382-X, Nagoya, Japan

Masuda, Y.; Fetters, MD.; Hattori, A.; Mogi, N.; Naito, M.; Iguchi, A.& Uemura, K. (2003) Physicians' reports on the impact of living wills at the end-of-life in Japan. *Journal of Medical Ethics,* Vol.29 (August 2003), pp.248-252, ISSN 0306-6800

Matsui, M. & Braun, K. (2010) Nurses' and care workers' attitudes toward death and caring for dying older adults in Japan. *International Journal of Palliative Nursing,* Vol.10, (December 2010), pp.593-598, ISSN 1357-6321

Matsui, M. (2010) Effectiveness of end-of-life education among community-dwelling older adults. *Nursing Ethics,* Vol.17, No.3, (May 2010), pp.363-372, ISSN1477-7330

Matsuda, S.& Yamamoto, M. (2001). Long-term care insurance and integrated care for the aged in Japan. *International Journal of Integrated Care,* Vol.1, No.1, (September 2001), pp.1-11, ISSN 1568-4156

Meek, SS. (1993) Effects of slow stroke back massage on relaxation in hospice clients. *Image-J Nurs Scholarsh* Vol.25, No.1, (Spring 1993), pp.17-21, ISSN 0743-5150

Ministry of Health, Labour and Welfare. [Current situation of main caregivers]. Comprehensive Survey of Living Conditions of the People on Health and Welfare 2010. (in Japanese) 02.08.2011. Available from http://www.mhlw.go.jp/toukei/saikin/hw/k-tyosa/k-tyosa10

Ministry of Health, Labour and Welfare (July 2004). [Report of the study on end-of-life care: future direction of end-of-life care in Japan]. (in Japanese) 02.08.2011. Available from http://www.mhlw.go.jp/shingi/2004/07/s0723-8.html

Morrison, RS. & Siu, AL. (2000) Survival in end-stage dementia following acute illness. *JAMA,* Vol.284, (January 2000), pp.47–52, ISSN 0098-7484

Morrison, RS. & Siu AL. A comparison of pain and its treatment in advanced dementia and cognitively intact patients with hip fracture. *Journal of pain and symptom management,* Vol.19,No.4, (April 2000), pp.240-248, ISSN 0885-3924

Nakao, H. ; Morita, H. ; Nakamura, H. ; Fujimura, T. ; Tsutsumi, M. ; Kobayashi, T. ; Nagakawa, T.& Obayashi, M. (2003) [A study on nursing professionals' awareness of ethical problems]. *Yamaguchi Kenritsu Digaku Kango Gakubu Kiyo,* Vol.8, (March 2003), pp.5-11, (in Japanese) ISSN 1343-0904

National Institute of Population and Social Security Research. *Population Statistics 2011,* (February 2011) 01.08.2011, Available from http://www.ipss.go.jp/syoushika/tohkei/Popular/Popular2011.asp?chap=0

National Advisory Committee (2000). A guide to end-of-life care for seniors. University of Tronto and University of Ottawa, ISBN0-9687122-0-7

Okuno, S.; Tagaya, A.; Tamura, M.& Davis AJ. (1999) Elderly Japanese people living in small towns reflect on end-of-life issues.*Nursing Ethics,* Vol.6, (July 1999) pp.308-315, ISSN 1477-0989

Okuyama, S. (2005). [Long-term care for elderly in rural area under the public long-term care insurance system—mainly through the case of rural area in Northwest rural Japan] . *Gendai Hogaku*, (March 2005), pp.55-90, (in Japanese) ISSN1345-9821

Rabow, MW.; Hardie, GE.; Fair, JM.& McPhee, SJ. (2000) End-of-life care content in 50 textbooks from multiple specialties. *JAMA*, Vol.283, No.6,(February 2000), pp.771-778. ISSN 0098-7484

Sally, J. & David, C. (2007) Assessing the impact of care management in the community: associations between key organisational components and service outcomes. *Age and Ageing*, Vol.36, No. 3, (March 2007), pp.336-339, ISSN 1468-2834

Sampson, EL. ; Ritchie, CW. ; Lai, R. ; Raven, PW.& Blanchard, MR. (2005) A systematic review of the scientific evidence for the efficacy of a palliative care approach in advanced dementia. *Int Psychogeriatr*, Vol.17, No.1, (March 2005), pp.31–40, ISSN 1041-6102

Sepúlveda, C.; Marlin, A.; Yoshida, T.& Ullrich, A. (2002) Palliative Care: the World Health Organization's global perspective. *Journal of pain and symptom management*, Vol.24, No.2, (August 2002), pp.91-96, ISSN 0885-3924

Shimizu, T. (2009). [Decision-making process in the elderly patients at end-of-life]. *Geriatric Medicine*, Vol.47, No.4, (April 2009), pp.439-442, (in Japanese) ISSN 1172-7047

Tsutsui, T.& Muramatsu, N. (2007) Japan's Universal Long-Term Care System Reform of 2005: Containing Costs and Realizing a Vision. *Journal of the American Geriatric Society*, Vol.55, (September 2007), pp.1458–1463, ISSN 0002-8614

Tsuruwaka, M.& Semba Y (2010). [Study on confirmation of intention concerning end-of-life care upon moving into welfare facilities for elderly requiring care]. *Journal of the Japan Association for Bioethics*, Vol.20, No.1, (September 2010) pp.158-164, (in Japanese) ISSN1343-4063

Uemura, K. (2000) [The terminal care in the elderly: a position statement from the Japan Geriatric Society--a draft of JGS Ethics Committee]. *Nippon Ronen Igakkai Zasshi*, Vol.37, No.9, (September 2000), pp.719-21, (in Japanese) ISSN 0300-9173

Weinrich, SP. & Winrich, MC. (1990) The effect of massage on pain in cancer patients. *Applied nursing research*, Vol.3, No.4, (November 1990), pp.140-145

WHO,World Health Statistics 2011 (May 2011). ISBN 9789241564199. Available from http://www.who.int/whosis/whostat/EN_WHS2011_Full.pdf